# THE CHILDREN'S HOSPITAL
## OF PHILADELPHIA

# GUIDE TO

# COMMON

# CHILDHOOD

# INFECTIONS

# ALSO BY THE AUTHORS

LOUIS M. BELL:
*What Every Parent Should Know About Vaccines*
*Breaking the Antibiotic Habit*

JANE BROOKS:
*Midlife Orphan: Facing Life's Changes When Your Parents are Gone*

MARION STEINMANN:
*The Children's Hospital of Philadelphia Parent's Guide to Allergies and Asthma*
*The American Medical Association Book of BackCare*
*Life & Health*
*Island Life*

# THE CHILDREN'S HOSPITAL
## OF PHILADELPHIA

# GUIDE TO
# COMMON
# CHILDHOOD
# INFECTIONS

**Louis M. Bell, M.D. Mary Lou Manning, Ph.D., R.N.**

**Jane Brooks and Marion Steinmann**

Macmillan • USA

MACMILLAN
A Simon & Schuster Macmillan Company
1633 Broadway
New York, NY 10019-6785

Macmillan Publishing books may be purchased for business or sales promotional use. For information please write: Special Markets Department, Macmillan Publishing USA, 1633 Broadway, New York, NY 10019.

Illustrations by Laura M. Robbins
Illustrations, pages 21, 22, 111 and 200, are based on those appearing in *Caring for Your Baby and Young Child: Birth to Age 5* by Steven Shelov Robert E. Hannemann. Copyright © 1991 by American Academy of Pediatrics. Used by permission of Bantam Books, a division of Bantam Doubleday Dell Publishing Group, Inc.

**Library of Congress Cataloging-in-Publication Data**

The Children's Hospital of Philadelphia guide to common childhood
  infections /Louis M. Bell . . . [et al.].
      p.    cm.
  Includes index.
  ISBN 0-02-860435-0
  1. Infection in children—Popular works. 2. Communicable diseases in children—Popular works. 3. Bacterial diseases in children—Popular works. 4. Children—Health and hygiene—Popular works. I. Bell, Louis M. II. Children's Hospital of Philadelphia.

RJ401.C47    1988
618.92'9—dc21                            98-18546
                                             CIP

Printed in the United States of America

10 9 8 7 6 5 4 3 2 1

# DEDICATION

*From Louis M. Bell, M.D.:*
To my children Sarah, Chris, Amy and Sue

*From Mary Lou Manning, R.N., Ph.D.:*
To Joe and Joe Jr.

*From Jane Brooks:*
To my sons Daniel and Andy

*From Marion Steinmann:*
To Charles

# CONTENTS

# FOREWORD

*By C. Everett Koop, M.D., Sc.D.*

This is a book about the common (and not so common) infections of childhood. But why have one from the folks at The Children's Hospital of Philadelphia? The answer is simple: The professional people there have a long history of research into the causes and cures for many of these ailments.

When the Children's Hospital was founded in 1855, smallpox, typhoid, typhus, and cholera were pandemic. Diphtheria, scarlet fever, measles, and whooping cough were epidemic as were tuberculosis and joint infections. But when I joined the Children's Hospital's staff in 1946, the nation's first hospital for sick children had already made inroads against some of these infectious diseases. A hyperimmune serum, for example, to protect children and pregnant women against whooping cough had been developed in 1936 by scientists at the Children's Hospital. This serum was manufactured in the Hospital's laboratory and then distributed in forty-eight states here, as well as abroad.

Three years before my arrival at the Children's Hospital, Drs. Werner and Gertrude Henle—who were to become internationally renowned during their forty-year association with Children's Hospital—developed the first convincing demonstration of vaccination against influenza and mumps. In the 1950s, Dr. Joseph Stokes, Jr., the Hospital's physician-in-chief, and his colleagues were the first to prove the effectiveness of gamma globulin in preventing paralytic polio, a disease known to the public as infantile paralysis. For this wonderful discovery, Dr. Stokes was awarded the Medal of Freedom by President Harry S. Truman.

After Dr. Stokes's initial success with gamma globulin, he focused more broadly on polio by inviting Dr. Lewis L. Coriell to conduct field trials for the prevention of the disease. This was the basis for the development of the Salk vaccine and, ultimately, the defeat of polio. Drs. Stokes and Coriell had established that a small amount of antibody prevented invasion of the spinal cord, thus inoculating against the infection that caused devastation among so many.

The Children's Hospital of Philadelphia also played a major role in the development of the new tool that was used in all infectious disease research: tissue culture, the growing of human cells in glass bottles. By the mid-1950s, Drs. T.N. and Susanna Harris made strides toward clarifying the role of lymphocytes, a component of the blood, in producing antibodies that fight disease.

Dr. Stanley A. Plotkin, another Children's Hospital physician specializing in infectious diseases, developed the rubella (German measles) vaccine in the 1960s with his colleagues at Philadelphia's Wistar Institute of Anatomy and Biology. Less than a decade later, working with other associates, Dr. Plotkin created a vaccine for cytomegalovirus, a cause of congenital mental retardation. He then helped to begin the research that ultimately led to a vaccine for rotavirus diarrhea. The group of researchers, including H Fred Clark, D.V.M., Ph.D., and Paul A. Offit, M.D. at the Children's Hospital, have developed a rotavirus vaccine that is expected to be available in the year 2003. The vaccine has the potential of saving tens of thousands of infants' lives annually, particularly in underdeveloped countries.

Although my professional responsibilities at Children's Hospital covered the growth of surgical subspecialties that saved or improved many children's lives around the world, there was an aura of excitement in the entire hospital whenever a new vaccine was developed. The interest in infectious diseases and their prevention or cure moved from one generation of physicians to another. It is a characteristic ingrained in the hospital's culture.

I left The Children's Hospital of Philadelphia some years ago to become Surgeon General of the United States at the request of President Ronald Reagan. But whenever I return, I find that the physicians involved with patient care are seeing children with ailments increasingly difficult to cure. The research people at Children's Hospital are now involved with more virulent infectious diseases such as AIDS, and the doctors educating medical students and young graduates have far more esoteric information to impart than they formerly had. The Children's Hospital's goal of preventing and curing infectious diseases is stronger than ever.

This book is a natural outgrowth of the hospital's concentration on the improvement of pediatric health through the defeat of many harmful conditions. It is directed to all those who care for children to enable them to understand common infections, as well as to learn more about infections that, while rare, are still so daunting to us. The book is written in an accessible manner and basic information is consistently organized for rapid access and understanding. With this essential resource, parents and other readers will have the information they need on common and not-so-common infections of childhood in order to make well-informed decisions that affect their children's health and safety.

# ACKNOWLEDGMENTS

We would like to thank Shirley Bonnem, Vice President of The Children's Hospital of Philadelphia for coordinating the making of this book.

Also at The Children's Hospital of Philadelphia, we would like to thank Mark Bagarazzi, M.D., Susan Coffin, M.D., Jill Foster, M.D., Richard Gesser, M.D., Jean O. Kim, M.D., Paul A. Offit, M.D., Barbara Watson M.D., and Jeff Weiser, M.D. for adding their knowledge and expertise to this book.

Thanks to Nancy Love, our agent, for her support and to Betsy Thorpe, editor, for her diligence, patience and wit.

Thanks to Janice Fisher, author of *Ear Infections—Outer Ears*, and *Scabies*; Maureen Haggerty, author of the *Ringworm* chapter; Martha Phan, author of the *Conjunctivitis* chapter; Patricia Gottlieb Shapiro, author of the *Pinworms* chapter, and Martha Jablow, for her contributions. We would like to thank Nancy W. Bauer, Ph.D., at the School of Arts and Sciences, University of Pennsylvania; Stephen M. Ostroff, M.D., Associate Director for Epidemiologic Science, National Center for Infectious Diseases, Centers for Disease Control and Prevention, U.S. Public Health Service, and the librarians at Scott Memorial Library, Thomas Jefferson University.

# INTRODUCTION

Children, particularly young children, catch infectious diseases far more frequently than adults do. That's a fact. And children do get sick often, as parents, day-care workers and teachers—those who live with or care for children—know well. You have probably noticed that babies and toddlers, especially, get many more colds and other illnesses than you do. Some babies seem to have continual colds for months at a time. Fortunately, there is much you can do to keep your child healthy.

This book provides you with the information you need about the common infectious diseases that your children are most likely to catch. The guide is intended to help you identify these illnesses and make educated decisions about when your child needs medical intervention or attention. Each disease entry covers the following topics: causes, how it spreads, incubation period (how long it takes for a child to get sick after infection), symptoms, when to call the doctor, diagnosis, and treatment. You will learn how to help *prevent* the disease and how to protect your family against the disease. Armed with this knowledge, you will feel more confident in your capacity as caretaker.

What, exactly, is an infectious disease? It is any illness that is caused by microscopic organisms, that is, germs. These microscopic organisms are invisible to the eye but capable of invading and multiplying inside our bodies. Most infectious diseases are caused by bacteria or viruses. However, other types of microorganisms, such as fungi and parasites, also cause infectious diseases.

So prevalent are infectious diseases in the United States that they cause children to miss more than 35 million days of school every year. At The Children's Hospital of Philadelphia, 60 percent of the children whose parents bring them in to see the pediatricians in our emergency department turn out to have an infectious disease.

There are some infectious diseases that your children are going to catch no matter what you do. A cold is one. But it may surprise you to learn that diarrhea is another common infectious disease. A child generally experiences some seven to fifteen episodes of diarrhea by the time he is five years old. Most young children develop conjunctivitis, a common eye infection. And about 80 percent of children have at least one middle-ear infection by the time they are three.

Why are young children so vulnerable to infectious diseases? One reason is that their immune systems are not yet fully developed. A child encountering germs for the first time does not yet possess the full array of antibodies and other weapons that the adult immune system uses to fend off germs. Adults have already developed some protective immunity to these germs, having met them long ago.

A young child's anatomy also contributes to the reason why he gets some infections. Babies and toddlers, for example, may develop croup—a barking cough caused by an obstruction of the airway—because their throats are so narrow. Young children get middle-ear infections because the tubes draining fluids from their ears slant in a way that does not allow fluid to flow out as easily as it does in older children and adults.

Hygiene also plays a big role in infectious diseases. You may have noticed that the hygienic practices of a young child leave something to be desired. Her hands are everywhere—in the sandbox, in her nose, in her food, in her diaper or panties. Then she puts her fingers in her mouth or rubs her eyes. It is not hard to see how germs spread.

With so many parents working outside the home these days, more than 11 million young children attend day-care facilities and are at greater risk for contracting infectious diseases, particularly respiratory or gastrointestinal diseases. This greater risk can be partly attributed to sheer numbers and the laws of probability— these children come in contact with so many other young children. The germs come home, where they are spread to sisters and brothers and other family members.

As children go off to school, their ever-widening circle of contacts exposes them to still other types of germs. Your child is most likely to catch the streptococcus bacteria that cause strep throat when he is in elementary school, or may be infected with the Epstein-Barr virus that causes mononucleosis (the so-called kissing disease).

\* \* \*

For a while it looked as if modern science had conquered infectious diseases. Early in the twentieth century, as water supplies were cleaned up and the pasteurization of milk became widespread, such killers as cholera and typhoid virtually disappeared from industrialized nations.

In the mid-twentieth century, the introduction of antibiotics meant that, for the first time, bacteria growing inside a person's body could be killed.

With the use of antibiotics, the number of people dying from bacterial pneumonia dropped dramatically. Today, as a result of taking antibiotics, considerably fewer children develop heart damage from rheumatic fever following a strep throat or lose their hearing as a result of complications from a middle-ear infection.

Vaccines, which prevent an individual from catching an infectious disease, have made a significant advance in our fight against these diseases. Diphtheria, which killed 15,000 Americans a year up through the 1920s, is no longer much of a threat in the United States. Remember when measles, mumps, and rubella (German measles) were a childhood rite of passage? No more. Parents no longer need to fear that polio will cripple their children, as it did so many during the 1940s and 1950s. And meningitis from *Haemophilus influenzae* type b bacteria is now mostly a disease of the past, thanks to the vaccine given in infancy.

Despite these advances, infectious diseases are far from conquered. As some types of infections have virtually vanished, other diseases have emerged to take their place. Lyme disease was first recognized in Connecticut in 1975, and it was only in 1993 that the infamous *E. coli* O157:H7 bacteria, which can contaminate raw hamburger, received widespread attention.

Improved detection techniques help us to discover more and more disease-causing organisms. Campylobacter bacteria, for instance, first identified as a cause of human disease in the 1970s, are now known to rival salmonella as a cause of food poisoning, particularly in young children. No doubt many more new or previously unknown germs will be identified in the future.

Unfortunately, some types of bacteria are now fighting back and developing resistance to antibiotics. In some communities, more than 30 percent of the common *Streptococcus pneumoniae* (pneumococcus) bacteria—which cause pneumonia, meningitis, sinusitis, and middle-ear infections in children—are resistant to penicillin. The overuse of antibiotics for viral infections, especially those of the upper respiratory tract, is the major reason for the emergence of resistant bacteria.

In developing countries, many diseases nearly eradicated from industrialized nations are still prevalent. Worldwide, infectious diseases are still the number-one cause of death. Tuberculosis kills more than 2 million people a year, and measles about another million, mostly infants and young children. Respiratory diseases as a group are responsible for the deaths of more than 4 million children under age five each year, and diarrhea kills another 3 or 4 million young children annually.

Even in the United States, infectious diseases remain one of the leading causes of death. The influenza viruses kill 20,000 Americans in an average year. What this tells us is that our work is not complete. Despite numerous and significant advances in fighting infectious diseases, we must still be vigilant.

Education is a good place to start. The Children's Hospital of Philadelphia hopes that you will use this book to educate yourself about these diseases and to arm yourself with the knowledge to help your child and to know when a call to the pediatrician is needed. We have included in this book the infectious diseases that most commonly afflict children.

We have also included some less common infectious diseases that you should know about for other reasons. There are ten diseases that your child should routinely be vaccinated against. See the *Vaccines* section, page 301, in the Appendices, for a listing of these diseases. Some other diseases—such as infections you can get from food or from your pets—are ones that you need to constantly guard against. And still other infectious diseases—such as epiglottitis and meningitis—we have included because they are life-threatening emergencies, for which you need to get medical attention immediately.

While you may not be able to prevent your child from catching a common infection of childhood, you can learn how to keep him comfortable and prevent the disease from worsening or spreading to others. Remember that, as a parent or child-care worker, you can make a significant difference in a child's health.

# SYMPTOMS INDEX

For your convenience in locating material in this book, here is a list of common (and some uncommon) symptoms that your child may experience from infectious diseases. After each symptom is a listing of diseases that may cause that symptom and page numbers indicating where they can be found.

**ABDOMINAL PAIN OR DISTENTION:** Campylobacter Diarrhea (page 60), Cryptosporidium Diarrhea (page 63), Diarrhea (page 52), E. coli Disease (page 97), Encephalitis (page 102), Food Poisoning (page 119), Giardia Diarrhea (page 67), Hepatitis A (page 136), Hepatitis B (page 140), Salmonella Infections (page 231), Shigella Diarrhea (page 72), Sore Throats (page 249), Strep Throat (page 262), Toxocariasis (page 9), Yersinia Diarrhea (page 77), Urinary Tract Infections (page 278)

**BACK PAIN, LOW:** Urinary Tract Infections (page 278)

**BREATHING DIFFICULTY:** Bronchiolitis (page 21), Croup (page 46), Diphtheria (page 80), Epiglottitis (page 105), Pneumonia (page 200), Rabies (page 6)

**BREATHING, RAPID:** Bronchiolitis (page 21), Fevers (page 109), Pneumonia (page 200)

**BURNING SENSATION WHEN URINATING:** Urinary Tract Infections (page 278)

**CHEEKS, SWOLLEN:** Mumps (page 191)

**CHEST PAIN:** Pneumonia (page 200), Tuberculosis (page 275)

**CHEWING TROUBLE:** Ear Infections—Outer Ears (page 93)

**CHILLS:** Cellulitis (page 256), Fevers (page 109), Urinary Tract Infection (page 278), Meningitis (page 183), Psittacosis (page 5), Rabies (page 6), Scarlet Fever (page 260), Tetanus (page 267)

**COMA:** Encephalitis (page 102), Meningitis (page 183)

**CONFUSION:** Encephalitis (page 102), Meningitis (page 183)

**CONVULSIONS:** Streptococcus Infections (page 254), Tetanus (page 267)

**COUGH:** Bronchiolitis (page 21), Common Colds (page 34), Croup (page 46), Encephalitis (page 102), Influenza (page 149), Measles (page 179), Pneumonia (page 200), Psittacosis (page 5), Rabies (page 6), Rubella (page 225), Sinusitis (page 242), Sore Throats (page 249), Toxocariasis (page 9), Tuberculosis (page 275), Whooping Cough (page 286)

**DEEP SLEEP:** Reye's Syndrome (page 217)

**DIARRHEA:** Campylobacter Diarrhea (page 60), Cryptosporidium Diarrhea (page 63), Diarrhea (page 52), E. c oli Disease (page 97), Food Poisoning (page 119), Giardia Diarrhea (page 67), Influenza (page 149), Listeria Infections (page 166), Rotavirus Diarrhea (page 69), Salmonella Infections (page 231), Shigella Diarrhea (page 72), Trichinosis (page 271), Urinary Tract Infections (page 278), Yersinia Diarrhea (page 77)

**DILATED PUPILS:** Reye's Syndrome (page 217)

**DIZZINESS:** Encephalitis (page 102), Meningitis (page 183), Toxic Shock Syndrome (page 257)

**DOUBLE VISION:** Botulism (page 16), Rabies (page 6), Trichinosis (page 271)

**MUSCLE ACHES:** Diarrhea (page 52), Influenza (page 149), Listeria Infections (page 166), Lyme Disease (page 170), Rabies (page 6), Scarlet Fever (page 260), Trichinosis (page 271)

**MUSCLE SPASMS:** Poliomyelitis (page 211), Tetanus (page 267)

**NAUSEA:** Bronchiolitis (page 21), Campylobacter Diarrhea (page 60), Cryptosporidium Diarrhea (page 63), Diarrhea (page 52), E. coli Disease (page 97), Food Poisoning (page 119), Giardia Diarrhea (page 67), Hepatitis B (page 140), Listeria Infections (page 166), Lyme Disease (page 170), Meningitis (page 183), Mumps (page 191), Pneumonia (page 200), Poliomyelitis (page 211), Rabies (page 6), Reye's Syndrome (page 217), Rotavirus Diarrhea (page 69), Salmonella Infections (page 231), Sore Throats (page 249), Strep Throat (page 262), Streptococcus Infections (page 254), Trichinosis (page 271), Urinary Tract Infections (page 278), Whooping Cough (page 286), Yersinia Diarrhea (page 77)

**NOSE, RUNNY OR CONGESTED, SNEEZING:** Bronchiolitis (page 21), Common Colds (page 34), Croup (page 46), Fifth Disease (page 115), Influenza (page 149), Measles (page 179), Mononucleosis (page 188), Pneumonia (page 200), Roseola (page 223), Respiratory Syncytial Virus (RSV) Infections (page 26), Rubella (page 225), Sinusitis (page 242), Sore Throats (page 249), Whooping Cough (page 286)

**NOSE BLEEDS:** Rheumatic Fever (page 258)

**PARALYSIS:** Botulism (page 16), Poliomyelitis (page 211)

**RASH:** Chickenpox (page 30), Fifth Disease (page 115), Hand, Foot, and Mouth Disease (page 134), Jock Itch (page 159), Lyme Disease (page 170), Measles (page 179), Mononucleosis (page 188), Rheumatic Fever (page 258), Ringworm (page 219), Roseola (page 223), Rubella (page 225), Scabies (page 237), Scarlet Fever (page 260), Strep Throat (page 262), Toxic Shock Syndrome (page 257), Toxocariasis (page 9), Toxoplasmosis (page 11)

**RASH, SCALY:** Jock Itch (page 159), Ringworm (page 219)

**RECTAL ITCHING:** Pinworms (page 197)

**SEIZURE:** Fevers (page 109), Meningitis (page 183), Rabies (page 6), Shigella Diarrhea (page 72)

**SENSITIVITY TO LIGHT:** Measles (page 179), Meningitis (page 183), Rabies (page 6), Trichinosis (page 271)

**SEVERE PAIN:** Necrotizing Fasciitis (page 257)

**SIDE PAIN:** Urinary Tract Infections (page 278)

**SKIN, BLISTERS, SORES, OR BUMPS:** Impetigo (page 147), Ringworm (page 219), Scabies (page 237), Warts (page 282)

**SKIN WOUND:** Necrotizing Fasciitis (page 257)

**SORE AREA ON SKIN:** Cellulitis (page 256)

**SORE GUMS:** Herpes Simplex Type 1 (page 144)

**SORE THROAT:** Botulism (page 16), Common Colds (page 34), Conjunctivitis (page 42), Diphtheria (page 80), Encephalitis (page 102), Epiglottitis (page 105), Fifth Disease (page 115), Hand, Foot, and Mouth Disease (page 134), Influenza (page 149), Lyme Disease (page 170), Mononucleosis (page 188), Poliomyelitis (page 211), Rabies (page 6), Rubella (page 225), Scarlet Fever (page 260), Sinusitis (page 242), Sore Throats (page 249), Strep Throat (page 262), Tetanus (page 267), Toxoplasmosis (page 11)

**SPEECH DIFFICULTIES:** Botulism (page 16), Encephalitis (page 102), Trichinosis (page 271)

**STIFF NECK:** Lyme Disease (page 170), Meningitis (page 183), Poliomyelitis (page 211), Tetanus (page 267)

**STRAWBERRY TONGUE:** Scarlet Fever (page 260)

**STOOLS, DISCOLORED :** Campylobacter Diarrhea (page 60), Giardia Diarrhea (page 67), Diarrhea (page 52), E. coli Disease (page 97), Food Poisoning (page 119), Hepatitis A (page 136), Salmonella Infections (page 231), Shigella Diarrhea (page 52)

# Common Childhood Infections

# ANIMAL-BORNE DISEASES

Also called Zoonotic Diseases.

Pets are a welcome addition to any household. Certainly we love our pets and encourage our children to delight in the joy of animals. At the same time, it's important to temper that enthusiasm with a healthy dose of caution.

As enjoyable as animals are, animal-related injuries are a reality. An animal may carry a disease that can infect your family. A dog may nip and bite and a cat can scratch, and after the incident the experience is usually forgotten. But infections may occur and knowledge will help prevent and/or identify them more quickly.

Zoonotic diseases, or zoonoses, are diseases that infect animals and can be transmitted to humans. You should know about these diseases because many of them have symptoms that are similar to those of other illnesses. For example, psittacosis (parrot fever) symptoms range from flulike to acute pneumonia. Often it is difficult to diagnose zoonotic diseases unless the physician is aware of the child's exposure to an animal.

This doesn't mean you have to give away your pet pooch. It simply means that you need to exercise caution. Teach your children to respect animals and to stay away from stray or unfamiliar animals. It's always important to practice good hygiene—but particularly so after contact with animals. Train your children to wash their hands after petting, feeding, or playing with an animal.

## *Cat Scratch Disease*

Your child should be seen by a doctor to be treated for cat scratch disease.

## SYMPTOMS

- Swollen glands
- Fever
- Headache
- General sick feeling
- Fatigue
- Loss of appetite

Cat scratch disease is an infection that causes swelling of the lymph nodes (small bean-shaped glands) after what may seem like a harmless animal scratch, often from a cat. Each year there are about 22,000 cases in the United States. More than 80 percent of cases of cat scratch disease affect children and young persons under age twenty-one. Typically, more than one family member gets this disease—it's not uncommon for siblings who share a pet to come down with cat scratch disease. For some reason we see more of this infection during the fall and winter.

After the animal scratches, a bump may develop. It's easy to mistake the bump or blister for an insect bite. About 75 percent of people with this infection have a mark from a cat scratch somewhere on their bodies, but by the time the swollen glands develop at the wound site, the primary sore has healed. It generally appears on the arms, hands, head, or scalp. Once you have cat scratch disease, you will be immune for the rest of your life.

Complications are rare, but when they do occur, the child may suddenly develop a high fever and convulsions. This can happen anywhere from one to six weeks after the swollen lymph nodes appear, and these symptoms may be short-lived or may last for one to two weeks. A child with such a severe case almost always recovers completely. For a typical case of cat scratch disease, your child should make a complete recovery within two to four months with no complications.

## Causes

Cat scratch disease is caused by *Bartonella henselae* bacteria and is transmitted through an animal (usually a cat) scratch.

## How It Spreads

This infection is not spread from person to person. It is transmitted from the scratch of an infected animal, most often a kitten. The animal does not appear sick but may carry bacteria in its blood and saliva for months.

## Incubation Period

It takes anywhere from seven to twelve days for a sore to appear at the site of a cat scratch. Swollen glands generally appear about two weeks after a cat scratch, but the range is from five to fifty days.

## Symptoms

Swollen glands near the area of the scratch are the main symptom in children and adolescents. The glands (or lymph nodes) may be painful to touch, and the skin over them may be warm and red. Your child may also have fever, a headache, and a general "sick" feeling. She may seem very tired and lose her appetite. The swollen glands usually disappear within two to four months.

## Diagnosis

The first clue to this disease is a history of exposure to a cat or kitten. If your doctor sees signs of an animal scratch and swollen lymph nodes, she will order a blood test for cat scratch disease, which has only recently become available. She may also want skin tests, blood tests, and additional cultures to rule out other causes of swollen lymph nodes.

### CALL YOUR DOCTOR

- If your child has swollen or painful lymph nodes in any part of the body.

- If your child has been scratched by a cat or kitten and develops swollen glands and fever accompanied by a general sick, achy feeling.

## Treatment

Your doctor may prescribe antibiotics, at least initially. Even without antibiotics, cat scratch disease will go away in time. Use acetaminophen to relieve any pain from swollen glands and to bring the fever down. You do not have to isolate your child because the disease is not contagious.

## Prevention

Avoid animal scratches and puncture wounds. Instruct your child to avoid stray or "strange" cats. Anytime your child is scratched by a pet, even your own, wash the injured area thoroughly with soap and water. You do not have to destroy your pet if someone in the family has caught cat scratch disease from your cat's scratch. You should ask about having your cat declawed.

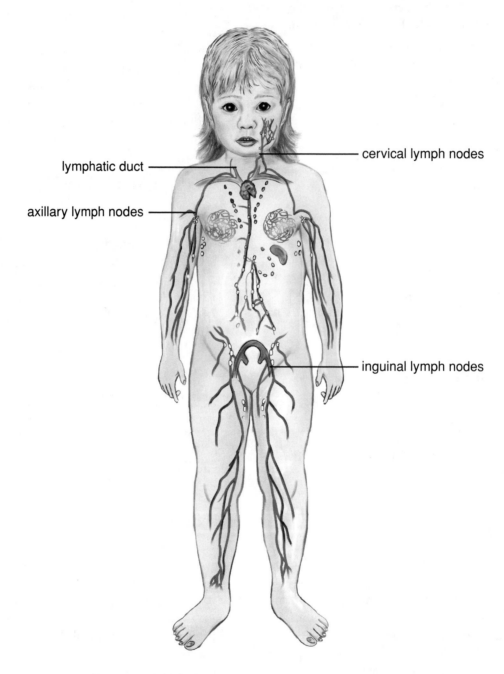

lymphatic duct —

cervical lymph nodes

axillary lymph nodes —

inguinal lymph nodes

*Swollen or painful lymph nodes are a symptom of animal-borne diseases.*

# *Psittacosis*

### *Psittacosis must be treated by a doctor.*

Also known as parrot fever.

| SYMPTOMS |
| --- |
| • Dry cough |
| • Fever |
| • Headache |
| • Chills |
| • Muscle and joint pain |
| • Gastrointestinal distress |

Psittacosis is also called parrot disease or parrot fever because its source is exotic birds such as parrots, parakeets, or finches. It can also be contracted from common fowl like turkeys and pigeons. The infection may cause a mild, flulike illness, or it can cause an acute pneumonia. (See *Pneumonia*, page 200.)

The birds themselves may or may not have symptoms, but they spread the organism among their colonies. Psittacosis may occur infrequently, or it may occur in clusters if a group of people comes in contact with the feces of infected birds. In the United States we see only about 100 to 200 cases each year. However, in the past twenty years there has been an increase in psittacosis cases, most likely because of an increase in the number of exotic birds imported as pets. Many of these birds are smuggled into the country and have not undergone the required quarantine period and treatment.

Psittacosis occurs primarily in adults, especially those who work with animals in occupational settings. For example, workers in poultry factories breathe in the bacteria from infected birds, carcasses, and secretions and from contaminated facilities.

When children get psittacosis, which they rarely do, it is generally from exposure to an infected bird in captivity, such as a pet parakeet or parrot.

## Causes

Psittacosis refers to an infection or disease in humans caused by *Chlamydia psittaci* bacteria.

## How It Spreads

People contract psittacosis by inhaling bacteria that are in the feces of infected domestic birds. A small number of cases of psittacosis are spread person to person. Lab workers who test birds for psittacosis have been known to get the disease.

## Incubation Period

Symptoms show up after an incubation period of seven to fourteen days.

## Symptoms

Psittacosis is often mistaken for other illnesses because its symptoms are so general. The most telling symptom is a dry cough (which may become productive). Your child may experience a headache, chills, and fever and will probably complain of muscle and joint pain. If your child has a severe case of psittacosis, he will probably experience gastrointestinal symptoms.

| CALL YOUR DOCTOR |
| --- |
| • If your child develops a cough, cold symptoms, or joint pains and has had recent contact with a bird. |

## Diagnosis

Be sure to tell your doctor if your child has been exposed to birds. If your doctor suspects psittacosis, she will order special blood tests to diagnose the infection.

## Treatment

Tetracycline is considered the drug of choice for psittacosis and is usually given for at least ten to fourteen days. Your doctor will prescribe erythromycin if your child is younger than nine.

## Prevention

One sure way to prevent psittacosis is to eliminate the infection in birds. Imported exotic birds must undergo quarantine and treatment with certain medicines and vaccines. Be certain to buy pet birds from a reputable dealer.

## *Rabies*

*In the event of a possible rabies exposure, a passive and long-lasting immunization is available to protect your child. Ask your doctor about vaccination.*

*Rabies exposure is an emergency and must be treated immediately by doctors in a hospital.*

Rabies is an extremely serious infection of the nervous system that is caused by a virus in the saliva of infected animals. It is usually transmitted by an animal bite. Although this disease is quite serious, it rarely occurs in humans if proper treatment is carried out immediately after exposure.

In almost all cases, we find that someone with a rabies infection was bitten by an animal about a month or two before the symptoms showed.

Throughout the world, rabid dogs present the highest risk to humans. In the United States, however, the vaccination of animals has largely eliminated canine rabies. Instead, it is bites from infected wild animals (such as raccoons or bats) that have caused most of the infrequent cases of human rabies that have occurred since 1960. Health departments continue to encourage the vaccination of pet dogs and cats so they do not become infected with rabies by a wild animal and then spread it to humans.

### SYMPTOMS

- Twitching or tingling at site of animal bite
- Fever, headache
- Malaise, muscle aches
- Loss of appetite, nausea, vomiting
- Sore throat, cough
- Exhaustion, irritability, agitation
- Hallucinations
- Seizures
- Muscle spasms
- Weakness or paralysis
- Sensitivity to light
- Double vision
- Difficulty swallowing, aversion to water
- Increased inability to swallow saliva ("foaming at the mouth")
- Coma

Dogs infected with rabies may exhibit the symptoms of either of two kinds of rabies. Most

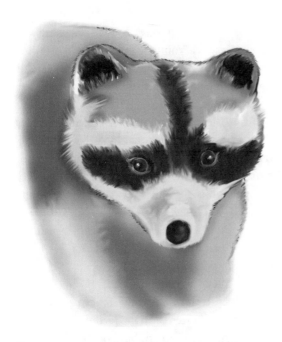

*Raccoons are one of the most common rabies carriers.*

oblivious to the car. After several minutes the wary driver maneuvered the car around the animal and went to her nearby home, where she called the police to report the raccoon's location and atypical behavior. Almost certainly the raccoon was rabid.

In the United States the most common rabies carriers are raccoons, skunks, bats, and foxes. A few cases have also been reported in wolves, coyotes, and ferrets. Rabbits and rodents (including squirrels) rarely if ever spread rabies, and their bites seldom if ever justify treatment. Although the number of cases of raccoon rabies has increased dramatically in the Mid-Atlantic states, raccoons are more likely to spread rabies to other species of animals than to humans. No human deaths have been attributed to raccoon rabies.

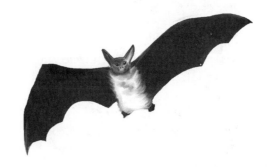

*Silver-haired bats have transmitted a form of rabies after minimal or insignificant contact.*

frequently described and known as the "furious rabies," this form is characterized by a kind of frenzied behavior and viciousness, followed by paralysis and death. "Dumb rabies" is characterized mainly by symptoms of paralysis. While rabid wild animals may show wild behavior, generally the behavioral changes are not very obvious. For instance, you may see a nocturnal animal (a bat, for instance) become active in the daytime.

One parent, riding home at night with her child in tow, encountered a raccoon in the middle of a street that ran through a popular suburban shopping center. She flashed her brights to get the raccoon to move. Instead, the raccoon remained in the street and began to walk in a circle. Thinking that the car had frightened the raccoon, the driver backed down the street and turned off her headlights, but the raccoon continued to move in an endless loop, seemingly

The form of human rabies, transmitted from silver-haired bats, is especially difficult to diagnose because its mode of transmission is unclear, but it is not from a bite or scratch. A person with this form of rabies may be unaware that he is at risk.

Recently, even insignificant exposure to bats, for example a bat flying in one's house, may warrant vaccination against rabies. Obviously, anyone who has been bitten by an animal suspected of having rabies must be evaluated and treated in a hospital. It is critical to try to safely capture the animal that caused the bite so it can be observed for signs of rabies.

## Causes

Rabies is a contagious infection caused by a virus that is present in the saliva of infected (rabid) animals. When the rabies virus enters the body, after a period of being dormant, it begins to multiply in the muscle surrounding the bite area. This explains why the first doses of the two antirabies medicines are usually injected right into the area around the animal bite. Eventually the rabies virus travels up a nearby nerve to the brain. When it reaches the brain, the virus infects many important areas of the brain and nerves, finally causing death.

## How It Spreads

Rabies is spread in the saliva of infected animals and usually infects humans through an animal bite or scratch. In rare cases the virus may spread to humans when an infected animal's saliva touches someone's mucous membranes (moist skin surfaces) or contacts an area of broken skin, such as a cut, scratch, or open wound.

## Incubation Period

The incubation period for a rabies infection can be anywhere from five days to one year but is usually one to two months. Once symptoms appear, chance of survival is rare. Without artificial life support, a person dies in four to twenty days.

## Symptoms

A merciless disease, rabies begins with an initial period of generalized symptoms that usually lasts for one to four days. The symptoms include fever, headache, malaise, muscle aches, loss of appetite, nausea, vomiting, sore throat, cough, and exhaustion. One unique symptom that exists in more than half the cases of rabies is a tingling or twitching sensation around the area of the bite.

After these first symptoms appear, the next stage brings symptoms that look like encephalitis. (See *Encephalitis*, page 102.) The infected person may have a very high fever with hallucinations. He will be extremely irritable and agitated, and may become very aggressive. You may witness seizures, muscle spasms, weakness or paralysis, and extreme sensitivity to bright lights, sounds, or touch.

The later stages produce symptoms that reflect the infection's destruction of many areas of the nervous system. The infected person may develop double vision or have problems moving his facial muscles and the muscles that control the diaphragm and breathing. Because it becomes difficult to swallow and there may be an increased production of saliva, it appears that the patient is "foaming at the mouth," the symptom usually associated with rabies.

In the final stage a patient may slip into a coma and stop breathing.

## Diagnosis

Your doctor needs to know about the history of any animal that bites your child—the type of animal, its health history (whether it was vaccinated or not), and whether or not the animal was provoked.

If the animal that bit your child is a pet and has no symptoms and can be contained, it will be held for observation. If the animal remains healthy for ten days, the veterinarian can conclude that it was not infectious when it bit your child and no treatment will be necessary. If however, the biting animal was rabid or a wild animal, it should be killed and its brain submitted to a laboratory for testing—a biting animal must be proved to have no infection if the bite victim is to avoid treatment.

## CALL YOUR DOCTOR

- If your child has recently been bitten by an animal.
- If your child has been exposed to an animal that might have rabies.

## Treatment

If your child is bitten by an animal, clean the wound with soap and water immediately and take her to the doctor. Your pediatrician will clean the wound thoroughly and check to see if your child's tetanus immunizations are up to date. If not, she may need a tetanus booster.

Possible rabies exposure requires immunizations as soon as possible to prevent infection. What used to be a series of painful injections into the stomach is instead now a series of intramuscular (into a muscle) injections. Two kinds of immunizations are given concurrently but not at the same site.

## Prevention

One of the best preventive measures is to clean the area of an animal-related wound aggressively and immediately with soap and water. Notify your doctor immediately. Once an infected animal has bitten a human, a rabies infection can be prevented by a series of immunizations.

If your child needs these shots, he will receive a series of five injections of human diploid cell vaccine and of human rabies immune globulin.

The human rabies immune globulin is given at the first visit. Thereafter, a single dose of human diploid cell vaccine is given on the first day of the bite and then repeated on days 3, 7, 14, and 28. Your doctor will decide whether or not to begin the series of prophylactic (disease-preventing) injections based on the circumstances of the bite, the type of animal that did the biting, whether the animal can be reliably observed, and the suggestions of local health authorities.

Persons who have a high risk of exposure to rabid animals sometimes have a series of rabies injections as a preventive measure.

A good way to prevent rabies in humans is to see that your pets are vaccinated. Report stray animals or animals with unusual or atypical behavior to local health authorities or the animal warden. Remind your child not to feed or touch stray animals.

## *Toxocariasis*

***Toxocariasis must be treated by a doctor.***

Also known as visceral larva migrans.

## SYMPTOMS

- Rash
- Cough or wheezing
- Stomach pain
- Lack of appetite
- Vision problems
- Swollen glands
- Enlarged liver
- Fever

Toxocariasis is an illness that usually affects children under ten years of age (usually one to four years of age), particularly those who like to put things in their mouths or those with pet dogs or cats. The disease is transmitted when a child unwittingly eats soil that contains the larvae or eggs of common parasites found in dogs and cats. It is also spread by exposure to a litter of puppies or by eating gravel or ice that has the larvae in it.

## Causes

Toxocariasis is caused when toxocara, common parasitic roundworms found in cats and dogs—especially puppies or kittens—infect humans. The larvae of these worms live in the intestines of dogs (*Toxocara canis*) and less commonly in cats (*Toxocara cati*). Eggs from these parasites pass into the stools of dogs and cats and then contaminate areas around the home. The eggs can be swallowed by young children who frequently put things in their mouths and may not wash their hands often. Once the toxocara eggs enter a child's body, they hatch into larvae that penetrate through the walls of her digestive tract and may move to her liver, lungs, eyes, and other parts of the body.

About 20 percent of dogs pass these eggs in their stools, which may be deposited, in turn, in sandboxes and play areas in public parks. How sick your child gets depends upon the number of larvae she ingested—something impossible to determine. Most children who are lightly infected do not experience any symptoms.

In older children the larvae may migrate to the eyes, causing ocular larva migrans.

## How It Spreads

Toxocariasis is spread by contact with the larvae of toxocara parasites. It is not spread from person to person. Puppies in the household are usually the cause of most infections.

## Incubation Period

Because the incubation period varies, it is not known exactly how long it takes to become ill. Symptoms may appear within weeks to months after a child swallows the eggs. You will probably not know that your child ingested the eggs until he has symptoms.

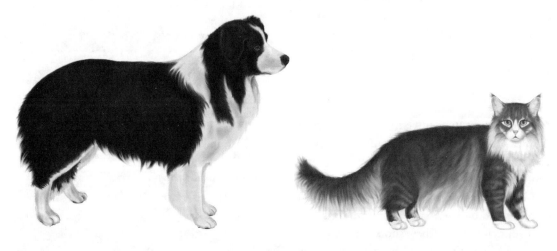

*The larvae of toxocara parasites live in the intestines of dogs (*Toxocara canis*), and less commonly in cats (*Toxocara cati*).*

## Symptoms

Most children have no symptoms or very mild ones. Your child may develop a fever, a cough or wheezing, abdominal pain, an enlarged liver or spleen, a rash that looks like hives, and swollen glands. He may lose his appetite and pick at his food. This disease may also affect his eyes, which may appear swollen or cross-eyed, or his vision may be impaired.

---

**CALL YOUR DOCTOR**

- If your child has played with kittens or puppies or in an open sandbox and has any of the symptoms of cat scratch disease (see page 2), or chronic symptoms including rash, cough or wheezing, stomach pain, diminished appetite, and vision problems.

---

## Diagnosis

Your doctor will examine your child and perform some blood tests to make a diagnosis of toxocariasis.

## Treatment

For a mild case your pediatrician may not prescribe anything. If your child has a severe case, the doctor may prescribe medication to kill the toxocara larvae. If the infection reaches the lungs or if the central nervous system has been affected, your child may also be given anti-inflammatory drugs.

## Prevention

One of the best ways to prevent toxocariasis is to keep pets away from the sandbox and cover it when it is not being used. Take your pets to the veterinarian to be dewormed, especially any puppies less than six months old. Remind your children to wash their hands frequently, especially after playing in the sandbox. Also remind them to keep their hands out of their mouths. Discourage them from eating dirt and snow.

# Toxoplasmosis

*Toxoplasmosis must be treated by a doctor.*

---

**SYMPTOMS**

- General "sick" feeling, fatigue

- Fever

- Sore throat and headache

- Rash

- Swollen lymph glands

---

Humans get toxoplasmosis infections through contact with soil or objects contaminated with cat feces that contain certain parasites. Another way that people get toxoplasmosis is by eating poorly cooked meat that contains these parasites.

The greatest risk is to an unborn baby whose mother contracts a primary infection during her pregnancy. If an infection occurs early in the pregnancy, an abortion may occur. When the infection occurs later in the pregnancy, the outcome may be a miscarriage, stillbirth, or a child born with a disease that can be fatal. In the last case symptoms may appear shortly after birth, but more often they become evident months or even years later.

Except for transplacental (across the placenta) infection from mother to fetus, toxoplasmosis is not spread from person to person. On rare occasions it is transmitted by a blood transfusion and from infected organ donors.

## Causes

Toxoplasmosis is caused by *Toxoplasma gondii,* a protozoan parasite that infects many species of warm-blooded animals. Members of the cat family are hosts for these parasites, which they get when they feed on infected animals, such as mice, or uncooked household meats. Cats then excrete the parasites in their stools.

## How It Spreads

Toxoplasmosis is not spread from person to person except from mother to fetus, which is the greatest danger of this disease.

## Incubation Period

The incubation period is approximately seven days, but it can range from four days to three weeks.

## Symptoms

Most people who have toxoplasmosis do not have any symptoms. When symptoms do develop, they are nonspecific and include a general "sick" feeling, fever, sore throat, and headache, similar to the symptoms of a mono infection (see *Mononucleosis*, page 188). There may be an accompanying rash. The symptoms are generally harmless and disappear without treatment.

In newborns, however, toxoplasmosis is quite a different story. Most infected newborns show no recognizable signs of infection at birth. Occasionally, a baby born to a mother who aquired toxoplasmosis early in her pregnancy may show severe manifestations of the disease at birth. An infant who is severely affected may have hydrocephalus (an enlarged head due to accumulation of fluid, also called water on the brain), chorioretinitis (inflammation of parts of the eye), and calcification in the brain. These manifestations

can lead to later convulsions, mental retardation, spasticity or palsy, deafness, or severely impaired vision. Unfortunately, a mild case of toxoplasmosis is often not recognized at birth, and symptoms (such as partial blindness) may not show until later, either months after birth, in early childhood, or even in early adulthood.

Babies of HIV-infected mothers or mothers with immunosuppressed systems who are chronically infected with toxoplasma may acquire congenital toxoplasmosis as a result of maternal parasites that get reactivated, as sometimes happens. The outcome is poor for children born with congenital toxoplasmosis acquired during the first trimester. These children often die in infancy or suffer severe damage to the central nervous system.

## Diagnosis

It is very difficult to diagnose congenital toxoplasmosis. If there is a suspicion of the disease prenatally, your doctor will take a blood sample and other tests to make a diagnosis. If the diagnosis of toxoplasmosis is suspected but unconfirmed at delivery, the doctor will order ophthalmologic and neurologic exams, a CAT scan of your baby's head, and blood tests on both you and your baby for comparison.

## Treatment

For infants with congenital toxoplasmosis, a treatment that uses certain drugs for a one-year period, has been shown to lead to significant improvement in their neurologic and developmental outcome. However, treatment needs to start early after birth to have the best effect.

## Prevention

Be sure to dispose of cat litter daily because the parasite eggs are not actively infectious during the first twenty-four to forty-eight hours after passage. Feed your cats commercially prepared cat food and do not let them roam outdoors. Also, do not let your pets eat raw or partially cooked kitchen scraps. Make sure to cook all red meats thoroughly, and if you are pregnant, eat only well-done meat. If you are pregnant and you have a negative or unknown toxoplasma titer (a test that analyzes whether or not you have toxoplasmosis), you should avoid contact with cat feces. This means you should stay out of the garden or any areas in the yard to which cats have access.

There are also some other diseases that—while not primarily spread by animals—your child can sometimes catch from a pet. See *Giardia Diarrhea,* page 67; *Ringworm,* page 219; *Scabies,* page 237; *Salmonella Infections,* page 231, and *Yersinia Diarrhea,* page 77.

And you can also catch Lyme disease from an infected deer tick that your dog or cat brings in. See *Lyme Disease,* page 170.

# ATHLETE'S FOOT

## SYMPTOMS

- Dry skin
- Itching and burning
- Scaling
- Inflammation
- Blisters
- Cracked skin

Athlete's foot belongs to a group of fungal skin infections referred to as tinea. These include jock itch (page 159), ringworm (page 219), and athlete's foot. The medical name for athlete's foot is *Tinea pedis*. Tinea infections can affect most skin types. Athlete's foot is most prevalent in older children, adolescents, and adults. It commonly affects the feet because shoes provide the kind of warm and moist environment that encourages fungal growth. The condition usually occurs between the toes, but it can also infect the toenails. Athlete's foot occurs throughout the world. It is contagious for as long as the infection is present.

There are other conditions that look like athlete's foot, such as eczema, psoriasis, and allergic reactions. If treatment is not working, another condition may be present and you should consult your child's physician.

## Causes

Athlete's foot is a skin disease caused by a fungus. This condition is so named because the fungi that cause it breed in warm, moist environments where athletes may be found—areas around swimming pools, showers, and locker rooms. Athlete's foot is seen most frequently in adolescents and adults. While your teenager may develop athlete's foot, it is unlikely that a young child will.

## How It Spreads

The process of how tinea spreads from one person to another is not well understood. Instruct your child not to touch any area that is actively infected on another person. Sometimes athlete's foot spreads either to the soles of the feet or to the toenails. If your child scratches the infection and then touches himself elsewhere, he can spread the fungus to other parts of the body, particularly the groin and underarms.

Your child can also spread the infection to other parts of the body from contaminated bed linens or clothing.

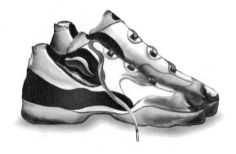

*Footwear can be a breeding ground for Athlete's foot fungus.*

## Incubation Period

The incubation period is not known.

## Symptoms

You will see any one of a number of symptoms or a combination of symptoms. These include dry skin, itching, scaling, inflammation, and blisters that often lead to cracking of the skin. When the blisters break, small raw areas of tissue are exposed, and your child experiences pain and swelling. As the infection spreads, the itching and burning increase.

---

### CALL YOUR DOCTOR

- If your child complains of itchy red skin or has patchy lesions.

- If your child's fungus condition does not respond to home treatment and does not show improvement within two weeks.

---

## Diagnosis

If the fungus condition does not respond to proper foot hygiene and care using over-the-counter remedies, you should consult your child's doctor. He or she can diagnose athlete's foot by observation. In certain cases the doctor may take a scraping and culture it to confirm that a fungus is causing the problem.

## Treatment

Most cases of athlete's foot are treated with anti-fungal ointments and creams that you can buy over the counter in the drugstore. These are generally applied topically two times a day. In rare instances, if bacteria has caused an infection on top of the fungal infection, the doctor may prescribe antibiotics.

## Prevention

It is difficult to prevent athlete's foot because your child usually contracts it in showers, locker rooms, and the area around swimming pools, where bare feet come in contact with the fungus. One of the most important things you can do is to instruct your child in healthy foot hygiene. The feet should be washed with soap and water and dried carefully, especially between the toes. Buy socks that keep the feet dry. If your child is prone to Athlete's foot, make sure she changes shoes and stockings or socks frequently to decrease the moisture and help prevent the fungus from infecting the feet. Encourage daily use of a good foot powder or talcum powder to absorb and decrease perspiration. Have your child wear light and airy shoes, particularly in hot weather. Encourage the use of shower shoes in public showers.

If your child has an active infection, she should avoid public areas that are conducive to transmission.

# BOTULISM

***Botulism is an emergency and must be treated by doctors in a hospital.***

## SYMPTOMS

- Muscle paralysis, particularly of head and throat
- Blurred or double vision
- In babies, constipation, not sucking normally, floppiness, weak cry

Botulism is a particularly severe—and life-threatening—form of food poisoning. It attacks a person's nerves and paralyzes his muscles. Even if the person survives, it can take months to recover.

Fortunately, botulism in humans is also rare. However, the germ that causes botulism is far from rare. It is very common in the environment around us.

You need to know what precautions to take to keep anyone in your family from getting botulism. *It is one of the reasons you should not let food sit out at room temperature. It is also the reason you should never feed honey to a baby.*

"Although there are very few cases of botulism poisoning each year," emphasizes the Public Health Service's Centers for Disease Control and Prevention, "prevention is extremely important."

## Cause

A bacterium called *Clostridium botulinum* is the culprit causing botulism poisoning. The name *Clostridium* comes from the Greek word for "spindle," which is what these bacteria look like under a microscope.

*C. botulinum* bacteria are so widespread because one of the ways they reproduce themselves is by forming tough, dormant cells called spores. Botulinus spores are commonly found in soils, both cultivated and not, and in sediments at the bottom of lakes, rivers, and ocean waters throughout the world. The spores are thus often present in the intestinal tracts of fish and other animals and on the surfaces of fruits and vegetables, and they float into our homes as part of the house dust.

*C. botulinum* can be deadly because when its spores germinate, the bacteria produce a powerful toxin. (A toxin is a poison made by a living organism.) Botulinus toxin is one of the most potent poisons known. A few billionths of a gram can make a person sick.

## How It Spreads

A person can get botulism poisoning in two different ways: from the toxin or the spores.

First, a person can develop botulism by eating food contaminated with botulinus toxin. Some twenty to fifty people in the United States get botulism this way each year, according to the Public Health Service.

Botulinus bacteria grow and produce their toxin only in places where there is little or no oxygen. In the nineteenth century one food that sometimes was a source of botulism was sausage; the nearly airless interiors provided the conditions the bacteria like for growth, and it was sausage that gave the disease its name. The word *botulism* comes from the Latin word for "sausage."

Today in the United States, the most common source of botulism food poisoning is improperly processed canned foods. Botulinus spores are so tough they are able to survive boiling for many hours. If foods are not heated to higher temperatures, high enough to destroy the spores, they can survive and produce their deadly toxin in the airless conditions inside a sealed can or glass jar.

Commercially canned foods are generally safe because manufacturers know they must routinely heat foods to temperatures high enough to sterilize them. When an occasional slip-up does occur, the Food and Drug Administration issues an immediate recall. Today the most common source of botulism food poisoning is improperly processed foods canned at home. While the bacteria can grow in almost any food, botulinus toxin forms most commonly in canned vegetables, including asparagus, corn, beets, peas, peppers, and green beans.

Several recent outbreaks of botulism food poisoning have been caused not by canned foods but by foods preserved in oil. Covering food with oil can provide the airless conditions these bacteria need to grow. In one incident seven people developed botulism after eating roasted eggplants in oil. In another, three people were hospitalized for botulism they got from the bottled garlic in oil they used to make garlic bread.

Botulinus bacteria are among the many germs that can grow in foods left out of the refrigerator at room temperature. In an outbreak in Illinois, twenty-eight people got botulism poisoning from sautéed onions a restaurant had left sitting out all day. A layer of margarine over the onions had kept out air and permitted the bacteria to grow and make their toxin.

Fish can sometimes be a source of botulism food poisoning. Fish intestines, you recall, are among the many places where botulinus spores can occur. In Hawaii one summer, three people got botulism from a fish they grilled at home. It turned out that the market had not fully cleaned the fish and then had not refrigerated it properly.

In another incident eight people got botulism from salt-cured, air-dried—and ungutted—whitefish they ate without cooking.

\* \* \*

The second way that people—in this case infants—can get botulism is by ingesting not the toxin but the spores themselves. Occasionally the spores can germinate in a baby's intestinal tract, where there is little oxygen, and produce botulinus toxin right there, on the spot, in the baby's own intestines. The baby does not eat the poison but makes his own, so to speak.

This infant botulism, as it is called, was discovered only in 1976 but is now recognized as the most common type of botulism poisoning that occurs in the United States. Some 60 to 100 cases are reported each year to the Public Health Service, twice as many as for foodborne botulism. At The Children's Hospital of Philadelphia, we see perhaps five to ten babies a year with infant botulism.

Just where and how these babies acquire botulinus spores is usually never discovered. One food that definitely can be a source is honey. In one study researchers found botulinus spores in 10 percent of honey samples they tested, and some babies who developed infant botulism are known to have eaten spore-containing honey. Other babies may simply have inhaled spores floating in house dust and then swallowed them. Spores may be released when construction is going on in a home or in the immediate area.

This infant form of botulism affects only babies under the age of one year and is most common in those under six months. The reason it targets this age group has to do with the other bacteria inhabiting the intestines of babies this young; there is probably a brief period of time when the spores are able to grow in a baby's intestine. Why some babies this age get botulism and most do not remains a mystery.

## Incubation Period

If a person ingests botulinus toxin in food, it usually will take twelve to thirty-six hours for her to develop symptoms, but it can take as few as six hours or as long as eight days.

For infant botulism, when a baby ingests not the toxin but the spores, the incubation period is three to thirty days.

## Symptoms

If a person eats botulinus toxin in food, the poison passes into the bloodstream and then spreads throughout the body. The toxin molecules attach themselves to his nerve cells at the places where nerve-cell endings join the muscles. This blocks nerve impulses from reaching and activating the muscles, thus paralyzing them.

Botulinus toxin first, and most severely, affects the nerves controlling the muscles of the head, face, eyes, and throat. As the poison paralyzes these muscles, the eyelids droop. The person develops double and blurred vision. He may have trouble speaking and swallowing. His mouth, tongue, and throat may become so dry that they hurt, and he will complain of a sore throat. He may feel dizzy.

The paralysis may then spread downward on both sides of the body. The arms and legs may become weak. If the intestines are affected, he may become constipated. The paralysis often weakens the respiratory muscles, and he may find it difficult to breathe. Severe botulism can completely paralyze him.

In babies who have the infant form of botulism, the first sign of the disease is usually constipation, several days in a row without a bowel movement. As the muscles that control the baby's sucking and swallowing become weakened, she does not feed as well as usual. Sometimes a mother who is breastfeeding notices that her breasts are becoming engorged. The baby's face may become expressionless, and her cry feeble. She may be unable to hold up her head and may become increasingly weak and floppy.

### CALL YOUR DOCTOR

- If your baby becomes constipated, is not sucking and swallowing normally, loses head control, and seems generally weak and floppy.

- If your child has droopy eyelids, blurred or double vision, or trouble speaking or swallowing.

## Diagnosis

If physicians suspect that a child or baby may have developed botulism, they have laboratory methods to detect botulinus toxin in his blood and in a sample of his stool. The lab also tries to culture (grow) the bacteria from a stool sample in order to identify them. This takes five to seven days.

If doctors suspect a child has ingested botulism toxin in food, they have a lab test the suspect food for the toxin and also try to culture the bacteria from the food. They try to locate any other people who may have eaten the food and find out whether they, too, have any symptoms of botulism.

If a baby turns out to have infant botulism, the hospital reports the case to the local health department. At Children's Hospital we always try to determine the source of the spores, and we ask the parents for information about the baby's diet.

## *Treatment*

Anyone who has botulism—whether a baby who has had the spores germinate in his intestines or someone who has ingested the toxin in food—must be hospitalized, usually in an intensive care unit where heart rate and breathing can be continuously monitored. If the throat muscles are affected and he is having trouble swallowing, he may need to be fed by tube. If the respiratory muscles are so weakened that he has trouble breathing, he needs to be on a mechanical respirator.

Children and adults who have contracted botulism from contaminated food are promptly given an injection of botulism antitoxin. This can neutralize any molecules of toxin not yet bound to his nerve endings.

In the early part of the twentieth century, botulism food poisoning killed about 70 percent of the people who had it. Today, even with modern medical care, two or three deaths from botulism food poisoning usually occur in the United States each year. Currently, there is no treatment for infant botulism other than careful support in an intensive care setting. There is research using a special immuniglobulin for treatment but it is not available at this time. With infant botulism fewer than 2 out of every 100 babies with the disease succumb to it. Survivors usually recover completely, but they may face a lengthy convalescence. A person fully recovers only when her damaged nerves grow new nerve endings, a process that can take many weeks or months. She may need to spend weeks in the hospital until she can breathe and eat on her own

again. One California baby had to spend ten months in the hospital.

## *Prevention*

Botulinus bacteria produce gas as they grow, and this may cause a can to bulge. Do not buy any swollen or dented cans of food, advises the U.S. Department of Agriculture (USDA). If you have any such damaged cans at home, do not eat the food. Throw it out.

Food tainted with botulinus toxin does not necessarily look or smell different from other food. However, if you do notice that food in a can or jar—or anywhere else—appears discolored or smells bad, do not even taste it. Just discard it, says the USDA.

And remember: botulinus bacteria are among the many germs that can grow in food left sitting out of the refrigerator at room temperature. The Food and Drug Administration and the Public Health Service both recommend that you not leave food out at room temperature for longer than four hours. The USDA, on the other hand, advises that you not leave food out for more than *two* hours. If you do make a mistake and leave food out, again, throw it out.

Make sure you carefully read the labels on canned, bottled, and other processed foods and follow the instructions about whether or not you need to refrigerate them.

If you do can foods at home, you need to use a pressure canner when processing most vegetables and many other foods in order to heat them to temperatures high enough (240° to 250°F) to kill any botulinus spores and sterilize the food. The exact times and pressures needed vary depending on the food, the way it is packed, and the size of the jars.

You can obtain detailed instructions from your local office of the Cooperative Extension Service about how to do home canning safely. You should be able to find it in the phone book under the name of your state's land-grant university. In Pennsylvania, for instance, the Cooperative Extension Service is part of Penn State University. In New York State it is run by Cornell University.

The Public Health Service suggests that if you do can foods at home, you might want to take another step. While botulinus spores are hard to kill, it is relatively easy to inactivate any botulinus toxin that may contaminate a food. You can destroy any toxin by boiling the food for ten minutes. "People who eat home-canned foods," says the Health Service, "should consider boiling the food before eating it to ensure safety."

If you prepare roasted vegetables in oil at home, the Health Service also warns, you "should be aware that this practice may be hazardous, especially if such foods are allowed to remain above refrigerator temperatures."

To prevent babies from getting infant botulism, the Public Health Service and the American Academy of Pediatrics both recommend that you do not feed honey to any child under twelve months of age. Honey "should not be placed on nipples before breastfeeding," says the academy, which also warns against corn syrup. "Although cases of infant botulism have not been linked to corn syrup, prudence indicates that infants should not be fed this nonessential food, which also has been reported to contain *Clostridium botulinum.*"

# BRONCHIOLITIS

*If your child is having difficulty breathing, he needs to be evaluated by a doctor.*

The ending *-itis* means "inflammation."

## SYMPTOMS

- Breathing difficulties
- Very, very runny nose followed by a worsening cough
- Coughing, sometimes followed by vomiting
- No fever to a high fever, 103° to 104°F

Bronchiolitis is a very common and potentially serious, sometimes life-threatening disease of a child's lower respiratory tract, the lungs. It is primarily a disease of babies.

Bronchiolitis is an inflammation of a child's bronchioles, which are the smallest air passageways in the lungs.

If you think of the respiratory tract as an upside-down tree, the windpipe (trachea) is the trunk, and the bronchial tubes are the main branches. (See figure below and on page 22.) The bronchioles are the very tiniest branches, the twigs that hold the buds and leaves, which correspond to the air sacs (alveoli). We have millions of bronchioles and air sacs in our lungs. In babies these bronchioles are so tiny that any infection causing inflamation can cause them to swell and be blocked off.

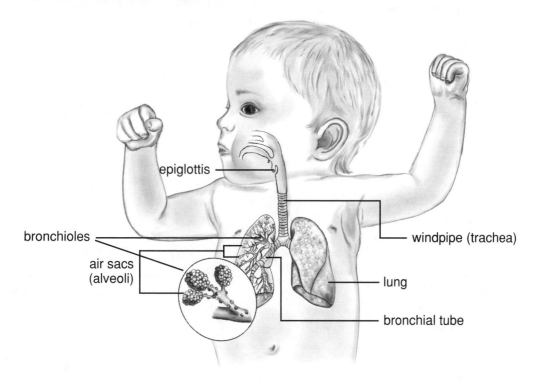

epiglottis

bronchioles

air sacs (alveoli)

windpipe (trachea)

lung

bronchial tube

*The respiratory tract.*

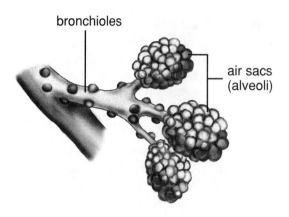

*Close-up of bronchioles and air sacs.*

More than 80 percent of children who develop bronchiolitis are babies in their first year of life. A baby is most likely to have bronchiolitis between the ages of two and six months. For some unknown reason, boys get it more often than girls.

Like so many respiratory infections, bronchiolitis is seasonal. Babies most often get it between the beginning of November and early February. During these months at Children's Hospital, we usually see five to ten babies a day with this infection.

## Causes

Ninety percent of the time, bronchiolitis is caused by an important and widespread virus called respiratory syncytial virus (RSV).

Respiratory syncytial virus is the number-one cause of serious lower respiratory tract disease in infants and young children. It is a major cause of childhood pneumonia as well as of bronchiolitis, and it can also cause croup, bronchitis, and ear infections. RSV appears on the scene in annual epidemics, which in turn are responsible for the seasonal peaks of bronchiolitis. Older children and adults can become infected with RSV, but it often causes just a common cold. See *Respiratory Syncytial Virus (RSV) Infections,* page 26, for more information about this major virus.

Other viruses that can also cause bronchiolitis include the parainfluenza viruses, influenza viruses, and adenoviruses. Like RSV, these are common viruses that also can cause a variety of other respiratory diseases. In older children and adults, they often just cause colds.

Your baby can thus get bronchiolitis from an older sibling or a grownup who merely has a cold.

## How It Spreads

Respiratory syncytial virus (RSV) spreads readily through families and day-care centers. People who are infected with RSV shed virus particles in the secretions from their nose and throat. If you are infected, you can get the virus on your hands when you blow your nose or when you help an infected child blow his nose. If you do not wash your hands afterward, you can carry RSV to another child.

If you set a used tissue down on a table, it is possible to leave RSV on its surface. RSV is a heardy virus. RSV particles can remain alive on such surfaces—such as a tabletop—for six to eight hours.

When another person touches the table, the RSV can get on the hands. RSV enters the body of this second person through the membranes lining the nose or the eye. When she touches her nose or eye, the virus can enter her body.

From the tip of the nose or eye, RSV particles multiply and can spread down along the windpipe and bronchial tubes into the lungs and bronchioles.

## Incubation Period

It usually takes about four to six days from the time your baby is infected with RSV until he starts to show symptoms, but it can take from as few as two days to as many as eight.

## Symptoms

For the first two or three days while the virus remains confined to a baby's upper respiratory tract (his nose and throat), he has just a very, very runny nose, with great quantities of clear mucus running out.

Then the baby's symptoms gradually worsen. By about day three, as the virus spreads down into his bronchioles, he starts coughing, three or four coughs in a row that may wake him up at night. After a bout of coughing, he may vomit; the coughing sets off a reflex that triggers vomiting. And he starts breathing much more rapidly. A baby in his first months of life usually breathes 30 to 40 times a minute. With bronchiolitis he may reach 70 or 80 times a minute. He may or may not have a fever, but it can become quite high, up to 103° or 104°F.

Bronchioles, it is important to remember, lead to the air sacs (alveoli); these are where oxygen passes into the bloodstream. As the virus continues to multiply in a baby's bronchioles, it causes the tissues lining these tiny tubules to become inflamed and swollen, thus narrowing these airways, and mucus and other secretions further clog them.

With your baby's bronchioles narrowed and clogged with mucus, he may develop respiratory distress: he has to work harder to breathe. He not only breathes faster but may also start to wheeze. As he tries to get more air, the sides of his nostrils may flare outward. He may use additional muscles to help him breathe, developing what physicians call "retractions": the muscles in the spaces between his ribs pull in (retract) with every breath, and you can see these spaces sinking in. You can also see him draw in the muscles in the spaces at the base of his neck, above his collarbone, with each breath, and he may use his abdominal muscles for breathing, causing his breastbone to sink down. You may hear him gasping if he is really struggling to breathe.

With less air getting to his air sacs, less oxygen is getting into his bloodstream and reaching his brain and other tissues. He may start turning blue or grayish around his mouth and at the tips of his fingers. His behavior may change. Instead of smiling and being playful, he may become limp and lethargic and less responsive as he concentrates just on breathing.

In severe cases of bronchiolitis, a baby can go into respiratory failure. He may pause from time to time in his breathing or even stop breathing entirely.

The babies who are most likely to suffer these more severe symptoms of bronchiolitis are those who have chronic heart or lung disease: babies who have congenital heart defects and especially babies who were born prematurely and spent time on a respirator in a neonatal intensive care unit. These infants may have some residual damage to their lungs, a condition called bronchopulmonary dysplasia. Their bronchioles may be smaller than those of other babies and clog even more easily.

## Diagnosis

When your doctor listens to your baby's lungs with a stethoscope, she may be able to hear sounds caused by mucus in the baby's lungs,

## CALL YOUR DOCTOR

- If your baby is breathing faster than usual, coughing, and also vomiting.

- If your baby has other signs of respiratory distress: he is working harder to breathe; his nostrils are flaring and he is retracting (pulling in) the muscles between his ribs and at the base of the neck as he breathes.

**CALL 911 or take your child to your hospital emergency room:**

- If your baby is struggling to breathe and gasping.

- If your baby has a bluish or grayish tinge around the mouth or at the tips of the fingers.

- If your baby is lethargic or unresponsive.

- If your baby pauses in his breathing for more than 10 seconds.

sounds caused by air flowing around the mucus clogging the bronchioles. Physicians call these distinctive sounds rales.

At Children's Hospital the actual amount of oxygen reaching a baby's bloodstream is measured with a device called a pulse oximeter, a light probe that fits on a baby's finger and gives the doctors an immediate reading.

On a chest X-ray, the lungs of a baby with bronchiolitis may look normal or somewhat more inflated than usual. In a baby with more severe disease, the lungs may have areas of visible mucus and also white patches where air sacs have collapsed because air is no longer reaching them. In very severe bronchiolitis a baby may have extensive collapsed areas on both sides of the lungs.

We test for respiratory syncytial virus (RSV) only if a baby is so sick that we must admit him to the hospital. Otherwise we do not need to know what virus is causing the bronchiolitis because the information does not affect treatment. It is important to know if a baby is being admitted to the hospital because our staff will

take special isolation precautions to keep the virus from spreading to other sick children in the hospital. To test for RSV, a small sample of mucus is suctioned from the baby's nose, and the laboratory performs a rapid test that tells us the answer within a few hours.

## Treatment

Most babies who have bronchiolitis have a mild illness and are cared for at home.

Your baby does not need to take any antibiotics. Antibiotics do not work against—that is, they do not kill—respiratory syncytial virus or any of the other viruses that can cause bronchiolitis.

Your pediatrician will probably suggest the following.

### Fluids

It is very important that you give your baby plenty of extra fluids to drink because babies this small can very quickly become dangerously dehydrated. Babies with bronchiolitis produce so much mucus that they lose a lot of fluid from their respiratory tract. They also lose fluid if they have a fever and when they vomit.

With babies under a year, however, you should never give plain water. You need to give them special fluids called oral rehydration solutions. See *Fluids*, page 290, in the Appendices for more about dehydration and also about these special fluids for babies.

## Medications

If your baby has a significant fever and is uncomfortable because of fever, you can give acetaminophen. Always follow the label directions.

## Humidity

Use a humidifier to increase the moisture content of the air your baby is breathing. This increased humidity will not reach down as far as the bronchioles, but it may help loosen mucus in the baby's nose and throat. See *Humidity*, page 293, in the Appendices for more information about humidity and humidifiers.

\* \* \*

If you have taken your baby to the doctor early in the course of bronchiolitis, on the first or second day of illness, you should know that the symptoms could get worse *after* your doctor has checked the baby over. Bronchiolitis tends to worsen over the first three or four days. Be prepared to call your doctor again if any of your baby's symptoms intensify. By the fourth day, however, the symptoms should start to taper off and slowly disappear. It can take up to two weeks for bronchiolitis to resolve completely.

Children generally do not develop bronchiolitis as severely a second time. It is mainly during the three-month RSV season each winter that babies get bronchiolitis. By the time the

next RSV season rolls around, the next winter, children are a year older, their bronchioles are bigger, and they may also have developed some immunity against RSV.

Babies who have severe RSV bronchiolitis may later develop asthma. It is uncertain, however, whether bronchiolitis increases a child's chances of getting asthma or whether children with a tendency toward asthma are more likely to get bronchiolitis.

## Hospitalization

About 13 out of every 1,000 infants with RSV bronchiolitis are sick enough and in such respiratory distress they must be admitted to the hospital. At Children's Hospital we are more likely to admit those babies who are less than three months old and those who were born prematurely.

In the hospital we continuously monitor the baby's heart and breathing rates and periodically measure the oxygen level in his blood. If he is vomiting a lot because he is coughing so much, we may give him extra fluids orally or intravenously. If his bronchioles are so blocked that he is not getting enough oxygen, he may get extra oxygen. If he needs assistance breathing, he can be put on a respirator in the intensive care unit.

Sometimes physicians give babies with very severe RSV bronchiolitis an antiviral medication called ribavirin. This must be administered by mist and only in the hospital, and it is not all that effective. At Children's Hospital ribavirin is used on a limited basis and usually for babies with chronic lung disease.

Bronchiolitis proves fatal for about 1 out of every 1,000 babies who are sick enough that they need to be hospitalized. These are usually infants who have other lung disease in addition to RSV bronchiolitis.

## Prevention

Respiratory syncytial virus is so widespread during its annual appearance that you really cannot keep your new baby away from everyone who might be infected. But remember that your baby can get an RSV infection from an older brother or sister or an adult who just has a cold. It is usually very difficult to keep older brothers and sisters away from a baby, so encourage everyone to wash their hands before touching the baby.

Since RSV particles spread primarily via nose and throat secretions from infected people, be careful—and teach your older children to be careful—about coughing and blowing your nose when you have a cold. Cover your mouth when you cough. Discard your used tissues in the trash can.

Wash your own hands before taking care of your children. And when you help young children blow their nose, wash your hands afterward.

## Respiratory Syncytial Virus (RSV) Infections

### SYMPTOMS

- Common cold, with very, very runny nose

- Bronchiolitis

- Croup

- Ear infection—middle ears

- Pneumonia

You may never have heard of respiratory syncytial virus (RSV), but it is a very common virus that we all catch again and again throughout our lives. In infants and young children, RSV is the single most important cause of serious infections of the lungs.

RSV is one of the most regular of respiratory viruses, causing epidemics every year. It appears on the scene every fall around the first of November and stays all winter, up through April.

It is so widespread and so contagious that your baby has about a fifty-fifty chance of becoming infected with it during the first winter of his life. And the younger a child, the more likely it is that an RSV infection will cause a significant problem; the most severe RSV disease occurs in babies two to six months old. By the end of the second winter of life, nearly all children have been infected.

During RSV season, at The Children's Hospital of Philadelphia, we see several dozen children every week with RSV disease of some kind.

## Cause

Respiratory syncytial virus gets its cumbersome name from what it does to cells as it grows: it causes them to fuse into masses called syncytia.

## How They Spread

Respiratory syncytial virus makes its home and multiplies in the respiratory tracts of humans, and it spreads *very* easily from child to child and from adult to child within families and in day-care centers and schools.

Children and adults who are infected with RSV shed virus particles in the mucus and other secretions from their nose and throat. These virus particles get all over their clothes, their bedding, their hands, and the tissues they use to blow their nose. When you help an infected child blow his nose, you get RSV particles on your hands. Touch a countertop or set a used tissue down on a bedside table, and you deposit RSV on the surface. When an infected person coughs, he gets

RSV particles on his hands or sprays them onto surfaces. RSV can remain alive on hard surfaces such as furniture for six to eight hours.

In hospitals a classic way RSV can spread is via bed railings. A baby infected with RSV gets virus particles all over his crib and bedding. When a staff member lowers the bed railing to take care of the baby, she gets RSV particles on her hands. If she does not wash her hands thoroughly afterward, she can easily carry RSV particles to another patient.

The virus enters the next person via the mucous membranes lining his nose or eyes. From there, as the virus grows and multiples, it spreads throughout his upper respiratory tract and often, in young children, down into his lungs.

## Incubation Period

It usually takes about four to six days from the time RSV enters a person's body until symptoms begin to appear, but it can take a little as two days or as long as eight.

## Symptoms

Your baby's first encounter with respiratory syncytial virus almost always causes her to have some symptoms. The virus may remain in her upper respiratory tract and cause her to have just a cold with a very, very runny nose. In many babies, however, the virus migrates down into the lower respiratory tract and causes severe lung disease, most commonly pneumonia.

RSV is the major cause of pneumonia in infants and young children. It is also responsible for 90 percent of cases of bronchiolitis, another potentially serious lung disease of babies. RSV can also cause bronchitis, croup, and middle-ear infections.

We do not develop full immunity to RSV, but we do develop some antibodies against the

virus, and your child's next encounter with RSV, during her second or third winter of life, is likely to be less severe. By the time your child is three, she is unlikely to get pneumonia or bronchiolitis from RSV.

However, RSV infections can be particularly severe in children of any age who have another underlying disease: children with congenital heart disease; children whose immune systems are not normal; and children who were born prematurely, spent time on a respirator, and thus have some lingering lung disease (a condition called bronchopulmonary dysplasia).

The older we become, the less likely RSV infections are to be severe. In adults, RSV usually causes only a cold and perhaps some coughing. This means that your baby can catch pneumonia or bronchiolitis from an older brother or sister or a grownup who has nothing more than a cold.

### CALL YOUR DOCTOR

- If your child shows symptoms of bronchiolitis (page 21).

- If your child shows symptoms of croup (page 46).

- If your child shows symptoms of middle ear infection (page 84).

- If your child shows symptoms of pneumonia (page 200).

## Diagnosis

At Children's Hospital we test a child for respiratory syncytial virus only if he is so sick that we must admit him to the hospital for bronchiolitis or pneumonia. Otherwise, we do not need to know whether he has RSV because this information does not affect his treatment. But if we have to admit a child to the hospital, we do need to know whether he has RSV because it spreads so easily. Our staff must take precautions to keep RSV from infecting other hospitalized children.

To test for RSV, we use a small catheter to suction a sample of mucus from the child's nose. The lab performs a rapid test that gives an answer almost immediately. During the height of the RSV season, our lab runs RSV tests several times a day.

## Treatment

When your child has an RSV infection, she does not need to take any antibiotics. Antibiotics are not effective against RSV. They do not kill RSV or any other virus.

You usually can treat your child at home with the same supportive care that you give for many other respiratory tract infections: extra humidity to loosen your child's nasal secretions and keep her irritated mucous membranes from drying out; extra fluids to keep her from becoming dangerously dehydrated; and acetaminophen to reduce her fever and help make her more comfortable. See "Treatment," page 38, in *Common Colds* and *General Treatments for Children*, page 290, in the Appendices.

### Hospitalization

However, some 13 out of every 1,000 babies with RSV infections are sick enough that they need to be hospitalized for additional treatment. In the United States, RSV infections cause 90,000 infants and young children to be hospitalized every year, according to the U.S. Public Health Service's Centers for Disease Control and Prevention (CDC). During RSV season, at Children's Hospital we admit about two to three babies a day for RSV diseases.

In the hospital our staff can monitor a baby's heart and respiratory rates. We can periodically measure the oxygen level of his blood and provide extra oxygen if he needs it. We can give extra fluids intravenously if he becomes too dehydrated. In very severe cases, a baby may need to be on a respirator in the intensive care unit.

For babies with severe RSV disease, pediatricians sometimes prescribe an antiviral drug called ribavirin. Ribavirin, in the form of a mist, must be administered in the hospital; however, it is not very effective. At Children's Hospital we reserve ribavirin for those babies who have chronic heart or lung disease or whose immune systems are not normal and for otherwise normal babies who have very severe RSV infections. We usually give ribavirin to no more than 1 out of every 100 babies we admit.

(Pregnant women and women of childbearing age should be aware that ribavirin can cause birth defects in animals and should avoid exposure to the mist during treatments.)

Most babies hospitalized with RSV can go home in two to four days. Deaths occur among babies who have a heart, lung, or immune-system disease. According to the CDC, RSV kills 4,500 American children a year.

## Prevention

Remember that your new baby can get a serious RSV infection—bronchiolitis or pneumonia—from an older brother or sister or a grownup who merely has a cold.

Respiratory syncytial virus is so widespread during its winter season that it is almost impossible to avoid. You cannot really keep your baby away from everyone with a cold. But since RSV does not spread much through the air but instead travels from person to person via nose and throat secretions, you can help prevent RSV from spreading within your family.

Although it is almost impossible, try to limit your new baby's contact with her older sisters and brothers when they have colds and other respiratory infections.

Since RSV particles can survive on surfaces for so many hours, avoid contaminating surfaces with nasal secretions from anyone with a cold. If you set a tissue with such secretions down on a dresser top, the virus particles can remain alive on that dresser long enough to infect the next person who comes along and touches it. Dispose of tissues carefully so that they will not spread the virus to others.

If you have a cold yourself, wash your hands thoroughly after blowing your nose and before touching your children. Also wash your hands between taking care of your older child with a cold and caring for your new baby.

At Children's Hospital we isolate children with RSV infections, housing them together in the same room, apart from other hospitalized children, to reduce the risk of the virus spreading to them. RSV-infected children usually have their own nursing staff, who take care of them only and thus cannot carry RSV particles to other children. Finally, there is active research going on to develop an RSV vaccine. Preliminary results look promising but a commercial vaccine is still years away.

# CHICKENPOX

*A vaccine is available to protect your child against chickenpox. See Vaccines, page 301, in the Appendices.*

## SYMPTOMS

- Fever
- Loss of appetite
- General malaise
- Red itchy rash
- Headache

At one time, itchy, scratchy chickenpox was a rite of passage for most children. But a vaccine and a changing perspective on the effects of the disease now aim to eliminate chickenpox from the list of common childhood illnesses. More than 95 percent of Americans get chickenpox before the age of fifteen. Chickenpox typically occurs in late winter or early spring in temperate climates.

Chickenpox is characterized by an itchy blister rash (pox) that covers the face, scalp, and trunk. For a couple of days before the rash appears, your child may be achy and feverish. With its accompanying headache, malaise, and loss of appetite, chickenpox is generally a very uncomfortable nuisance.

Because chickenpox is so contagious, infected children must avoid contact with others until all the poxes have crusted over, generally six to seven days after the rash appears. That means missing school, activities, and sometimes even vacations. If one of your children has chickenpox, there is a 90 percent chance that your other susceptible children will catch it.

One parent recalls, "I was a virtual prisoner in my house for more than a month when my kids had chickenpox. First the six-year-old came down with it, then his younger sister had it, and then two weeks later, the baby had a fever. After a few cranky days, she broke out in the rash. During those four weeks I went outside only to walk to our mailbox."

The chickenpox rash is characteristically blisters surrounded by a red ring best described as a "dew drop on a rose petal." The rash begins ten to twenty-one days after being exposed, with

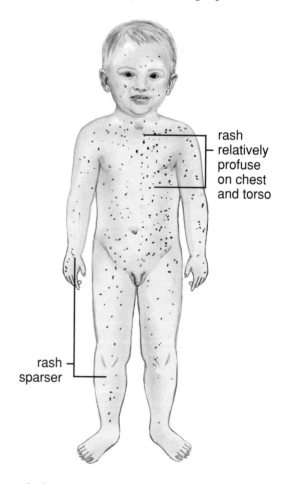

rash relatively profuse on chest and torso

rash sparser

*Chickenpox (varicella).*

an itchy rash of small red bumps on the scalp, face, or trunk, and spreads to the back or stomach, but this can vary from person to person. The rash breaks out in successive crops over a two- to four-day period, so your child will have poxes of varying stages at the same time—some will be crusting while others are just forming. Generally, by the fourth day the lesions stop forming, and crusting of all lesions stops by the sixth day. Once all of the poxes crust over, your child is no longer contagious and can resume activity. It can take two weeks for the scabs to fall off.

Complications from chickenpox are rare. Nonetheless, of the estimated 4 million cases of chickenpox each year, more than 9,000 people—mostly children—are hospitalized for complications. In particular, a child with a suppressed immune system can experience serious complications from chickenpox. These can include pneumonia and neurologic problems, including encephalitis, or staphylococcus and streptococcus bacterial infections.

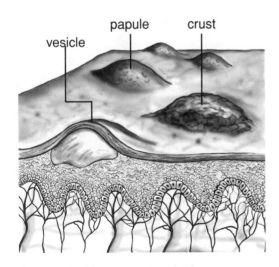

*Simultaneous stages of lesions in chickenpox.*

The most common complication is bacteria-infected areas around the rash. If your child scratches and breaks the skin, any bacteria on the hands or skin can infect the pox blisters. If you see pus around the scabs, call your doctor. If some of the poxes become infected or are removed prematurely by scratching, for example, there may be some scarring.

The possibility that complications from chickenpox may require hospitalization increases with age. But in general, your teenager will experience chickenpox much the same as younger children.

## Causes

Chickenpox is caused by varicella zoster virus (VZV), a highly contagious virus.

## How It Spreads

Chickenpox is so contagious in its early stages that an exposed person who is not immune to the virus has a 70 to 80 percent chance of catching the disease. It is spread by direct person-to-person contact and by airborne droplets from coughing, sneezing, a runny nose, or just breathing. It is also easily spread directly from exposure to the fluid from open pox sores, so it is important to isolate children with chickenpox.

Once a child gets chickenpox, the varicella zoster virus remains dormant in his body in the nerve endings for the rest of his life. If reactivated, it can cause herpes zoster, or shingles. An adult with shingles can spread the virus to someone who hasn't had chickenpox, and that person will develop chickenpox.

Chickenpox gives a person lifelong immunity; that is, a child can get it only once. There is an exception: children who get chickenpox before developing leukemia have lifelong immunity, but if they get it after they are on leukemia treatments, their immune system may not be able to protect them from future infections and will be susceptible to chickenpox every time they are exposed.

## Incubation Period

The incubation period is generally fourteen days, although secondary cases may be seen from as soon as ten to as much as twenty-one days following exposure. This period may be shorter for a child who is immunocompromised or longer if the child has received a postexposure medicine—for example, some children, such as cancer patients, receive varicella zoster immune globulin (VZIG) to prevent or minimize the symptoms.

Your child is most contagious for one to two days immediately before the appearance of the rash until all lesions are crusted, usually five to six days from onset.

## Symptoms

Your child may be "out of sorts" for a couple of days—with a slight fever, loss of appetite, and general malaise. Then a red rash appears, spreading from the scalp and face to the trunk of the body and finally out to the arms and legs. Most of the lesions will appear on the face and on the central part of the body. There may be some in the mouth or genitalia, which can be painful.

## Diagnosis

Chickenpox is easy to diagnose because its rash is so distinctive. Because the disease is highly contagious, your doctor may not want you to bring your child to the office. Given the symptoms and the appearance of the rash, it is fairly easy to

### CALL YOUR DOCTOR

- If your child develops red, tender skin or red streaks or a speckled red rash.
- If your child has a high fever for more than four days.
- If the itching is so severe that it doesn't respond to treatment.
- If you see pus around the lesions or under the scabs.
- If your child has swollen, painful glands under his arms, in the neck area, behind the ears, or in the groin area.
- If your child has severe vomiting, trouble breathing, or problems standing or walking.

diagnose a case of chickenpox. There will be multiple small red bumps that become thin-walled water blisters, then cloudy blisters or open sores, and finally dry, brown crusts, all within a twenty-four-hour period.

## Treatment

Unfortunately, there is not much you can do for chickenpox except let it runs its course. Fever should be treated with acetaminophen (*not* aspirin). Because of the rare but serious complication known as Reye's syndrome, it is very important that you do not give aspirin to a child with chickenpox. Reye's syndrome affects the brain and liver and has occurred in a higher rate among children with chickenpox who have received aspirin during their illness.

Generally, treatment is aimed at relieving uncomfortable symptoms. Your child may have a poor appetite for a few days, so be sure to give her plenty of fluids to prevent dehydration. You may want to offer foods that soothe the mouth (cold liquids, ice cream, frozen desserts) if she has sores in her mouth or in her throat. Stay away from salty or spicy foods like chips, which can irritate sores. If mouth lesions are troublesome, give your child one teaspoon of an antacid solution to gargle or swallow four times a day after meals. If the genital area is irritated, apply some $2^{1}/_{2}$ percent Xylocaine (available over the counter) to the genital ulcers every four hours to relieve pain.

Change underwear, pajamas, and linens frequently to prevent bacteria from entering the rash. Have your child wear loose clothing and try to prevent her from perspiring, which can cause bacterial growth.

Keep your child's fingernails short and clean. Some parents put mittens or cotton socks on a young child's hands if the child continues to scratch lesions. Be sure your child washes his hands several times a day. You can show your child how to apply pressure to the itchy area instead of scratching.

To relieve the itch, let your child soak in a lukewarm oatmeal bath three or four times a day for at least fifteen minutes. Do not rinse the skin afterward. Pat dry and apply calamine lotion to the itchy areas.

Give a medication such as Benadryl (diphenhydramine hydrochloride compound) for severe itchiness. This nonprescription antihistamine may make your child drowsy. Do not give it to children under two years old. Never use both Caladryl, which can be absorbed into the body through an open or seeping wound, and Benadryl together (your child may overdose on diphenhydramine, the active agent in both of these medications).

Acyclovir is an oral, antiviral drug that can be used to treat chickenpox; however, it only helps if started within twenty-four hours of the appearance of the first lesions. Because research shows that acyclovir has mild benefits, it is not recommended, and most physicians don't treat normal, healthy children with acyclovir. They do agree that certain children—those with compromised immune systems, those taking steroids, and those with chronic skin or lung disease—should receive acyclovir. It is also recommended for teenagers and adults if started within the first twenty-four hours of the appearance of lesions.

## Prevention

With the recent FDA approval of a new varicella vaccine, chickenpox now joins the other common childhood illnesses that can be prevented with inoculation. The FDA guidelines call for children from twelve months to twelve years of age who have not had chickenpox to receive a single injection of the vaccine. Adolescents who have not had the disease will receive two doses given one to two months apart. This drug underwent a ten-year clinical testing phase during which nearly 10,000 children, along with 1,600 adolescents and adults, were treated and followed. The studies confirmed the safety of the vaccine. The most common side effects were related to pain and swelling at the injection site, as is the case with many vaccines. Although most experts expect immunity following vaccination to be lifelong, it is possible that booster shots may some day be recommended.

# COMMON COLDS

Also called URIs (for upper respiratory infections) and rhinitis. *Rhin-* means "nose," and the ending *-itis* means "inflammation."

## SYMPTOMS

- Runny nose
- Sneezing
- Congested nasal passages
- Sore throat
- Cough
- Possible fever

Colds—virus infections in the upper respiratory tract that are centered in the nasal passages—are probably the most common of all the infectious diseases. Rarely do any of us, children or grownups, get through a winter without the familiar nuisance of a head cold.

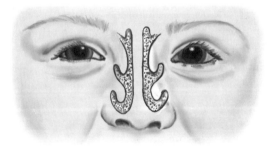

*Nasal passages.*

The important thing to know about colds, however, is that they go away on their own, usually in a few days, leaving us with no lasting harm.

Your child may be cranky and miserable for a few days, but colds are not something that you need to worry much about.

The question, of course, is when might your child's "cold" not be a cold at all but something else, some other disease that could be more serious and that could require different treatment. For information about signs that a "cold" might be more than a cold, see the "Call Your Doctor" box on page 37.

Children catch many more colds than adults do, as you probably have noticed. Children get an average of three to eight colds every year, and if your child attends a day-care center, you can expect that she will get even more.

Babies catch so many colds, starting when they are about two or three months old, that it often seems to parents that they have had a continuous cold for months and months. Parents may worry that this means something is wrong with the infant's immune system.

If you pay close attention to your baby's cold symptoms, however, you will probably find that they are actually not continuous but instead do come and go. They are not all symptoms of the same cold. Your baby has been infected by a series of different cold viruses, and he is having different colds, one after the other. It is quite normal for infants to have so many colds.

As your child grows older, and he encounters and develops some immunity to more and more different cold viruses, he will catch fewer colds. By adulthood, people get only about half as many colds each year as children do.

## *Causes*

Many, many different, common respiratory viruses can cause colds.

The most common culprits, particularly in children, are the rhinoviruses. Rhinoviruses take their name from where they live: in the nasal passages. As mentioned, *rhin-* means "nose." The word *rhinovirus* is thus a relative of *rhinoceros.* There are more than 100 different strains of rhinoviruses, and they cause some 30 to 50 percent of all colds. Your child is most likely to catch a rhinovirus cold during the spring, summer, or fall.

Other respiratory viruses that commonly cause colds include the parainfluenza viruses (which are also the most common cause of croup), the coronaviruses (there are several dozens of these), and a very common virus with a long name: the respiratory syncytial virus (RSV). See *Respiratory Syncytial Virus (RSV) Infections,* page 26.

Your child is most likely to catch a parainfluenza-virus cold in the fall or spring and a coronavirus cold from midwinter to early spring. She is most likely to catch an RSV infection from November through April.

Still other viruses that sometimes cause colds are the adenoviruses (there are dozens of these too; they are also a common cause of sore throats), the enteroviruses (again, there are dozens of these), and the influenza viruses.

The fact that so many common viruses can cause colds is the reason why we all catch colds again and again throughout our lives. We recover from encounters with one cold virus after another and develop some immunity to those viruses, but there is always another cold virus coming around the corner to which we are not yet immune.

## How They Spread

Children can catch one of these cold viruses from someone who has a cold, of course, but they can also catch one from a person who appears perfectly well but is coming down with a cold and does not yet have any symptoms. A person infected with a cold virus sheds great quantities of virus particles in the secretions from the nose and throat. Children shed even more virus and for longer periods of time.

When an infected person sneezes or coughs or even just talks, he can spew cold-virus particles directly onto anyone in his path or onto any nearby surfaces. If he gets virus particles on his hands, he can deposit virus on anything he touches. Parainfluenza-virus particles can survive on such surfaces for up to ten hours; respiratory syncytial virus, for six to eight hours.

When your child touches a contaminated surface, he can get virus particles on his hands. You can get virus on your hands when you help an infected child blow her nose. You touch your nose, and you can become infected. Some cold viruses can even enter your body through your eyes. It may sound strange, but you really can catch a cold by rubbing your eyes.

Once inside your child's or your nose, cold-virus particles settle down in the nasal passages and proceed to grow and multiply.

## Incubation Period

Once a cold virus starts growing in your child's nose, it usually takes two to five days for the child to develop symptoms.

## Symptoms

As the cold virus multiplies in your child's nasal passages, the mucous membranes lining the nose swell and become inflamed, and they produce more and more mucus and other secretions.

Your child's nose runs and runs. He may sneeze again and again. The secretions coming out of his nose may be watery and clear, or they may become thick and yellow or even turn greenish. The excess secretions may clog his nasal passages, causing his nose to become congested and his head to feel stuffed up. As the mucus drips down, it may become encrusted inside and around the end of his nose. And he has to blow and wipe his nose so often that the outside often becomes red and raw.

The excess mucus may run down the back of his throat—in what is called a "postnasal drip"—and make his throat sore and also cause him to cough. And when he lies down to sleep at night, this mucus tends to pool in his throat. His cough is thus usually worse at night, and between his cough and his stuffed-up nose, he may find it hard to sleep.

Your child may or may not have a fever with his cold. His temperature could remain normal, or it could go up as high as 104°F, and he could still have nothing more serious than a cold. He may have a headache and be achy and uncomfortable.

Your child may still feel alert and energetic enough to carry on his usual activities, or his energy level may be way down and he may want to sleep more than usual.

Babies especially have a hard time when they have colds. Because their nasal passages are so tiny, they become congested more readily than older children. And below the age of about three months, a baby cannot breathe through her mouth. A stuffed-up nose thus interferes with her breathing even more than it does with an older child. And even with a baby who can breathe through her mouth, a cold can interfere with her feeding since she has to stop sucking for a moment to take each breath.

But all this will pass by itself. Your child's immune system will gradually produce enough antibodies to kill off all the virus particles. This usually takes three to five days, although some colds—depending on the virus—may last as long as seven to ten days.

## Complications

Although colds are usually mild, they can sometimes pave the way for an infection elsewhere in the body than in her nasal passages. As the virus multiplies in her nose, it may damage the tissues lining her upper respiratory tract. This may allow bacteria to invade spaces in her head that are normally sterile.

In young children bacteria may spread into the middle ear and cause an ear infection. Middle-ear infections are extremely common in babies and toddlers, affecting millions of American children every year. See *Ear Infections— Middle Ears*, page 84.

In older children and adults, bacteria may spread into the sinuses. Bacterial infections of the sinuses are much less common than middle-ear infections and are rare in children under the age of two. See *Sinusitis*, page 242.

And in babies and young children particularly, a cold virus itself may sometimes spread downward into the lower respiratory tract and cause a more serious disease of the lungs, such as bronchiolitis or pneumonia. See *Bronchiolitis*, page 21, and *Pneumonia*, page 200.

If you think that what your child has is just a cold, you do not usually need to call your pediatrician at all. Small babies, with their tiny nasal passages, normally sneeze a lot and breathe noisily, particularly at night. If your baby seems otherwise happy and playful and is eating well, he probably does not need to see the doctor.

What often does prompt parents to call their pediatrician is that a child is coughing so much at night that she is keeping not only herself but everyone else in the house awake. Parents want her to stop coughing so everyone can get their sleep.

## *Diagnosis*

Most people recognize the symptoms of a cold. But if you do have to take your child to see your pediatrician, she will check your child for more serious lung disease, such as bronchiolitis, pneumonia, or asthma. (Asthma is not an infectious disease.)

If your child needs to visit the doctor, your doctor will listen to the sounds of his breathing with a stethoscope, count how fast he is breathing, and observe whether he is having any trouble breathing. If the doctor suspects that your child has a lung disease, she may ask for an X-ray of his chest.

Many other diseases (influenza, measles, whooping cough, and bronchiolitis to name a few) can also cause runny noses, particularly at first, but among the disorders most often mistaken for colds are nasal allergies.

Nasal allergies are what your doctor probably calls allergic rhinitis and most people call hay fever. These allergies are not an infectious

Although you do not need to call your doctor when your child has just a cold, the following are signs that what she has may be something else. These are not signs of a cold; these are signs that it may *not* be a cold. The list to follow indicates possible signs of pneumonia or other lung disease.

### CALL YOUR DOCTOR

- If your child—particularly a child under three months old—has a cough that is getting worse or is not getting better over a three- or four-day period.

- If your child is breathing faster than usual or you are concerned about the way she is breathing. With just a cold, a child usually does not breathe faster.

- If your child is working harder to breathe or is showing signs of respiratory distress: her nostrils are flaring out and she is pulling in (retracting) the muscles between her ribs and at the base of her neck as she breathes.

**Also consult your doctor if your child's "cold" symptoms last longer than a cold should:**

- If your child has a very runny nose, particularly with a greenish discharge, that lasts for more than two weeks, and he also complains about a headache or pressure behind his face. These may be signs that he has a bacterial infection in his sinuses. See "Symptoms," page 242, in *Sinusitis*.

- If your child has a runny nose with a clear, watery discharge that lasts several weeks, particularly if his eyes and nose are also itchy. These may be signs that he has nasal allergies.

disease but instead are due to a child's sensitivity to some airborne substance or substances. With such allergies, your child's runny nose lasts longer than with a cold, the secretions usually remain clear and watery, and his nose often itches. Another tip-off is if your child tends to get a "cold" at about the same time every year. If so, he may be allergic to certain pollens. The peak seasons for pollen allergies and for colds are different: pollen allergies peak in spring, summer, and fall, while colds more often occur in winter. However, your child could be allergic to other substances—such as animal dander or dust mites—that could cause him to have a runny nose the year around.

Allergic rhinitis affects about 10 to 15 percent of the American population, but it is not common in children under about five. If your child is going to develop nasal allergies, she will probably do so before she is out of her teens.

And of course, it is quite possible for your child to have allergic rhinitis and a cold at the same time.

## *Treatment*

For a cold your child does not need to take any antibiotics. Antibiotics do not work against colds; they do not kill any of the respiratory viruses that cause colds. In addition, antibiotics do not prevent the child with a cold from getting a bacterial infection.

While your child's immune system fights off the virus, there are some things you should or can do to help.

## Fluids

It is very important that you make sure that your child drinks plenty of extra fluids to keep him from becoming dehydated. He is losing more

fluid than usual via the extra secretions running out of his nose, and if he has a fever, he is also losing more fluid. Dehydration can be very dangerous, even life-threatening; babies particularly can become dehydrated very quickly because they are so small.

Keeping the tissues in your child's nose well hydrated and moist will also actually help fight the cold virus. The more mucus your child produces in his nose, the more antibodies he has right there in his nose to kill the virus.

Offer your child a variety of liquids, and yes, you can include chicken soup. Chicken soup really does help fight colds; studies show that it actually increases those antibodies in the nose. With a baby under a year, however, you should never give plain water. You need to give special fluids called oral rehydration solutions. See *Fluids*, page 290, in the Appendices for more about these special fluids and also what fluids to give and not give older children.

## Feeding

If your child does not have a fever, her appetite probably remains as good as usual. If she does have a fever, she may lose her appetite some, and a young child may lose interest in solid foods. You do not need to worry about this. Your child may lose a little weight, but as soon as she recovers from her cold and feels better, she will gain the weight right back again. See *Feeding*, page 292, in the Appendices for information about what foods to give and not give your child when she is sick.

## Humidity

With colds and other respiratory infections, extra humidity in your child's room helps moisten and soothe the inflamed tissues inside his nose. The extra humidity also helps liquefy and loosen the excess mucus that is clogging his nose. See *Humidity*, page 293, in the Appendices for more information about humidity and humidifiers.

## Nose Drops

When your baby's nose gets so crusty that she has trouble breathing through her nose—remember that babies under about three months cannot breathe through their mouth—you can help clear her nasal passages by using saline (salt-water) nose drops that you can make yourself. Saline nose drops can also be purchased in your local drugstore. Saline drops are less irritating to the mucous membranes lining her nose than plain water would be.

---

### SALINE NOSE DROPS

Boil 1 cup of water for 3 minutes. Then add $^1/_2$ teaspoon of ordinary salt and stir until the salt is dissolved. Cool the solution to room temperature before you use it. You need to make this saline solution each day to prevent it from becoming contaminated with bacteria.

With a bulb syringe, gently put a few drops of this saltwater solution into your baby's nostrils and then carefully suck out as much of the mucus as you can. An older child can help by blowing out some.

---

## Rest

If your child has a fever (101°F or more), she should stay home from her day-care center or school.

If your child does not have a fever, you can be guided by how she feels and how she is acting. If she feels well enough and her energy level is normal or near normal, she can go to day-care or school if she wants to.

You do not have to be concerned about your child spreading her cold to the other children and adults. These cold viruses are so common and so widespread that people are going to encounter them anyway.

But if your child's energy level is down and she feels tired and sleepy, let her take a day or two off and rest. Resting more and sleeping more will help her body overcome the cold virus and also make it less likely that she will develop pneumonia or some other complication.

## Medications

If your child has a fever or headache or is achy and uncomfortable, you can give her acetaminophen, which will both reduce her fever and relieve her achiness. Always follow the directions on the label. However, you should not give acetaminophen to a baby under about three months old because your pediatrician should be advised if she does have a fever. A fever in a child that young could be a sign of something more serious.

You should never give your child aspirin when she has a cold. If a child is infected with an influenza virus, taking aspirin is associated with the development of a very rare but very serious, life-threatening, neurologic disease called Reye's syndrome. And since you can never be sure that your child's cold is *not* due to an influenza virus, it is prudent to avoid giving her aspirin. The American Academy of Pediatrics "strongly advises" that you "not give your child or teenager aspirin or any medications containing aspirin when he has any viral illness." See *Reye's Syndrome*, page 217, for more about this disease.

There are hundreds of cold medicines on the market, so many that they are confusing. Some are sold over the counter; others are available only by prescription. These cold medicines generally contain various combinations of four different types of medications: a pain- and fever-relieving medicine such as acetaminophen (discussed above), a nasal decongestant, a cough medicine, and sometimes an antihistamine.

None of these medications can cure a cold—that is, kill any of the cold viruses—or shorten the duration of your child's symptoms, but they may help make her more comfortable while the cold is running its course.

At Children's Hospital, however, we usually do not give any of these combination cold medicines to babies under about ten to twelve months of age. These medicines usually do not help children that young, and some of the ingredients in these preparations can actually hurt them. In general, before giving any medication to your child, you might want to check with your doctor, especially during the first two years of your child's life.

For an older child, a nasal decongestant can help him breathe more easily. Decongestants can open up your child's nasal passages and reduce the swelling and inflammation in his nose by constricting the tiny blood vessels in the membranes lining the nose. A commonly used nasal decongestant is pseudoephedrine. In babies, however, the side effects of nasal decongestants outweigh any benefit.

The cough medicine component of the combination cold medicines is usually a cough suppressant. The one that physicians most commonly suggest for children is dextromethorphan.

However, you do not necessarily want to suppress your child's cough completely. Coughs are useful. A person coughs because excess mucus and other secretions are clogging the air passages to the lungs, and coughing is the body's way of getting rid of those extra secretions.

Another reason for not suppressing a cough for too long is that a persistent cough could be a sign that a child (or adult) may have some other disease, something more serious than a cold that needs to be identified and treated.

However, if your child's cough is interfering with sleep, a bedtime dose of cough suppressant might be indicated. As mentioned, you should call your doctor if your child's cough lasts more than three to five days or is getting worse.

The antihistamine component of these combination cold medicines is one of the types of medications used to treat allergies. Antihistamines block a substance in the body called histamine, which is a main cause of allergic reactions. Antihistamines are thus sometimes also called histamine blockers. Antihistamines may help your child if she has allergic rhinitis along with his cold.

The most common side effect of many antihistamines is that they may make your child sleepy. This can be helpful before she goes to bed at night, but it is not so good before she goes to school (if she feels well enough to go to school) or during the day at school. Nor is it good idea for a teenager or an adult to take an antihistamine that makes him drowsy if he needs to drive a car.

Another consideration with these combination cold medicines is that a given combination may not target the exact combination of your child's symptoms. If your child's nose is not congested, she does not need a nasal decongestant. If she is not coughing, do not give a cough suppressant. And it is never a good idea to give your child a medicine she does not need. It is an unnecessary expense, for one thing, and all medications can have possible adverse effects.

You need to read the label carefully to select a cold medicine that matches your child's symptoms. Or you can search for a brand that contains just the one ingredient your child actually needs.

At Children's Hospital, for children older than a year who are having trouble sleeping and are coughing, we often suggest that they take a cold medicine—with a nasal decongestant, cough suppressant, and perhaps an antihistamine—just at bedtime and just for the three to five days while they are getting over the worst of the cold. We usually do not suggest that they take the medicine during the day unless they are coughing a lot and their symptoms are really bothering them.

If your child or teenager is sleeping well at night without a lot of coughing, he may not need any cold medicine at all.

No matter what you do, what medicine you give or not give, your child's cold will last as long as it lasts and will then disappear in its own time. And your child will have developed some immunity to that cold virus and probably will not be as sick the next time he meets it.

## *Prevention*

The many viruses that cause colds are so common and widespread that your child cannot avoid them entirely. Children are going to encounter most of these viruses, sooner or later, at some point during their lifetime.

Remember, however, that a common way cold viruses are spread is via the hands. You can reduce the odds of your children catching a cold virus by teaching them to wash their hands—frequently. It is particularly important that they wash their hands before eating.

Also teach your children not to sneeze or cough onto other people. They should learn to cover their nose and mouth with their hand or a tissue. You can also suggest to children that they sneeze or cough onto their arm. This keeps the virus particles off of their hands.

Remember, too, that babies and young children can get pneumonia or another serious lung disease from some common viruses that only cause colds in older children and adults. If you do have a cold, wash your hands before touching your baby.

# CONJUNCTIVITIS

Also called pinkeye. The ending *-itis* means "inflammation."

## SYMPTOMS

- Pink or red eyes
- Discharge from the eyes

The most common type of eye infection in children is conjunctivitis. This is an inflammation of the conjunctiva, the thin, clear membrane that covers the whites of the eyes and also lines the inside surfaces of the eyelids. If the whites of your child's eyes turn pink or red, she probably has conjunctivitis, which is also aptly called pinkeye.

The incidence of conjunctivitis tends to be highest in preschool children, and virtually all children have at least one episode of conjunctivitis by the time they are eight years old. Fortunately, while conjunctivitis can be uncomfortable, it is rarely serious.

## Causes

Many different germs can cause conjunctivitis in children, both virus and bacteria. Two types of bacteria are the most common causes: *Haemophilus aegyptius* and *Streptococcus pneumoniae* (also called pneumococcus and strep pneumo).

Among viruses, the most frequent causes are the adenoviruses. There are dozens of these, and they also cause sore throats, colds, croup, and other respiratory diseases.

Conjunctivitis can also result from causes other than infections. It can be caused by a foreign body in the eye or an allergic reaction to a substance such as eye makeup, aerosol-spray fumes, or pollen floating in the air. It can also occur when a toxic substance such as a household-cleaning product, hair spray, or hair dye gets in the eye. Adolescents and adults who wear contact lenses can develop conjunctivitis from the products they use to clean their lenses.

## How It Spreads

Whether caused by bacteria or a virus, conjunctivitis is highly contagious. Children most

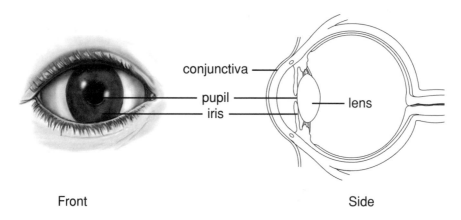

Front          conjunctiva  pupil  iris  lens      Side

*Parts of the eye: front and side views.*

commonly introduce the bacteria or virus particles into their eyes by touching or rubbing them with their hands.

These are very common germs. Many healthy children carry strep pneumo in their nose and throat, and adenoviruses are the most common causes of viral sore throats. There are plenty of opportunities for children to pick up these germs on their hands.

Children who are infected with these germs shed them in the secretions from their noses and throats. When they cough or sneeze, they can deposit the germs on nearby surfaces such as toys and furniture. Adenovirus is so hardy that it can survive on inanimate objects for several hours. When other children touch the toy or furniture, they get the germs on their hands. They touch their eyes, and they become infected. Conjunctivitis germs can also spread from child to child when they share such items as pillows, towels, washcloths, and blankets

While we all touch our eyes more than we realize, young children develop conjunctivitis more easily simply because they more often touch their eyes with unclean hands.

Adenoviruses can also spread from person to person in swimming pools that are not adequately chlorinated; you may have heard the term *swimming-pool conjunctivitis*. Teenagers can spread conjunctivitis germs from one to another if they use each other's eye makeup.

If a pregnant woman is infected with certain germs, she can transmit these germs to her baby at the time of delivery. These germs can cause serious eye infections, including conjunctivitis, in newborns; such eye infections in the nineteenth century used to be a major causes of blindness.

## Incubation Period

Although the length of time depends on the particular germ involved, a child usually develops symptoms of conjunctivitis within two to seven days of being exposed.

## Symptoms

The most common symptoms include a discharge from the eyes along with pink or red eyes. With a virus infection, the discharge is likely to be watery. With a bacterial infection, it is more likely to be thick, yellow, and sticky. A child may wake up in the morning with his eyelids and eyelashes stuck together by dried pus. His eyelids and the skin surrounding his eyes may become red, swollen, and irritated. His eyes often burn and tear. Some children complain of pain in their eyes.

These symptoms frequently begin in just one of the child's eyes but almost inevitably spread to both eyes within a day or two.

Your child can have conjunctivitis alone or as part of an upper respiratory infection, a cold. Conjunctivitis caused by an adenovirus is often accompanied by a sore throat or a fever. By itself, conjunctivitis does not usually reduce your child's energy level.

The American Academy of Pediatrics recommends that children with "purulent conjunctivitis"—that is, pink or red eyes accompanied by white or yellow eye discharge—be excluded from day-care until they have seen a doctor.

## Diagnosis

It is usually not necessary for your pediatrician to find out exactly which bacterium or virus is causing your child's conjunctivitis.

## CALL YOUR DOCTOR

- If the whites of your child's eyes become very red, and her eyelids and the area surrounding her eyes become swollen.

- If your child has large amounts of discharge from her eyes when she wakes up in the morning that remain even after you clean her eyes.

- If your child's eyelashes are matted together when she wakes up.

- If your child has severe pain in her eye, becomes extremely sensitive to light, or develops blurred or double vision.

- If your child has a fever, that is, a temperature of 101°F or more.

**It is particularly important that you talk with your doctor if your newborn baby develops any of these symptoms.**

If the doctor does need to identify the germ, a swab will be used to collect a sample of the eye discharge. This takes only a few seconds and is relatively painless. A laboratory then attempts to grow the organism from the sample.

## *Treatment*

If your child's pinkeye is caused by a virus, he does not need to take an antibiotic. Antibiotics do not work against viruses. Your child's infection must simply run its course while his own immune system overcomes all the virus

particles. This usually takes eight to ten days. Children with viral conjunctivitis are infectious as long as there is a discharge present coming from their eyes.

If your child's conjunctivitis is caused by bacteria, your doctor may prescribe an antibiotic to kill the bacteria. It is important to note, however, that there are no clear standards by which to prescribe antibiotics. Your doctor will make a decision based on the severity of your child's symptoms, how long they have lasted, and a variety of other factors.

Eye drops interfere less with your child's vision than an eye ointment does. Depending on the prescription, you usually apply the eye drops or ointment two to four times a day.

You can relieve the matting on your child's eyelids by using use warm compresses (a clean washcloth soaked in warm water).

Because conjunctivitis is so contagious, keep your infected child's towels, washcloth, and pillow separate from those used by other members of your family, and be sure to change these items every day.

Your child is considered infectious until she has received twenty-four hours of antibiotic drops or ointments. You should keep your child home from her day-care center or school during this twenty-four-hour period. Antibiotics cure most cases of bacterial conjunctivitis within five to seven days.

If your child has viral conjunctivitis and is thus not taking an antibiotic, you should keep her home until the discharge from her eyes starts to resolve.

You should call your doctor if your child's eyes show no signs of improvement after seven to ten days. Notify your doctor sooner if your child's

## HOW TO ADMINISTER EYE DROPS

It is scary for anyone—much less a small child—to hold his eye open and see a little eye dropper poised above it. Here are some tips that might help you administer eye drops to your child:

1. Make sure that both of you wash your hands thoroughly before starting.

2. It is easier to administer eye drops to someone who is lying down or reclining.

3. Let a young child hold his own eyes open to give him some sense of control. An older child may be able to apply the eye drops herself.

4. For a child who cannot keep his eyes open, apply several drops on his lashes and then tell him to open his eyes. The drops should roll in. An alternative method is to apply the drops to the inner corner of his eye and then have him tilt his head.

5. Wash your hands thoroughly afterward.

6. Keep applying the eye drops until your child wakes up two mornings in a row without any sticky discharge.

7. The American Academy of Pediatrics emphasizes, "Never put previously opened medication or someone else's eye medication into your child's eyes. It could cause serious damage."

eyes become redder, more swollen, or itchy after you apply the eye drops because the medication may be causing an allergic reaction. If your child's eyes continue to have a pussy discharge despite the drops, it may mean that she is infected with bacteria that are resistant to that antibiotic. Your doctor may give you a prescription for a different antibiotic.

Unfortunately, children do not acquire any immunity to conjunctivitis infections. Your child can develop them over and over again.

## Prevention

Because children most commonly spread conjunctivitis germs to their eyes from their hands, you can help keep your children from developing conjunctivitis by teaching them to wash their hands frequently. Also try, as much as possible, to have them keep from rubbing or touching their eyes.

Adolescents should be cautious about sharing eye makeup.

# CROUP

*If your child is having difficulty beathing, a
doctor should be consulted.*

### SYMPTOMS

- Sudden, barking cough at night

- Breathing difficulties

Croup is an infection of a child's lower throat
that usually starts abruptly at night with a dramatic—and frightening—barking cough.

If your child awakens with this croupy cough,
you may well want to call your doctor in the
middle of the night. Very, very rarely croup is
life-threatening because it can potentially interfere with a child's breathing. However, be reas-
sured that croup is rarely as serious as it sounds.
The bark of croup is far worse that its bite.

Your child is most likely to develop croup when
he is between the ages of six months and three
years. It is unusual in babies under a month old
and most common in toddlers between the ages
of one and two years. In this age group croup
strikes about one out of every twenty children.
For unknown reasons, boys are about one-and-a-
half times more likely to get croup than are girls.

Like so many respiratory infections, croup is
seasonal. Your child is most likely to get croup during the months from late fall through early spring.
During croup season at the hospital, we usually see
several children a week with the disease.

## Causes

Croup is usually caused by a virus, most often
one of the parainfluenza viruses or the respiratory syncytial virus (RSV). Less often croup is
caused by one of the influenza viruses, an adenovirus, or a bacterium called *Mycoplasma
pneumoniae.*

Parainfluenza viruses are widespread.
Throughout our lives we all have parainfluenza
infections. These viruses are not related to influenza viruses; they do not belong to the same virus family but are named *para*influenza viruses
because they cause somewhat similar diseases.
While croup is the disease that they frequently
cause, they also cause bronchiolitis, bronchitis,
and pneumonia and are common causes of colds
in both children and adults.

Respiratory syncytial virus (RSV), which can
also cause croup, is a very widespread virus and
the single most important cause of serious lung
infections—bronchiolitis and pneumonia—in
infants and young children. It is also a common
cause of ordinary colds in older children and
adults. For more about RSV, see *Respiratory Syncytial Virus (RSV) Infections,* page 26.

The fact that the parainfluenza viruses and
RSV are the most common causes of croup
explains its seasonal pattern. Parainfluenza
viruses are the usual causes of croup in the fall.
RSV causes croup from about the first of
November through the end of January. Then, in
the spring, a different type of paraflu virus often
shows up and causes more croup.

All of these viruses, as well as the bacterium
*Mycoplasma pneumoniae,* normally make their
homes in the respiratory tracts of humans, both
children and adults.

## *How It Spreads*

Since the parainfluenza viruses and respiratory
syncytial virus (RSV) are common causes of
colds, your baby or toddler can get croup from
an older sibling or grownup who merely has a

cold. People infected with these viruses shed virus particles in the secretions that come from their nose and throat.

When an infected person blows his nose, he gets virus particles on the tissue and on his hands. When he coughs or sneezes and covers his nose and mouth with his hand, he also gets virus on his hands. When you help an infected child blow her nose, you get virus on your hands. If you then touch your baby or toddler, you can infect her with the virus.

If you fail to wash your hands, you can also leave virus particles on any surface you touch: a chair, a toy, a doorknob. You can also contaminate a table if you set a used tissue down on it. Or if you cough or sneeze without covering your nose or mouth, you can spray virus on any nearby surface. Paraflu virus can remain alive on such surfaces for up to six to ten hours; RSV, for six to eight hours.

When your baby or toddler comes along and touches the toy or table, she can get virus particles on her own hands. When she touches her nose or mouth or eyes, she can infect herself with the virus, which then multiplies in the tissues lining the respiratory tract. In this manner, an adult's simple cold can easily become a child's croup.

## Incubation Period

Your child, when infected with a parafluenza virus, will usually develop symptoms in two to six days. With respiratory syncytial virus (RSV), the period is usually four to six days.

## Symptoms

Croup usually starts abruptly in the middle of the night. During the day your child has been playing and eating as usual. A slight cold may be present for a day or two, with a runny nose and perhaps a low fever.

While croup can start at any time of day or night, it most often strikes in the middle of the night, out of the blue, without warning. Your child suddenly wakes you at twelve o'clock, two o'clock in the morning with an alarming, dry cough. Most parents and physicians compare it to the barking of a seal. To one mother it sounded like a dog choking on something caught in its throat. The cough is so distinctive that even new parents sometimes say, "I'd never heard it before, but I knew immediately what it was, that it was croup."

Your child may also be making another, more ominous sound. As the child breathes in with each breath, you may hear a harsh, sometimes high-pitched and loud sound called stridor. (The word comes from the Latin for "harsh noise.") Stridor is a sign that your child has an obstruction in his upper airway in the region of the lower throat near the vocal chords.

What's happening inside your child's throat is that the virus has spread downward and is causing inflammation and swelling in the middle respiratory tract, in the tissues of his larynx (voice box) and trachea (windpipe). This swelling has reduced the diameter of the air passageway to his lungs. Mucus and other respiratory secretions are also clogging the airway, further narrowing it and obstructing the flow of air to the lungs. The infection and swelling may also spread downward as far as your child's bronchial tubes. Your doctor is likely to use the term *acute laryngotracheobronchitis* for croup, meaning that it has affected the larynx (*laryngo-*), the trachea (*-tracheo-*) and bronchial tubes (*-bronch-*). The ending *-itis* means "inflammation."

One reason croup is a disease of babies and toddlers is simply the size of their windpipe. A one-year-old's windpipe is so tiny that it does not take much in the way of swelling or secretions to clog it. Your child can get croup more than once, from different viruses, particularly if he has a small windpipe. An older child or an adult who has an infection in the same part of the throat would have only a sore throat, laryngitis, or a cold.

Why some children get croup while others do not remains a mystery. The virus causing croup are so common that they infect everyone; yet only a minority of children get the disease. It may have something to do with differences in their anatomy—the diameter of their airways— or perhaps with differences in the strains of viruses that happen to infect them.

Croup usually starts in the middle of the night partly because when your child is lying down to sleep, mucus and other respiratory secretions tend to pool in the throat. Also, as your child sleeps, the throat muscles become relaxed and do not keep the airway open as much.

Although croup almost never leads to problems, rarely a child with croup may need hospitalization. The danger of croup is that your child will develop what is called respiratory distress. Her larynx and windpipe may become so swollen and her airway so clogged with mucus that she must work harder to breathe. To get more air, her nostrils may flare outward at the sides. She may also develop what are called retractions: she must use extra muscles, ones she does not usually use for respiration, to help her breathe, and each time she takes a breath, you can actually see these muscles pulling in (retracting) in the spaces between her ribs and at the base of her neck above the collarbone.

If less air is getting to her lungs, less oxygen may be passing into her bloodstream and reaching the brain and other tissues. She may start to

## CALL YOUR DOCTOR

Or take your child to your hospital emergency room for the following:

- If your child awakens with a barking cough and is also making the harsh sound called stridor.

- If your child shows other signs of respiratory distress: he is working harder to breathe, his nostrils are flaring out, and he is retracting the muscles between his ribs and at the base of his neck.

CALL 911 or take your child to your hospital emergency room:

- If your child is really struggling to get her breath and is concentrating only on breathing.

- If your child is turning blue around her mouth and at the tips of her fingers.

- If your child has become limp, lethargic, and unresponsive.

turn bluish or grayish around the mouth and also at the tips of her fingers. Her behavior may also change. Instead of smiling and playing, she may become limp and lethargic and less responsive. She concentrates on breathing.

## Diagnosis

When you call your doctor, she may ask you to bring your child to the phone—or take a portable phone to your child's bedside—so she can hear the alarming sounds for herself. She may be able to say on the phone that it sounds like croup and may also make a preliminary evaluation of how serious it seems.

By the time you and your child reach your doctor's office or the emergency room, do not be surprised if your child has stopped the terrible coughing and seems fine and happy. This is a common scenario with croup. There is no reason for you to feel embarrassed.

The physician will assess the severity of your child's croup and his degree of respiratory distress. At Children's Hospital, if we can hear a child's stridor only with a stethoscope, for instance, we consider his croup moderately severe. But if a child has stridor loud enough that we can hear it with the unaided ear while he is quiet and resting comfortably, his croup may be serious enough that admission to the hospital for close observation and treatment is needed.

We can measure the actual amount of oxygen that is getting into a child's bloodstream and thus reaching his brain and other tissues. We use a light-probe device called a pulse oximeter, which fits over his finger and gives an immediate reading of his blood oxygen level. This does not hurt or bother your child and takes only a minute.

If it is decided to admit the child to the hospital, an X-ray made of the airways of his neck and chest may be obtained to make sure he does have croup and not something more serious.

Your doctor probably will not try to find out exactly which virus is causing your child's croup because the identity of the virus does not affect the treatment. At Children's Hospital a test for the virus is done only if a child is being admitted. A small sample of mucus is taken from the child's nose and the laboratory performs a viral testing. The staff will also take special precautions to keep the virus from spreading to other sick children in the hospital.

# Treatment

When you call your doctor, he may suggest that you first try treating your child at home, even before taking her to the office or to the emergency room, with the following treatments.

## Humidity

The main treatment for croup is mist therapy, that is, more moisture in the air your child is breathing. The extra humidity helps liquefy and loosen the mucus and other secretions that are clogging your child's throat. The humidity also helps moisten and soothe the inflamed tissues in the respiratory tract.

One way to give your child extra humidity quickly is to take her into the bathroom, close the door, and turn on the hot water in the shower to fill the room with warm moisture. Be sure to stay in the bathroom with her. Your doctor may tell you to try this for a certain length of time and then call him back.

## Outdoor Air

The air inside houses and apartments is often very dry, particularly in winter, when heating systems are running. If you take your child outdoors, where the air may be considerably more humid, it may help relieve the coughing.

One reason your child may be much better by the time you get her to the emergency room is that you have taken her outdoors and driven for a while through cool, moist night air.

## Medical Treatments

In the emergency department at Children's Hospital, we start treating a child with mist therapy while we evaluate the severity of his croup symptoms. Sometimes ten to twenty minutes of mist therapy causes a child's stridor to disappear.

Depending on the severity of your child's symptoms, your pediatrician may give him a corticosteroid medication. Corticosteroids reduce the inflammation and swelling in your child's throat, allowing him to breathe more easily. The doctor may give him a single injection of corticosteroid, or she may prescribe a short course of oral corticosteroids for him to take by mouth over the next two days.

Doctors also sometimes prescribe a medication called racemic epinephrine. This is delivered directly to the larynx in the form of a mist. Epinephrine also tends to reduce the swelling in a child's throat and open up his airway, an effect that lasts about an hour or so. At Children's Hospital we usually reserve racemic epinephrine for children whose croup symptoms are moderate to severe.

Your child usually does not need antibiotics for croup, since most croup is caused by viruses and antibiotics are not effective against viruses.

* * *

Most children with croup can be treated at home. Once you get your child back home, you may find that he seems fine during the day; he runs around and plays and does all the things he usually does. Then at night, and only at night, when he lies down to sleep, the cough comes back. You can expect about three similar nights of barking coughs.

Continue to give your child extra humidity in the air he breathes by using a humidifier in his room. See *Humidity*, page 293, in the Appendices, for more information about humidity and humidifiers.

If your child has some fever and is uncomfortable, you can give him acetaminophen.

You need to make sure that you are giving your child extra fluids to prevent dehydration because your child is losing more fluid than usual in his mucus and other secretions and also because of any fever he may have. Babies especially can become dangerously dehydrated very quickly, and you need to give them special fluids called oral rehydration solutions. See *Fluids*, page 290, in the Appendices for more about dehydration and these special fluids and also what fluids to offer older children.

By the third day of croup, your child should be much better. His symptoms may not have disappeared completely, but he usually is improved enough you do not need to worry about him so much.

## Hospitalization

Occasionally a child with croup needs to be hospitalized. About 20,000 children in the United States are hospitalized for croup each year. During croup season at Children's Hospital, we need to admit about one or two children a month for croup. In the hospital the staff continues to treat the child with mist therapy, often in a so-called croup tent. We monitor the child's heart and breathing rates and also the oxygen level in her blood, and we generally give her extra oxygen and intravenous fluids if needed. We give her corticosteroid medication and, if she needs it, racemic epinephrine. Very rarely a child may need to be on a respirator in the intensive care unit, but this is generally the case only for children who already have a chronic lung condition or other disease. Most children are well enough to go home after two or three days.

## *Prevention*

The parainfluenza viruses and respiratory syncytial virus are so widespread during their seasons that it is impractical to keep your baby or toddler away from everyone who might be shedding these viruses. However, try to limit the exposure of your baby or toddler to her older siblings and other children or grownups when they have colds.

When you yourself have a cold, cover your nose and mouth—and teach your children to cover theirs—whenever you must sneeze or cough. When you blow your nose or help children blow their noses, be careful about how you discard the tissue. After you sneeze or cough or blow your nose, wash your hands carefully before you touch your baby or toddler.

# DIARRHEA

## SYMPTOMS

- Increased frequency of bowel movements

- Bloody, watery, or mucus-containing stools

- Possible vomiting, fever, abdominal cramps, headache, muscle aches

Diarrhea is one of the most common of all infectious diseases affecting children. Most of the time your child will recover uneventfully, but in extreme cases diarrhea can be life-threatening.

You almost certainly will be dealing with episodes of diarrhea in your child at some point. Diarrhea is among the diseases that most frequently spread among children who attend day-care centers. By the time children in this country are five years old, each of them has experienced some seven to fifteen bouts of diarrhea, according to the U.S. Public Health Service's Centers for Disease Control and Prevention (CDC). Altogether, children under five have 20 to 35 million episodes of diarrhea each year, says CDC, prompting 2 million to 3.5 million visits to doctors. Diarrhea is responsible for 9 percent of all hospitalizations of children under five—200,000 hospitalizations a year. Most of the children who must be hospitalized are infants in their first year of life.

At Children's Hospital diarrhea is one of the most common complaints in the emergency department, and an average of one or two children a day are evaluated for diarrhea.

In the nineteenth century diarrhea was a major cause of death in children in the United States. Today diarrhea still kills 300 to 500 children in this country every year. Most of these deaths occur in infants under a year old. In developing countries diarrhea ( and dehydration) kills 4 million children each year—more than 10,000 children a day.

## *Causes*

Diarrhea can be caused by many, many different organisms. The most common causes in children are viruses, and the virus most commonly responsible is one called rotavirus. Rotavirus causes one-fourth of all diarrhea episodes among young children in the United States, 3.5 million cases a year. Rotavirus is also one of the germs that most readily spreads from child to child in day-care centers. It is also the number-one cause of deaths from diarrhea among children. See *Rotavirus Diarrhea*, page 69, for more about this type of diarrhea.

Other viruses commonly causing diarrhea in children include the Norwalk virus (which more often affects older children and adults), the adenoviruses, and the enteroviruses.

Among bacteria, the most common causes of diarrhea are salmonella, which makes an estimated 2 to 4 million Americans sick each year; shigella, another germ that frequently spreads among children in day-care centers; campylobacter, and *Yersinia enterocolitica*. See *Salmonella Infections*, page 231; *Shigella Diarrhea*, page 72; *Campylobacter Diarrhea*, page 60, and *Yersinia Diarrhea*, page 77.

*E. coli* bacteria are the most common cause of so-called traveler's diarrhea, which can strike children and adults visiting developing countries. One particularly dangerous strain of *E. coli* (O157:H7) received a lot of publicity recently after it killed several children in the Northwest. See *E. coli Disease*, page 97.

Two protozoans—microscopic, single-celled animals related to amebas—are also common causes of diarrhea in children: giardia and cryptosporidium. Giardia is another germ that often spreads in day-care centers, and cryptosporidium also causes day-care outbreaks. See *Giardia Diarrhea,* page 67, and *Cryptosporidium Diarrhea,* page 63.

In some parts of the world, cholera (caused by the bacterium *Vibrio cholerae*) is a major cause of diarrhea. However, cholera is rare in the United States, and most of the time when people here do have the disease, they have caught it outside the country.

## *How It Spreads*

Organisms that commonly cause diarrhea in children travel from person to person primarily via what is called the "fecal-oral" route—which often involves a partly hand-to-mouth route.

Most of these germs live and multiply in the intestines of infected humans, including children, who shed the germs in their stools. What's sneaky about these germs is that people can harbor them in their intestines and shed them in their stools without knowing it, without being sick or having any symptoms at all.

If an infant is infected and shedding germs, you can get them on your hands when you change her diapers. Or babies and toddlers can get the germs on their fingers as they explore their bodies; small children who are not toilet trained are a major source of diarrhea-causing germs. Or if you are infected, you can get the germs on your hands when you go to the toilet. Toilet paper is not enough to protect your hands.

If you fail to wash your hands after using the toilet, you may then deposit the diarrhea-causing organisms on anything you touch: doorknobs, tabletops, lightswitches, chairs, telephones, clothing, books, pens, pencils, crayons, toys, children's hands or faces.

When someone comes along and touches an object you have touched—a toddler picks up a toy, for instance—he can get the organisms on his own hands. Then when the infant or toddler puts the toy—or his fingers—in his mouth, he may become infected with the germs.

As few as ten individual shigella bacteria can make a child sick with diarrhea, and rotavirus particles can live on inanimate objects and surfaces for up to a week; giardia, for three months. It is no wonder that these three germs cause so many outbreaks of diarrhea among children attending day-care centers.

If you get diarrhea-causing organisms on your hands—because you touched a contaminated object or diapered an infected baby or are infected yourself—and fail to wash your hands before handling, preparing, or serving food, you can deposit the germs on the food and thus transmit them to anyone who eats the food. Shigella bacteria are among the many germs that can spread this way, as are *E. coli* bacteria.

Salmonella, campylobacter, and *E. coli* bacteria live and multiply in the intestines of many infected farm animals, including cattle and chickens. Red meats, poultry, eggs, and other foods of animal origin can thus be contaminated when you buy them at the store. If you do not handle and cook these foods carefully, they, too, can cause your child to develop diarrhea.

Flies can deposit diarrhea-causing organisms—particularly shigella and salmonella bacteria—on foods if they first land on animal or human feces containing the germs. Flies can carry bacteria attached to their legs, or they can get them in their gut and shed them in their own feces.

Some pets—birds, cats, lizards, and turtles—can carry salmonella bacteria in their intestines and shed them in their feces. If the stools contaminate objects and surfaces, infants and toddlers can get the bacteria on their fingers and into their mouths.

Some diarrhea-causing organisms—particularly giardia, cryptosporidium, and shigella bacteria—can spread in water, and your child can get infected from drinking or swimming in contaminated water. Malfunctioning sewage systems occasionally spill contaminated fecal matter from livestock or humans into rivers, lakes, or drinking-water supplies. Infected children who are not toilet trained can contaminate unchlorinated wading and swimming pools. In wilderness areas, infected wild animals (such as deer) sometimes contaminate streams and ponds with giardia.

Once diarrhea-causing germs get into a child's mouth, they are swallowed, pass through the stomach, and into the intestines.

## Incubation Period

How long it takes for your child to get sick after he ingests diarrhea-causing germs varies with the organism. Diarrhea due to salmonella can appear in as few as six hours. Rotavirus and shigella diarrhea usually appear in anywhere from one to four or five days or more, while diarrhea due to giardia may take several weeks to develop.

## Symptoms

In your child's gastrointestinal tract, these organisms all cause gastroenteritis, that is, an inflammation of the stomach and intestines. The most common symptom of gastroenteritis is diarrhea—an increase in the frequency of your child's bowel movements. (The word *diarrhea* comes from the Greek for "flowing through.") If your child has a moderate case of rotavirus diarrhea, she may have seven to ten bowel movements a day. If she has a severe case, she may reach up to fifteen bowel movements a day.

You should become familiar with your child's usual pattern of bowel movements so that you will be able to detect any significant increase in their frequency. Children may normally have one to two bowel movements a day. A newborn, during the first month of life, may normally have from one to four movements a day. *However, there is a wide range of normal.* What is important is whether your child is having more bowel movements than usual.

Along with the increase in frequency, the consistency of your child's stools usually changes. They may become very watery, to the point where they ooze or run freely out of her diapers. Stools may also contain blood if certain bacteria are involved. Shigella, campylobacter, *E. coli,* and yersinia bacteria all can cause bloody stools. (Bloody diarrhea is also called dysentery.) The blood may occur in clots, streaks, or flecks. And the stools may also contain mucus, similar to what comes out of your nose when you have a cold. Some mothers speak of a child having "cold in the stool."

Often with gastroenteritis and diarrhea, your child may also be vomiting, sometimes as often as every half hour or more. And she may also have a fever (sometimes high) or chills, bloating or cramping in her abdomen (which can be painful), a headache, muscle aches and pains, and a general feeling of being sick. And with a queasy stomach, a child usually loses her appetite and may lose some weight.

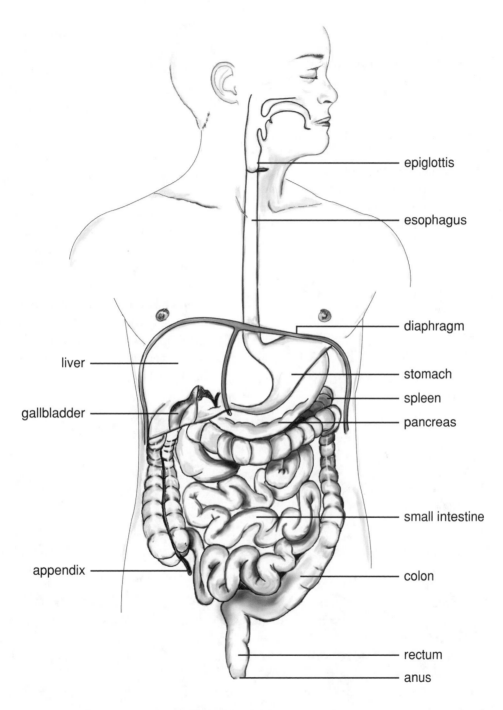

*Gastrointestinal tract.*

## Complications

The danger of diarrhea is dehydration—that your child will lose too much fluid from his body through his frequent bowel movements and vomiting and through increased evaporation from his skin due to fever. Dehydration can be life-threatening.

Dehydration is particularly dangerous for infants, and the smaller a baby, the more quickly he can become dehydrated. Eighty-five percent of children who die from diarrhea are infants in their first year of life. Rotavirus can kill a child from dehydration within a day.

See *Fluids*, page 290, in the Appendices for more about dehydration.

## Diagnosis

When you call your doctor, he is likely to ask you when your child's diarrhea began, how many stools he is passing per day and what do the stools look and smell like.

If your child's stools are just watery—with no blood or mucus in them—and his diarrhea has lasted no longer than five days, the chances are that the diarrhea is caused by a virus, either rotavirus or another of the common gastrointestinal viruses. Physicians do not usually need to order laboratory tests to find which one because whatever the virus, the treatment is the same.

If the pediatrician does not see blood in your child's stools, she may test for hidden, microscopic blood by placing a small sample of stool on a card and adding a liquid. If there is blood in the stool, it will turn blue.

If your child *does* have blood or mucus in his stools or his diarrhea has lasted more than five days, the chances increase that the diarrhea is caused by a bacterium or other microorganism. At Children's Hospital we then order lab tests

## CALL YOUR DOCTOR

- If your child has diarrhea and is under twelve months of age.

- If your child is having watery bowel movements more than ten times a day. She may be becoming dehydrated.

- If you see any blood or mucus in the stools of your child of any age. She may need treatment with an antibiotic.

- If your child has diarrhea with severe abdominal pain for more than one hour.

- If your child is showing any signs of dehydration. One of the clearest signs is if she is not urinating as much or as often as usual. Another sign is dryness of the mucous membranes, particularly the inside of the mouth, which may feel sticky or tacky rather than moist. The most important sign of possible dehydration, however, is if your child is not behaving normally: if she is less active than usual, lying around, sleeping more, and not playing as much.

    Dehydration due to diarrhea usually does not develop so fast that it requires a middle-of-the-night phone call to your pediatrician, but if your child is listless and lethargic, *call your doctor immediately*, whatever the time of day or night.

on a sample of a child's stool in order to identify the organism.

To identify the organism, the lab must isolate and culture (grow) them. The Children's Hospital lab routinely cultures diarrhea stool samples for the four bacteria that most commonly cause diarrhea: salmonella, shigella, campylobacter, and *Yersinia enterocolitica*. It may take up to five days to get the results.

If a child with diarrhea has recently returned from a developing country such as Mexico, a pediatrician may ask that the lab test for the type of *E. coli* that commonly causes traveler's diarrhea.

If a child has had diarrhea for a prolonged period of time, longer than ten days, particularly if he has recently visited a wilderness area, a pediatrician would request a test for giardia.

## Treatment

Your child does not usually need to take any medication when she has diarrhea and gastroenteritis.

There are no antiviral drugs that work against or kill the gastrointestinal viruses, which are the most common causes of diarrhea in children. Diarrhea due to viral infections usually goes away on its own after about three to five days.

If your child's diarrhea is caused by a bacterial infection, she still may not need any medication. Most of the time, antibiotics do not help, and sometimes they can actually hurt. With most salmonella infections, for instance, antibiotics can prolong the time your child carries the bacteria in her intestines and sheds them in her stools.

Pediatricians usually do prescribe antibiotics for diarrhea due to shigella bacteria or giardia. In infants under three months, physicians may prescribe antibiotics for salmonella infections

because the disease can be more serious in babies this young. Doctors may also prescribe antibiotics for campylobacter or *Yersinia enterocolitica* infections if they are causing a child to have diarrhea for a prolonged period of time. See the "Treatment" section in the chapter about each of these diseases or organisms.

Pediatricians do not usually prescribe or advise the use of antidiarrheal drugs for babies and young children. So-called antimotility drugs, such as loperamide, reduce diarrhea by slowing muscle movements in the intestines and thus slowing the passage of fluids and wastes through the intestines. With salmonella and shigella infections, this could hurt a child by prolonging the time the bacteria remain in her intestines.

## Replacing Fluids
### Oral Rehydration Therapy

The main treatment for a child's diarrhea—whatever the cause—is replacing the fluids that he is losing through his watery stools, vomiting, and fever so that he does not become dangerously dehydrated. The smaller your baby, the more important it is to replace these fluids.

First try giving him extra fluids by mouth; this is often called oral rehydration therapy. If your baby is under a year, you should not give him plain water. Babies this young, with their immature kidneys, are also losing essential salts along with fluids, and you need to replace these salts as well. Physicians advise giving babies special fluids called oral rehydration solutions. These solutions generally contain glucose (sugar) and also the necessary salts. For more information about these special fluids, see *Fluids*, page 290, in the Appendices.

*The U.S. Public Health Service's Centers for Disease Control and Prevention recommend that all families with infants and small children keep a supply of oral rehydration solution at home at all times as a staple of their medicine chest and start giving a child the solution when he first has diarrhea. Having the solution on hand could be lifesaving.*

When we see an infant with diarrhea at Children's Hospital, we evaluate his degree of dehydration and calculate how much oral rehydration solution he needs, depending on his weight and state of dehydration. We then give his mother a specific goal: try to get him to drink a certain number of ounces of rehydration solution over the next so-many hours.

This can be a tedious and time-consuming job. If you give your baby an eight-ounce bottle of solution all at once, he is likely to vomit it up. The key is to give him the fluid slowly, in very small amounts, over a period of time: one or two ounces at a time, in a bottle or with a spoon or medicine dropper. Then wait twenty minutes to let this fluid pass through his stomach and into his intestine so that he will be less likely to vomit it up. Then one or two ounces more and again wait twenty minutes, one or two ounces more and so on.

You can get some idea of whether you are indeed getting enough fluid into your baby by paying attention to his urination. If he is wetting his diaper as much as usual, you are probably giving him enough.

With a child over the age of one year, whose kidneys are more mature and better able to retain salts, you can be more free about what fluids you give. You can offer her a variety of clear fluids such as fruit juices, punches, broths and, yes, chicken soup. You can even make it fun and tempt her with different flavors of water ices and her favorite soft drinks. With carbonated sodas, however, you should first stir out the bubbles because carbon dioxide can irritate the stomach and intestines.

The main nonclear fluid to avoid is cow's milk. Cow's milk and other dairy products can make diarrhea worse (see below). Also avoid orange and grapefruit juices, which are harder to digest.

If your child is still losing fluid faster than you can replace it, if you cannot get enough fluid into your baby or get your older child to drink enough—and if she's having fifteen watery bowel movements a day and is also vomiting, it can be difficult—your doctor may need to give her fluid intravenously in his office or the hospital emergency department.

## Feeding

When your child has diarrhea and is vomiting, he usually is not very interested in eating: his stomach is upset, he may have some cramping in his intestines, and he does not feel well. You can continue to offer him whatever he is used to eating, but you do not need to worry too much if he does not eat it. If your child does want to eat, it is generally okay to keep feeding him whatever he is used to eating.

If you are breastfeeding your baby, continue to nurse him. Breast milk is very easy for infants to digest, and your milk may also contain antibodies against the germs causing his diarrhea. These antibodies may help reduce his symptoms.

Cow's milk and cow's milk formulas, however, are different in composition from human breast milk and harder for your baby to digest. Pediatricians usually do advise that you stop giving formula to your baby when he has diarrhea. With an older child, if you give him any milk products, he may actually have more diarrhea, have more trouble with gas in his intestines, and be more uncomfortable.

However, try to get your child back onto his regular diet as quickly as possible. For children who are old enough to be eating solid foods, you can start with bland foods (which are easier to digest) such as bananas, rice, applesauce, toast, and crackers. This is sometimes called the BRAT diet: B for bananas, R for rice, A for applesauce, and T for toast.

In addition to avoiding milk, also avoid giving him foods that are high in sugar or fat. Too much sugar can make his diarrhea worse, and fats are harder to digest. French fries, pizza, or spicy or heavy foods are not the best foods to start with when your child has had an upset stomach.

Parents are often very concerned when diarrhea and vomiting cause a child to stop eating solid food. You do not need to be too concerned. As your child's symptoms ease and she feels better, she will start to eat normally again. She may lose some weight during the illness, but she will gain it right back afterward. You do not need to force food into your child the way you need to force fluids. Drinking is the important thing; pushing fluids is what you should focus on. Eating solid food can come later.

## Skin Care

Because stools are acidic, diarrhea can cause your child's skin to become irritated and encrusted. To prevent this, wash her bottom with soap and water after each bowel movement. If the area gets irritated, try leaving the diaper off so that the air can circulate.

## Hospitalization

If a child's diarrhea cannot be controlled, or if the child is becoming seriously dehydrated, admission to the hospital may be warranted. The major reason for admission is to replace lost fluids by giving fluids intravenously. Sixty-five percent of the children who need to be hospitalized for diarrhea are babies under a year. At Children's

Hospital we then measure the amounts of different salts the infant is losing and make up an intravenous rehydration fluid tailored specifically to his needs. Babies admitted for diarrhea usually need to stay in the hospital for one to three days.

## *Prevention*

The single most effective thing you can do to help prevent your child from getting diarrhea and gastroenteritis—and spreading it within your family—is to wash your hands often and thoroughly.

Wash them immediately after changing your baby's diapers, helping an older child at the toilet, or going to the bathroom yourself. You or a child can be carrying—and shedding—diarrhea-causing germs without knowing it, without being sick.

Also wash your hands before handling, preparing, serving, or eating food. You never know what diarrhea-causing (or other) germs you may have picked up on your hands from touching a doorknob, a telephone, a child's toy, or another object.

You should wash your infant's or toddler's hands before letting her pick up food with her fingers. And as soon as your children are old enough, teach them to wash their own hands after going to the toilet and before eating or touching food.

Make sure you change your baby's diapers well away from where you prepare or eat food. Keep food out of the diapering area and dirty diapers out of the kitchen. This may seem obvious, but a newspaper column recently recounted two incidents of mothers who changed their babies' diapers on dining-room tables in public restaurants. When one diner complained, the mother rejected the complaint, saying, "It's no big deal." But it was a big deal. Both mothers were potentially exposing everyone who ate or worked in these restaurants to whatever germs their babies might be shedding in their stools.

Since diarrhea-causing germs occur so frequently in meat, poultry and eggs, you need to handle these foods carefully. See "Prevention," page 125, in *Food Poisoning* for tips on how to store and cook these foods safely so as to keep you and your family from getting sick.

For day-care centers, both the U.S. Public Health Service and the American Academy of Pediatrics have issued detailed recommendations for reducing the spread of diarrhea and other infectious diseases. See *Recommendations for Day-Care Providers,* pages 297–300, in the Appendices.

## *Campylobacter Diarrhea*

Also called campylobacteriosis. The ending *-osis* means "disease."

### SYMPTOMS

- Diarrhea, possibly watery or bloody
- Fever
- Abdominal cramps
- Vomiting
- Headache
- Muscle aches

You may never have heard of campylobacter, but these bacteria are one of the most common causes of diarrhea due to food poisoning, probably as common as the more familiar salmonella bacteria.

Long known to produce disease in animals, campylobacter was first recognized as a cause of human disease in the 1970s. Today, with better methods of detecting the bacteria available, it has

become apparent that they are a major cause of human illness. The U.S. Public Health Service's Centers for Disease Control and Prevention estimates that two to four million Americans may develop campylobacter diarrhea every year.

Campylobacter diarrhea is most common among babies and young children under the age of five. Curiously, it is also more common in a second age group: teenagers and young adults between the ages of fifteen and twenty-nine.

### Cause

The full name of the campylobacter species that mostly commonly causes diarrhea in humans is *Campylobacter jejuni.* You pronounce the name with the stress on the first and fourth syllables: cam'-py-lo-bac'-ter. The name comes from the Greek for "curved rod," which is what the bacterium looks like under a microscope.

Campylobacter bacteria live and multiply in the intestines of a wide variety of farm animals, including chickens, turkeys, cattle, pigs, and sheep. The bacteria can also infect the intestines of dogs and cats. Infected animals may be obviously sick with diarrhea, or they may appear perfectly healthy.

### How It Spreads

Infected animals shed campylobacter bacteria in their feces, and your child can become infected when she gets the bacteria in her mouth and swallows them.

People usually catch campylobacter from raw or undercooked meat or poultry, most commonly from chicken. One-third to one-half of the raw chicken on the market in the United States is contaminated with campylobacter bacteria, according to the Public Health Service. Your child can become infected by eating chicken that is not thoroughly cooked.

Your child can also become infected if you allow bacteria from chicken or meat to get onto other objects in your kitchen—a countertop, cutting board, knife, your hands. From there the bacteria can easily get into other food. If you use the same knife, for instance, to cut up vegetables for a salad, the bacteria could contaminate the salad.

Dairy cows often carry campylobacter without showing any signs of sickness, and the bacteria can get into milk directly, or milk can become contaminated from the cows' feces. Your child can become infected from drinking raw, unpasteurized milk. Outbreaks of campylobacter diarrhea have occurred when schoolchildren visited dairy farms on field trips and were given raw milk to drink. In one such outbreak 106 children developed diarrhea.

Your child can also get campylobacter diarrhea by drinking water polluted with animal or human feces. In Bennington, Vermont, one spring, 3,000 people—19 percent of the town's entire population—became sick with diarrhea when the bacteria somehow got into the water supply. People have also contracted campylobacter diarrhea after drinking water from mountain streams that looked clear.

*Campylobacter jejuni* is one of the many organisms that can cause people to develop traveler's diarrhea because they eat contaminated food or drink polluted water while traveling in developing countries.

Once in a person's mouth, the bacteria pass through the stomach and settle down in the intestinal tract, where they grow and multiply.

## Incubation Period

Diarrhea usually develops in one to seven days after campylobacter bacteria are consumed, but it can take longer.

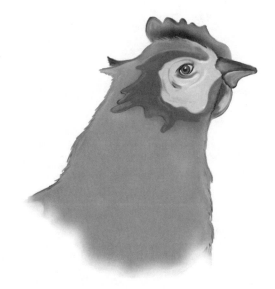

*Raw poultry may be contaminated with campylobacter.*

## Symptoms

As the bacteria grow in his intestinal tract, your child may experience no symptoms at all, or he may have mild diarrhea with a few loose stools for a few days. Or he may have more severe diarrhea, with ten or more watery bowel movements a day and stools streaked with blood.

Along with diarrhea—and often hours before it begins—a child may run a fever. He may have intense cramps in his abdomen, sometimes resembling the pain of appendicitis. He is often nauseated and vomiting; he may have a headache, and his muscles may ache.

The danger of any diarrhea is that it can cause your child's body to become dehydrated. He is losing extra fluid through frequent stools, through any vomiting, and if he has any fever, through increased evaporation from his body. Babies particularly, because they are so tiny, can very quickly develop serious—even life-threatening—dehydration.

See *Fluids*, page 290, in the Appendices for more about dehydration.

---

**CALL YOUR DOCTOR**

- If your child has diarrhea and is under a year old.

- If your child has any blood or mucus in her stools or has diarrhea with severe abdominal pain.

- If your child is having watery bowel movements more than ten times a day.

- If your child shows any signs of dehydration: if she is not urinating as much as usual; if her mouth is dry, or if she is less active than usual.

---

## Diagnosis

To find out whether campylobacter or some other germ is causing a child's diarrhea, physicians take a sample of his stool and have a laboratory try to culture (grow) and identify the organism. Usually it is not necessary to do this because most of the time children recover from diarrhea on their own.

At The Children's Hospital of Philadelphia, we order tests on a child's stool sample if the child has any blood or mucus in his stools or has had diarrhea for more than five days. Our lab routinely tests stool samples for campylobacter and also the three other bacteria (salmonella, shigella, and *Yersinia enterocolitica*) that most commonly cause diarrhea in children. It may take up to five days to get the results.

## Treatment

Whenever your child has diarrhea, whatever the cause, the main treatment is to make sure that

he drinks enough extra liquid to replace the fluids he is losing through his frequent stools and any vomiting or fever. If your baby is under a year old, pediatricians advise that you give him special fluids called oral rehydration solutions.

See *Fluids*, page 290, in the Appendices for more about these fluids, how to give them, and what fluids to offer and not offer older children. See also "Treatment," page 57, in *Diarrhea*, for information about what else to do and not do when your child has diarrhea.

If your child's diarrhea is due to campylobacter bacteria, your pediatrician may or may not prescribe an antibiotic for her. At Children's Hospital we usually do not prescribe antibiotics for children with campylobacter diarrhea because by the time we find out four or five days later that campylobacter is the cause, a child's diarrhea has usually disappeared.

However, campylobacter infections sometimes cause a child to have diarrhea that persists for several weeks. In that case—or if a child's symptoms are particularly severe—we may prescribe an antibiotic, usually erythromycin, by mouth, for five to seven days.

## Prevention

You can easily kill any campylobacter bacteria that may be present in the meat and poultry you purchase by cooking them thoroughly. The U.S. Department of Agriculture recommends that you cook meat to an internal temperature of 160°F to destroy any campylobacter and cook chicken to an internal temperature of 180°F to 185°F— which is the way most people like it anyway.

And remember that up to 50 percent of raw chicken has campylobacter on it. When you are working with raw chicken in your kitchen, be careful that it does not contaminate any other food. Clean up any chicken juices that may spill on your counter. Wash everything the raw chicken has touched—the cutting board, knife, bowl, platter, your hands—thoroughly with soap and water before you let them touch anything else. Do not put the cooked chicken back on the platter or board that held the raw chicken; either scrub the platter first or use a different, clean platter to serve the chicken.

Carelessness in handling raw chicken because of inexperience may explain why teenagers and young adults develop more campylobacter diarrhea. "The predilection of this infection for young adults," the Public Health Service suggests, "may be related to their cooking habits as they leave their childhood homes and begin cooking for themselves."

For more tips about how to handle and cook meats and poultry safely, see "Prevention," page 125, in *Food Poisoning.*

Pasteurization kills any campylobacter bacteria as well as other germs that may be present in milk. The possibility of contracting campylobacter diarrhea is one of the many reasons not to drink—or give your children—raw milk.

Chlorination destroys any campylobacter that may get into municipal drinking-water supplies. However, it is wise not to drink—or let your children drink—untreated water from lakes or streams. Even clean-looking water may be contaminated with animal feces and contain campylobacter or other disease-causing organisms.

## *Cryptosporidium Diarrhea*

Also called cryptosporidiosis or crypto. The ending *-osis* means "disease."

Many people first heard of the germ cryptosporidium in 1993 when it caused an

**SYMPTOMS**

- Diarrhea, possibly containing mucus, possibly persistent for weeks
- Possible abdominal cramps
- Vomiting
- Low-grade fever

estimated 403,000 men, women, and children in Milwaukee, Wisconsin, to become ill with acute watery diarrhea.

Cryptosporidium has long been known to produce diarrhea in farm animals, but it was not until the 1980s—as better methods of detecting the organism became available—that doctors realized it is also a significant cause of human disease.

Diarrhea due to cryptosporidium most frequently affects young children between the ages of six months and two years, and it is a cause of diarrhea outbreaks in day-care centers. In a typical episode, in Philadelphia, over a period of two months one summer, twenty-three of the fifty-three children attending one day-care center developed diarrhea due to cryptosporidium.

## Cause

Cryptosporidium is a microscopic, single-celled animal related to amebas. Its full name is *Cryptosporidium parvum.* The word *cryptosporidium* comes from the Greek and Latin for "hidden small spore."

Cryptosporidium organisms live in the intestinal tracts of a wide variety of animals—particularly young animals—including many farm animals (cows, horses, sheep, goats), wild animals (deer, elk), domestic animals (dogs, cats), and humans. The organisms undergo a complex, multistage life cycle and produce their equivalent of eggs, which are called oocysts.

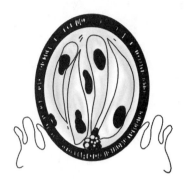

*Cryptosporidium oocyst.*

## How It Spreads

Animals and humans who are infected with cryptosporidium shed these oocysts in their feces. A child can become infected if the oocysts get into the mouth and are swallowed.

In day-care centers cryptosporidium oocysts may spread among babies and toddlers who are not toilet trained. Infected children may get oocysts from their stools on their hands. They can then spread the oocysts directly to each other as they play. They can also leave oocysts on anything they touch: a toy, a drinking cup, a book, a tabletop. Another baby or toddler puts the toy in her mouth—and she becomes infected. Or a child picks up the book, gets oocysts on his own hands, puts his fingers in his mouth—and he becomes infected.

People who work with animals, such as farm workers and veterinarians, can catch cryptosporidium directly from the animals, which are not necessarily sick themselves. Cryptosporidium organisms are present on more than 90 percent of dairy farms in this country, the Public Health

Service estimates, and 50 percent of dairy calves shed oocysts in their manure.

In one outbreak, in Maine, cryptosporidium oocysts in calf manure apparently contaminated apples on the ground. The fruit was then pressed into cider without being adequately washed, and 160 elementary and high school students developed diarrhea after they drank the unpasteurized cider at a school fair. Cryptosporidium oocysts can also get into food from a person's hands.

The biggest outbreaks of cryptosporidium diarrhea, however, have been caused by drinking polluted water. Cryptosporidium is one of the disease-causing organisms that people most commonly can catch from contaminated water.

Drinking water was the source of the cryptosporidium that sickened so many people in Milwaukee. The organisms presumably got into the city water supply from feces from infected farm animals or from human sewage. This Milwaukee outbreak was the largest outbreak of any waterborne disease ever recorded to date in the United States.

People have also contracted cryptosporidium diarrhea by swallowing contaminated water in swimming pools, wave pools, and water slides. And in tests of lakes, rivers, and streams around the country, researchers have detected cryptosporidium oocysts in 65 to 97 percent of the waters they sampled.

Once a person swallows cryptosporidium oocysts, the oocysts pass through the stomach into the intestines. There they hatch, so to speak, each releasing four sporozoites, the next stage in their life cycle. These sporozoites invade cells lining the intestines and there undergo several more stages of development, dividing and also reproducing sexually. Eventually they form more oocysts—which an infected person or animal excretes in feces.

## Incubation Period

An average of about seven days passes from the time a person ingests cryptosporidium oocysts until he develops diarrhea, but the incubation period can range from two to fourteen days. In the apple cider outbreak in Maine, some children became sick in as little as ten hours.

## Symptoms

As the cryptosporidium organisms grow and reproduce in your child's intestinal tract, she may have no symptoms at all. Usually she has mild diarrhea—several watery, foul-smelling bowel movements a day that usually contain mucus but no blood. Rarely, she may develop more severe diarrhea, up to ten stools a day, and her diarrhea may persist for weeks.

Along with diarrhea, your child may have abdominal cramps and excessive gas in her intestines. She may be nauseated and vomiting and have a low fever, 101° to 102°F. In the apple cider outbreak, a number of children experienced vomiting without any diarrhea.

The danger of any diarrhea, whether due to cryptosporidium or another germ, is that it can cause your child's body to become dehydrated. She is losing extra fluids through her frequent, watery bowel movements and also through her vomiting and any fever. Babies especially, because they are so small, can very quickly become dangerously dehydrated. See *Fluids*, page 290, in the Appendices for more about dehydration.

## Complications

In children and adults whose immune systems are not normal, cryptosporidiosis can be more serious. This includes people who have had organ transplants, are being treated for cancer, or whose immune systems are otherwise not normal.

### CALL YOUR DOCTOR

- If your child has persistant diarrhea and is under twelve months of age.

- If your child is having watery bowel movements more than ten times a day. He may be becoming dehydrated.

- If your child has any mucus in his stools or has diarrhea with abdominal pain for more than an hour or two.

- If your child shows any signs of dehydration: if he is not urinating as much as usual, if his mouth is dry, or if he is less active than usual.

- If your child has diarrhea that does not get better in five days.

## Diagnosis

To identify what organism, cryptosporidium or another germ, is causing a child's diarrhea, pediatricians have a laboratory examine a sample of her stool. To determine what germ is causing the diarrhea, a sample of the stool might be obtained by your doctor. However, this is usually not necessary because most of the time children recover from diarrhea on their own.

At Children's Hospital we might examine a child's stool for cryptosporidium if her diarrhea has persisted for more than five days. However, we would routinely test a stool for cryptosporidium in any child with diarrhea whose immune system is not normal. The lab studies the child's stool sample under a microscope, looking for cryptosporidium oocysts.

## Treatment

If your child's diarrhea is indeed due to cryptosporidiosis, he does not need to take any antibiotics or other medications if he has a normal immune system. *There are no drugs known that can kill cryptosporidium effectively.*

Whenever your child has diarrhea, whatever the cause, the most important treatment is to make sure he takes in enough extra liquids to replace the fluids he is losing through his frequent stools and also through any vomiting or fever. If your baby is under a year old, pediatricians advise that you give him special fluids called oral rehydration solutions.

See *Fluids,* page 290, in the Appendices for more about these fluids and how to give them, what fluids to offer and not offer older children.

See also "Treatment," page 57, in *Diarrhea* for information about what else to do and not do when your child has diarrhea.

In children and adults with normal immune systems, their bodies manufacture anti-cryptosporidium antibodies, which in time kill off all the cryptosporidium organisms. This usually takes seven to fourteen days. However, diarrhea due to cryptosporidium, even in normal people, can last four or more weeks and sometimes goes on for months.

### Hospitalization

Occasionally children with normal immune systems are sick enough with cryptosporidium diarrhea that they need to be hospitalized, primarily for treatment of dehydration. In the apple cider outbreak in Maine, only three out of the 160 children had to be hospitalized and only for a few days. Most often these children need to be treated with intravenous fluids for dehydration.

## Prevention

The most important thing you can do to keep cryptosporidium oocysts and other germs from spreading in your home is to wash your hands—and teach your children to wash their hands—frequently. You should always wash your hands immediately after you go to the toilet or change your baby's diapers or help a toddler go to the bathroom. Always wash your hands before you prepare food and before you eat.

For day-care centers the U.S. Public Health Service and the American Academy of Pediatrics has issued detailed recommendations for reducing the spread of diarrhea-causing and other disease-causing organisms. See *Recommendations for Day-Care Providers,* page 297, in the Appendices.

Since cryptosporidium also spreads in water, children and adults who have diarrhea should be kept out of swimming pools and other public bathing areas, says the Public Health Service, and they should remain out for at least two weeks after they are over their diarrhea. If your child has diarrhea, you should also keep her away from anyone who has an immune deficiency. This includes people, as mentioned, who have had organ transplants or are being treated for cancer.

You can kill any cryptosporidium oocysts that may be present in drinking water—as well as other disease-causing organisms—by bringing the water to a full, rolling boil for one minute, according to the Public Health Service and Environmental Protection Agency. If oocysts do appear in municipal water supplies, cities sometimes issue "Boil Water" alerts, instructing residents to boil all water intended for drinking. During the big Milwaukee outbreak, people had to boil their drinking water because the water supply was not cleared for eight days.

Cryptosporidium oocysts are very resistant to chlorine and other disinfectants commonly used to purify drinking water. The microscopic oocysts must be physically removed from water supplies by filtering. Millions of Americans, however, live in cities—including New York, Boston, and San Francisco—that do not filter their water supply.

## Resources

You can obtain more detailed information about preventing cryptosporidiosis from the Public Health Service's Centers for Disease Control and Prevention (CDC) by calling their toll-free Voice and Fax Information System at 1-888-232-3228 or by connecting to CDC on the Internet at http://www.cdc.gov.

# Giardia Diarrhea

**Your child must be seen by a doctor to be treated for giardia diarrhea.**

Also called giardiasis.

### SYMPTOMS

- Severe diarrhea
- Mild diarrhea (but lasts for a few weeks)
- Abdominal cramps
- Distended (abnormally large) belly
- Gas
- Nausea and vomiting
- Low-grade fever
- Weight loss

Giardia diarrhea is an intestinal illness found throughout the world. In some developing countries this illness is endemic (found in people who live there). Over two-thirds of those people may have no signs or symptoms of the illness even though they have the parasite that causes it in their intestines. Now recognized as a leading cause of diarrhea illness in child-care environments, giardia is spread person to person. It usually spreads from the contaminated hands of the children or their care providers to the families and the extended community.

In the United States giardia is the most common cause of diarrhea from contaminated water. The parasite can survive the routine chlorination of most community water supplies and live for more than two months in cold water. It takes only about ten parasites in one glass of water to initiate a severe case of giardia. While giardia infects mostly humans, it also can infect dogs, cats, beavers, deer, and other animals.

Children are three times more likely to have giardia than adults, which leads us to believe that we may develop some immunity as we get older. By adolescence the incidence seems to drop. However, we do see giardia occurring within families—some member will have severe symptoms; others will have a mild case. We find that babies who are breastfed by a mother with an immunity to giardia seem to acquire a passive immunity. Individuals with cystic fibrosis have an increased frequency of giardiasis, as do those whose immune systems are suppressed.

## Causes

This disease is caused by a microscopic parasite called *Giardia lamblia*. The infection is limited to the small intestine or/and biliary tract (bile ducts or gallbladder). The parasites attach to the

lining of the small intestines and make it difficult for the body to absorb fats and carbohydrates from digested food.

## How It Spreads

Giardia passes so easily from person to person
that it can become epidemic. You can even get
giardia from your family dog. Infected individuals and animals pass the parasite in their stools,
which can contaminate public water supplies,
swimming pools, and natural water sources like
streams and brooks. If you rinse uncooked foods
in contaminated water, you may also spread the
infection.

Giardia is easily spread in day-care centers,
where workers care for children who are not toilet trained or need bathroom assistance. Giardia
spreads either indirectly from contaminated food
or water or directly from hands that touch contaminated material, usually fecal matter, and then
go into the mouth.

## Incubation Period

Giardia occurs anywhere from one to four weeks
after a person is exposed, with the average incubation period being about eight days.

## Symptoms

Giardia begins with severe bouts of diarrhea.
Because the parasite affects the body's ability to
absorb fat, the feces contain unabsorbed fats. and
typically the diarrhea floats and is shiny and smells
quite foul. Your child will have abdominal cramps,
a distended (abnormally large) belly, and a lot of
gas. Nausea and vomiting result in a loss of appetite. Sometimes there will be a low-grade fever.
The symptoms can last for five to seven days or
longer. If longer, your child may lose significant
weight and show signs of malnutrition.

### CALL YOUR DOCTOR

- If your child has a lot of diarrhea,
  especially with a fever or stomach pain.

- If your child has occasional bouts of
  diarrhea that lasts for several days (or
  weeks) and is gradually losing weight.

## Diagnosis

Your doctor will want a stool sample to confirm
the diagnosis. Often several samples are required
before the parasite can be found and identified.
Although a single stool specimen detects 50 to
75 percent of infections, the rate increases to 95
percent with three specimens. You can collect
samples of your child's stools at home in conve-
nient childproof containers that preserve the
specimens. It will take from three to five days to
get results. A new, rapid test that gives results in
one to two days is now available and is very
accurate.

## Treatment

Your doctor will most likely prescribe an antiparasitic medication to speed up recovery. This
medication also shortens the contagious period.
Typically your child will take a liquid medicine
for seven to ten days. Some of these medications
may have side effects, so ask your doctor about
them.

See that your child drinks plenty of liquids to
offset dehydration from the loss of fluid. You do
not want your child to have any caffeinated
drinks like soda or iced tea because they make
the body lose water faster. If you wish to give
your child over-the-counter drugs for cramps or
diarrhea, ask your doctor first because these

preparations may mask symptoms and interfere with treatment or make the infection worse.

The biggest danger with giardia diarrhea is dehydration, especially with small babies. See *Fluids*, page 290, in the Appendices for more about dehydration and replacing fluids.

## Prevention

Encourage family members to wash their hands frequently, especially after going to the bathroom and before eating. If someone in your family has giardiasis, wash your hands often as you care for your child.

Some experts question whether infants and toddlers should be allowed in swimming pools. Certainly if your child has loose stools that cannot be contained in his diaper, keep him out of the pool.

If your child has diarrhea, keep him home from day-care until the treatment is finished and he has no more diarrhea. If there is an outbreak of giardia diarrhea in the day-care center, everyone should be screened. Anyone who is infected should be treated with an antiparasitic drug. Children and workers who have symptoms should stay home until the treatment is complete and the diarrhea is resolved. Carriers of the infection who have no symptoms may continue to attend. See *Recommendations for Day-Care Providers*, page 297, in the Appendices for information on preventing the spread of outbreaks.

If you are outdoors, boil all water from streams and lakes before drinking.

## *Rotavirus Diarrhea*

Rotavirus is the most common cause of diarrhea in infants and young children.

Your child will almost certainly be infected with rotavirus within her first few years of life,

### SYMPTOMS

- Very frequent, very watery bowel movements
- Vomiting
- Possible high fever, 102° to 104°F

probably when she is between six months and two years old. Virtually every child in this country—or any country—has been infected by the age of three. We all were infected with rotavirus before we were old enough to remember.

Rotavirus causes one-fourth of all episodes of diarrhea and gastroenteritis among children in this country, and it is one of the germs that most often spreads among children attending day-care centers. According to the U.S. Public Health Service's Centers for Disease Control and Prevention (CDC), 3.5 million American children have rotavirus diarrhea every year. Worldwide, rotavirus diarrhea affects some 80 to 130 million children a year.

One out of every eight American children sees a physician at some point for rotavirus diarrhea; the virus is responsible for 500,000 doctor visits a year. And one out of every 40 children is hospitalized with rotavirus; the virus sends 70,000 to 100,000 children to the hospital a year, at a direct medical cost of more than $500 million, it is estimated, and an indirect cost (counting such items as parents having to miss work) of over a billion dollars.

Most of the time rotavirus infections are mild, but they can be life-threatening. Rotavirus is the number-one cause of deaths due to diarrhea among children. In the United States, according to the CDC, rotavirus diarrhea is responsible for the deaths of 75 to 125 children every year. Worldwide, it kills about 873,000 children a year.

Like so many other infections, rotavirus diarrhea is seasonal. It starts each year in California in early October and then sweeps its way eastward across the country. It usually reaches Philadelphia at the end of December or in early January, peaks in February and March, and lasts until about mid-May. Rotavirus season finally finishes up in eastern Canada in late spring. No one knows why the virus behaves this way.

During rotavirus season, in the emergency department at Children's Hospital, we usually see 35 to 40 young children a day who have rotavirus diarrhea and gastroenteritis, and we need to admit up to three a day to the hospital.

## Cause

The organism that causes rotavirus diarrhea gets its name from its shape. In photographs taken with an electron microscope, the virus particles resemble tiny wheels. *Rota-* comes from the Latin for "wheel."

The usual home of rotavirus is the intestines of young children, where it lives and multiplies inside the cells of the tissues lining the intestines.

## How It Spreads

Rotavirus spreads easily from child to child in day-care centers and within families because infected children shed billions and billions of virus particles in their stools.

When you—or a staff member at a day-care center—change an infected infant's diaper or help a toddler go to the toilet, you can get rotavirus particles on your hands. And you never know when a child may be infected and shedding virus particles. Children shed virus particles up to two days before they have any symptoms. Or a child can be infected without being sick herself. About half of infected children never

show any symptoms; yet they can pass the virus on to others.

If you do not wash your hands after changing the diaper or helping the toddler, you can deposit rotavirus particles on anything you touch: doorknobs, tabletops, books, toys, drinking glasses, eating utensils, dishes, clothes. Or children can get rotavirus on their own fingers as they explore their bodies and then leave the virus on anything they touch. Rotavirus particles are very hardy; they can survive on such surfaces and objects for as long as a week.

Then other children come along, touch these objects or surfaces, and get rotavirus particles on their hands. They put their fingers in their mouth, as young children do—or put a contaminated toy in their mouth—and they, too, become infected. The rotavirus particles pass through their stomach and settle down in the cells lining their intestines, where they grow and multiply.

## Incubation Period

If your child is infected with rotavirus, he usually will start having diarrhea and gastroenteritis—if he is going to have symptoms at all—within one to three days.

## Symptoms

As the virus multiplies, it causes inflammation and irritation of your child's stomach and intestines (that is, gastroenteritis). The main symptom is very frequent, very watery bowel movements. If your child has a moderate case of rotavirus, he may have seven to ten bowel movements a day. With a severe case, he may have twelve to fifteen loose stools a day. The stools usually do not contain any blood or mucus, but they may have a foul smell.

About three-quarters of children with rotavirus diarrhea also vomit frequently, sometimes as often as every half hour or even more often. About half have a fairly high fever, 102° to 104°F.

The danger with rotavirus diarrhea—as with any diarrhea—is that it can cause a child to become dehydrated as he loses fluids through his frequent bowel movements and vomiting and also by evaporation from his skin due to fever. Dehydration is how rotavirus can kill a child. Rotavirus can dangerously dehydrate a child within twenty-four hours; death can occur within a day of the first symptoms. See *Fluids*, page 290, in the Appendices for more about dehydration.

---

### CALL YOUR DOCTOR

- If your child has diarrhea and is under a year old.

- If your child, at any age, has more than ten bowel movements a day.

- If your child is not urinating as frequently as usual or is listless and lethargic. These may be signs of dehydration.

NOTE: See "Symptoms," page 52, in *Diarrhea*, for other signs that should prompt you to consult your physician if your child has diarrhea.

---

## Diagnosis

If your child has watery diarrhea that has lasted no more than five days, with no blood or mucus in her stools, she probably has a gastrointestinal virus. And if she is under three years of age and it is during the winter and she is also vomiting and has a fever, she probably has rotavirus.

Your doctor probably will not need to order any specific laboratory test to confirm this (unless admitted to the hospital) because whatever virus is causing your child's diarrhea, the treatment is the same.

## Treatment

Your child usually will not need any antibiotic or other medication when he has rotavirus diarrhea and gastroenteritis. There are no drugs available that can kill rotavirus particles.

The main treatment for rotavirus diarrhea is the same as for diarrhea due to other germs: you need to make sure that your child takes in enough extra fluid to prevent him from becoming dangerously dehydrated. If your baby is under a year, you need to give him special fluids called oral rehydration solutions. See *Fluids*, page 290, in the Appendices for more about these fluids, how to give them and what fluids to offer and not offer older children.

See also "Treatment," page 57, in *Diarrhea* for more information about what else to do and not to do when your child has diarrhea.

If you are not able to get enough fluid into your child fast enough with oral rehydration therapy—and if he is having fifteen bowel movements a day, it can be difficult—your child may need to get additional fluids intravenously in your doctor's office or in the hospital emergency department. Or he may need to be admitted to the hospital.

Diarrhea due to rotavirus usually lasts one to four days and then goes away on its own. In more severe cases vomiting can last three to five days; fever, four to five days; and diarrhea, seven to nine days.

Once your child recovers from rotavirus diarrhea, he is unlikely ever to be as sick with it again. He can get infected with rotavirus particles over and over again, but he will have developed some immunity and the infections will be much less severe.

We all probably get infected with rotavirus over and over again. The degree to which you will be infected is probably the degree to which you are exposed to small children. When you are caring for a child with rotavirus, you probably will develop more antibodies to the virus, but you rarely will have any symptoms. You get rotavirus most severely when you are a six to twenty-four-month-old child.

## Prevention

As with diarrhea due to other organisms, the single most important thing you can do to prevent the spread of rotavirus in your home is to wash your hands immediately after changing your baby's diapers or helping a toddler go to the toilet. Remember, that your baby can be infected with rotavirus and show no symptoms.

For day-care centers, the U.S. Public Health Service and the American Academy of Pediatrics have set forth many detailed recommendations for reducing the spread of diarrhea-causing and other germs. See *Recommendations for Day-Care Providers,* page 297, in the Appendices.

A vaccine against rotavirus should be available within a few years. Two groups of researchers—one at the National Institutes of Health and the other, headed by Paul A. Offit, M.D., and Fred Clark, D.V.M., Ph.D., at The Children's Hospital of Philadelphia and the Wistar Institute—are currently developing such a vaccine.

The Children's Hospital vaccine is made from a live, weakened bovine rotavirus, genetically engineered so that it contains some human genes. Once it becomes available, infants will take the vaccine by mouth so that it will induce antibodies right on the spot in their intestines. They will get three doses, at the ages of two, four, and six months. Since the disease primarily affects children between six and twenty-four months, they need to be immunized by the time they are six months old.

The Children's Hospital group is testing their vaccine on thousands of infants in a number of American cities, including Salt Lake City; Cincinnati; Rochester, New York; Providence, Rhode Island; and Philadelphia. So far the vaccine appears to be well tolerated and very safe and protects about 75 to 80 percent of the vaccinated infants against rotavirus diarrhea.

## *Shigella Diarrhea*

### *Shigella diarrhea must be treated by a doctor.*

Also called shigella dysentery and shigellosis. The ending *-osis* means "disease."

### SYMPTOMS

- Diarrhea, possibly watery, bloody, or with mucus

- Possible fever

- Possible abdominal cramps

The word *dysentery* means "bloody diarrhea," that is, diarrhea in which the stools contain blood. Shigella bacteria are among the major causes of dysentery throughout the world.

Hundreds of thousands of people in the United States develop shigella dysentery every year, according to the U.S. Public Health Service's Centers for Disease Control and Prevention (CDC) in Atlanta, and in recent years the number of people getting shigella infections has been increasing.

Shigella diarrhea occurs most frequently in toddlers and young children between the ages of twelve months and four years. Shigella is one of the diarrhea-causing germs—along with rotavirus and giardia—that most commonly spread among children in day-care centers. In one study in Kentucky, children who attended day care developed shigella diarrhea ten times more often than children who were cared for at home. At The Children's Hospital of Philadelphia, we see some 100 children a year with diarrhea due to shigella.

Shigella bacteria are also a leading cause of diarrhea or dysentery in developing countries. In many countries in central Africa, for instance, shigella causes recurrent outbreaks and epidemics of severe bloody diarrhea.

## Causes

There are four different species of shigella bacteria—*Shigella sonnei, S. flexneri, S. dysenteriae,* and *S. boydii*—that cause diarrhea. Shigella bacteria take their name from a Japanese researcher named Shiga, who discovered them in the late nineteenth century. These bacteria live primarily in human beings, where they grow and multiply in the intestinal tract.

## How They Spread

People who are infected with shigella bacteria shed them in their stools, and your child can become infected when she gets the bacteria in her mouth and swallows them.

Shigella bacteria are among the most infectious of all microorganisms; your child can get sick from ingesting only a few individual bacterial cells. People can also carry the bacteria in their intestines without having any symptoms

of diarrhea. Your child can catch shigella diarrhea from another child or adult who is not sick at all.

In day-care centers, shigella bacteria can spread readily from child to child and from child to adult. Toddlers who are infected and not yet toilet trained can get the bacteria on their hands. They can leave the bacteria on anything they touch: a toy, a crayon, a tabletop. Another toddler picks up the toy, gets the bacteria on his hands, puts a hand to his mouth, and becomes infected with shigella.

Older children and adults who are infected can get shigella on their hands when they use a toilet. Toilet paper is not enough of a barrier to keep the bacteria off their fingers. If they do not wash their hands afterward, they can deposit shigella on a doorknob, a telephone, a pen, or other surface. When another person turns the doorknob or talks on the phone, he can get the bacteria on his hands. He puts a hand to his mouth—and we all touch our faces more than we realize—and he can become infected. Shigella is so infectious that you could catch it from an infected person who loaned you his pen just long enough for you to sign your name.

Shigella is one of the germs that frequently spread among family members. Children carry the bacteria home from day care or elsewhere, on their fingers or in their intestines, and pass them on to the rest of the family. Parents can get the bacteria on their hands as they change a toddler's diapers. Shigella infections are also more common among people in their child-bearing years.

Your child can also catch shigella from eating contaminated food. An infected person who prepares food without washing her hands can leave bacteria in the food, and shigella can survive in many common foods for up to thirty days. At a music festival in Michigan one summer, 3,137 people got shigella food poisoning from a tofu salad contaminated by infected food handlers. More than 100 people were sick enough that they needed to be hospitalized.

In another incident, hundreds of passengers—including twenty-one members of a professional football team—who flew on one airline over a period of several weeks caught shigella from sandwiches and other foods contaminated by infected people in the airline's central kitchen. Passengers on more than 200 flights to twenty-four states and four foreign countries were affected.

Shigella bacteria can also be deposited on food by flies, which can carry the bacteria in their own gut or pick them up on their legs when they land on contaminated human feces.

Your child can also get shigella diarrhea by drinking or swimming in water polluted with human feces from sewage or other sources. The bacteria can survive in water for six months or more, and because so few organisms are needed to cause infection, your child does not have to swallow much water to get sick. At one lake sixty-one swimmers became ill—and six had to be hospitalized—after a single infected child had defecated in the water.

Shigella bacteria are among the many germs that cause people to develop traveler's diarrhea when they eat contaminated food or drink polluted water while traveling abroad in developing countries.

Once swallowed, the shigella bacteria pass through the stomach and settle down in the intestines, where they grow and multiply.

## Incubation Period

If your child becomes infected with shigella bacteria, it usually takes from two to four days for him to develop diarrhea—if he is going to have any symptoms—but it can take anywhere from twelve hours to as long as a week.

## Symptoms

As the shigella bacteria multiply in your child's intestinal tract, she may have no symptoms at all, or she may just have a few loose bowel movements, nothing worth calling your pediatrician about.

Or she may have typical shigella diarrhea, with frequent bowel movements that contain both blood and mucus, accompanied by a fever and severe cramps in her abdomen. With shigella, a child's stools tend to be smallish, and she may find that they are painful to pass.

Your child may or may not experience profuse watery diarrhea for a day or two before her stools turn bloody. Or her stools may never become bloody at all; she may just continue to have watery diarrhea.

The danger of any diarrhea, whether due to shigella or another germ, is that it can cause your child's body to become dehydrated. She is losing extra fluid through her frequent bowel movements and, if she has any fever, through increased evaporation from her skin. Babies particularly, because they are so small, can very quickly develop serious—even life-threatening—dehydration. See *Fluids*, page 290, in the Appendices for more about dehydration.

## Complications

Some strains of shigella bacteria produce a toxin (poison) that can spread to a child's brain and cause him to have a seizure: he becomes unresponsive for a few seconds or minutes, his arms and legs usually flail rhythmically, and he may fall to the floor. Seizures have many, many possible causes in addition to shigella.

Seizures due to shigella toxin usually afflict babies or toddlers and are uncommon. At Children's Hospital we rarely see a child with shigella seizures each year. Occasionally a child has a seizure from shigella toxin before he displays any symptoms of diarrhea.

In developing countries, where so many children are malnourished, shigellosis can be particularly severe. Children can develop repeated bouts of dysentery that last for months, and the disease may kill 10 to 30 percent of them.

## CALL YOUR DOCTOR

- If your child has any blood or mucus in her stools or has diarrhea with abdominal pain for more than an hour or two.

- If your child is having watery bowel movements more than ten times a day.

- If your child has diarrhea of any kind and is under a year old.

- If your child shows any signs of dehydration: if she is not urinating as much as usual, if her mouth is dry, or if she is less active than usual.

NOTE: You do not need to call your pediatrician if your child just has a few loose bowel movements.

CALL 911 or immediately take your child to your hospital emergency room:

- If your child has a seizure.

## Diagnosis

Whenever a child with diarrhea has any blood or mucus in his stools, at Children's Hospital

we routinely have our laboratory test a sample of his stool for shigella bacteria as well as for the three other bacteria (campylobacter, salmonella, and *Yersinia enterocolitica*) that most commonly cause diarrhea in children. Our lab cultures (grows) the bacteria in order to identify them, and it may take up to five days to get the results.

## Treatment

If your child's diarrhea does turn out to be caused by shigella, your pediatrician will prescribe an antibiotic for her to kill the bacteria in her intestinal tract.

Shigella bacteria are among the few germs commonly causing diarrhea in children for which treatment with antibiotics is helpful. Physicians prescribe antibiotics both to shorten the duration of a child's diarrhea and also to stop her from shedding bacteria in her stools and spreading them to others. Without antibiotic treatment a person may shed shigella for as long as a month. For children doctors usually prescribe a five-day course by mouth of trimethoprim-sulfamethoxazole.

When your child has any diarrhea, whatever the cause, it is important to make sure that she drinks enough extra liquids to replace the fluids she is losing through her frequent bowel movements and through any fever. If your baby is under a year old, pediatricians advise that you give her special fluids called oral rehydration solutions. See *Fluids*, page 290, in the Appendices for more about these fluids, how to give them and what fluids to offer and not offer older children. See also "Treatment," page 57, in *Diarrhea* for information about what else to do and not do when your child has diarrhea.

Pediatricians generally do not advise giving babies or young children nonspecific anti-diarrhea drugs. Some over-the-counter drugs reduce diarrhea by slowing down muscle movements in the intestines; this slows the passage of wastes through the intestines. With shigella infections, however, this could actually hurt a child by prolonging the time the bacteria remain in her intestines.

Once your child starts taking the antibiotic, her fever will usually drop within twenty-four hours, and her diarrhea will usually disappear within two or three days. She also will stop shedding the bacteria in her stools within a day or two and will no longer be able to transmit the germs to others.

Since shigella bacteria spread so readily and people can be infected without having any symptoms, at Children's Hospital, when a child has shigellosis, we also do stool cultures on all the other members of his family, his parents and any other children in close contact. If any of them are infected with shigella, we have them also take an antibiotic to stop their shedding of the bacteria.

## Prevention

The most effective thing you can do to reduce the chances of your children getting shigella dysentery or other diarrhea—or spreading it to other members of your family—is to teach them to wash their hands frequently with soap and running water and to wash your own hands often.

Always wash your hands immediately after going to the toilet. You can be infected with shigella, remember, and not have any symptoms. Also wash your hands after changing your baby's diapers or helping your toddler go to the bathroom. Insist that your older children also wash their hands after they have used the toilet.

Also always wash your hands before you eat or prepare food for yourself or others. You never know what germs you may have picked up on your fingers as you went about your daily rounds, opening doors, buying groceries, touching countertops. Make sure your children wash their hands before they eat.

"Because young children are most likely to be infected with shigella and are also most likely to infect others," the Public Health Service emphasizes, "a strict policy of supervised handwashing for young children after they have defecated and before they eat is particularly important." In Kentucky, when the local health department started a hand-washing campaign for day-care centers and schools, within a few weeks the number of children developing shigella dysentery dropped substantially.

For day-care centers, both the U.S. Public Health Service and American Academy of Pediatrics have issued additional, detailed recommendations for reducing the spread of diarrhea-causing and other disease-causing organisms. See *Recommendations for Day-Care Providers*, page 297, in the Appendices.

If a person has diarrhea, he should not work at a job that involves preparing or serving food that other people will eat. If you have diarrhea, you should make sure that you are doubly careful about washing your hands before you fix food for your family. For more information about how to keep disease-causing germs from spreading in your kitchen, see "Prevention," page 125, in *Food Poisoning*.

Since shigella bacteria also spread so readily in water, children and adults who have diarrhea, warns the Public Health Service, should be kept out of swimming pools and other public bathing areas.

# Yersinia Diarrhea

***Also called yersiniosis. The ending -osis means "disease."***

## SYMPTOMS

- Diarrhea, sometimes bloody, watery, or with mucus

- Fever

- Abdominal cramps

You probably have never heard of yersinia bacteria, but these germs are among the most common causes of diarrhea due to food poisoning, especially in preschool-age children. At The Children's Hospital of Philadelphia, we probably see twenty to thirty children a year with yersinia diarrhea.

## Cause

The full name of the bacterium causing this type of diarrhea is *Yersinia enterocolitica.* (The organism was named in honor of Swiss scientist Alexandre Yersin.) It has been known since the 1930s that *Y. enterocolitica* can produce disease in humans.

This bacterium is unusual in that it multiplies readily in cold conditions. Most other bacteria causing diarrhea grow best in warm weather. Yersinia, however, can actually grow in your refrigerator, and children are more likely to get yersinia diarrhea during the winter months.

*Y. enterocolitica* bacteria are widespread throughout the world, and they most often cause disease in other animals. They can live and grow in the intestinal tracts of a wide variety of animals: wild mammals (including deer, rabbits, squirrels, raccoons, foxes, and beavers); birds (pigeons, doves, and pheasants); domestic animals (dogs and cats), and also many farm animals (cows, horses, goats, and turkeys). The major sources of the strains of yersinia bacteria that produce diarrhea in humans, however, are pigs.

## How It Spreads

Animals that are infected with *Y. enterocolitica* shed the bacteria in their feces. Your child can become infected with yersinia when he gets the bacteria in his mouth—usually from contaminated food or drink—and swallows them.

Yersinia bacteria can contaminate meats and poultry, particularly pork. Your child can develop yersinia diarrhea by eating tainted pork that is not thoroughly cooked. In Belgium, which has the highest incidence of yersiniosis disease in the world, people get the infection because they often eat pork raw.

In this country children have caught yersinia from chitterlings (also called chitlins), or pork intestines, which are considered a delicacy in the South. In an outbreak in Atlanta, fifteen children—fourteen babies and a ten-year-old boy—became ill from chitlins, seven of them sick enough that they needed to be hospitalized. The infants did not eat the chitlins themselves but were infected with bacteria from the hands of their caretakers. Before chitlins are cooked, the raw intestines must be painstakingly cleaned of fecal material. While the women were cleaning the intestines, they also tended the babies and spread the bacteria to them. The ten-year-old boy became infected when he handled raw chitlins but did not wash his hands afterward.

Yersinia bacteria are among the many germs that can get into raw, unpasteurized milk. In an outbreak in the state of New York, yersinia contaminated chocolate milk at a processing plant. The milk was delivered to school cafeterias, and over a period of months, hundreds of children and school employees became ill. Thirty-six children were sick enough that they needed to be hospitalized.

People have also become infected with yersinia bacteria from eating contaminated seafood, vegetables, and tofu (soybean curd). Sixteen people in North Carolina caught yersinia disease from a litter of puppies that had diarrhea.

Once your child swallows *Y. enterocolitica* bacteria, they pass through the stomach and settle down in the intestinal tract, where they multiply.

## Incubation Period

It usually takes about four to six days from the time a person ingests yersinia bacteria until symptoms appear, but it can take anywhere from one to fourteen days.

## Symptoms

As yersinia bacteria multiply in your child's intestines, he may not have any symptoms, or he may have diarrhea that can range from mild to severe. He may have up to ten bowel movements a day. His stools may contain blood and mucus, and they may be watery.

Along with his diarrhea, your child may be vomiting. Typically he will have a fever, which may reach as high as 104°F. He usually will have painful abdominal cramps, often in the lower right section of the abdomen. The location of the pain and its severity sometimes cause yersinia infections to be mistaken for acute appendicitis.

A danger of any diarrhea, whatever its cause, is that it can dangerously dehydrate your child's body. He is losing extra fluid through his frequent stools, through any vomiting, and if he does have a fever, through increased evaporation from his skin. Babies particularly, because they are so tiny, can very quickly develop serious—even life-threatening—dehydration. See *Fluids*, page 290, in the Appendices for more about dehydration.

## CALL YOUR DOCTOR

- If your child has diarrhea and is under twelve months old.

- If your child of any age has any blood or mucus in her stools.

- If your child is having watery bowel movements more than ten times a day.

- If your child has diarrhea with abdominal pain for more than an hour or two.

- If your child shows any signs of dehydration: if she is not urinating as much as usual; if her mouth is dry; or if she is less active than usual.

## Diagnosis

To find out what germ is causing a child's diarrhea, physicians can take a sample of her stool and have a laboratory try to culture (grow) any organisms that may be present. Usually doctors do not need to do this, however, because most of the time children recover from diarrhea uneventfully, on their own.

At Children's Hospital we ask for tests on a child's stool sample if she has any blood or mucus in her stools or if she has had diarrhea for more than five days. Our lab routinely tests stool samples for *Y. enterocolitica* as well as for the three other bacteria (campylobacter, salmonella, and shigella) that most commonly cause diarrhea in children. It may take up to five days for us to get the results.

## Treatment

Whenever your child has diarrhea, the main treatment is to make sure he drinks enough extra liquid to replace the fluid he is losing through his more frequent stools and through any vomiting or fever. If your baby is under a year old, pediatricians advise that you give him special fluids called oral rehydration solutions.

See *Fluids*, page 290, in the Appendices for more about these fluids and how to give them and what fluids to offer older children.

See also "Treatment," page 57, in *Diarrhea* for more about what else to do and not do when your child has diarrhea.

If your child's diarrhea is indeed caused by *Y. enterocolitica* bacteria, your pediatrician may or may not prescribe an antibiotic. At Children's Hospital we usually do not prescribe antibiotics for children with yersiniosis because by the time we find out—four to five days later—that yersinia bacteria are the cause of a child's diarrhea, the diarrhea has usually disappeared. If a child's symptoms are particularly severe, however, or he continues to have diarrhea for a prolonged period, we may prescribe an antibiotic by mouth.

## Prevention

You can easily destroy any *Y. enterocolitica* bacteria and other germs that may contaminate pork and other meat or poultry by cooking them thoroughly. The U.S. Department of Agriculture recommends that you cook meat to an internal temperature of 160°F and cook poultry to a temperature of 180°F to 185°F. The Public Health Service, on the other hand, recommends that you cook pork to 170°F.

Be sure to wash your hands after you handle any raw pork or other meat or poultry and wipe up any juices that may have spilled on your kitchen counter. Also thoroughly wash the knife, cutting board, platter, and anything else that meat or poultry has touched before you use these items again or let them come in contact with other foods.

If you do prepare chitlins, the Health Service advises that you not allow children to touch the raw pork intestines and that you wash your hands carefully before you touch a child or anything used by a child, such as a toy or bottle.

Both the Health Service and the American Academy of Pediatrics recommend a further precaution. "Because the potential for transmission of the agent is strongest from foodhandlers to children," says the Health Service, "someone other than the foodhandler should care for children while chitterlings are being prepared." The Academy of Pediatrics agrees that "persons handling pork intestines should not simultaneously care for infants."

Since *Y. enterocolitica* bacteria and many other germs can contaminate raw, unpasteurized milk, the Health Service and the Academy of Pediatrics both advise that people avoid drinking unpasteurized milk.

For more recommendations about how to keep your family from contracting food-borne diseases, see "Prevention," page 125, in *Food Poisoning*.

# DIPHTHERIA

*A vaccine is available to protect your child against diphtheria. See* **Vaccines**, *page 301, in Appendices for a complete listing and the schedule of all the vaccines your child needs.*

*Diphtheria must be treated by a doctor in a hospital.*

## SYMPTOMS

- Severe sore throat

- Fever

- Very swollen neck

- Difficulty breathing

Diphtheria is potentially a very severe disease, particularly among children. Fortunately, it can be prevented by vaccination. Your baby should routinely get diphtheria shots starting at six to eight weeks of age.

In the early part of the twentieth century, up through the 1920s, diphtheria infected about 150,000 people a year in the United States and killed about 15,000. Most of its victims were children under the age of four.

A legacy of those days still lingers. In 1925 a diphtheria epidemic struck Nome, Alaska, and teams of sled dogs and mushers relayed diphtheria antitoxin across 675 miles of snow and ice to save the children. The lead dog on the last leg was named Balto; a statue of Balto stands in New York's Central Park, and he has been the hero of Hollywood movies. And every year Alaska's famed dog-sled race, the Iditarod, retraces the route the antitoxin took to Nome.

Today, however, diphtheria has virtually disappeared from the United States and other developed countries. Only a handful of cases of diphtheria are reported each year to the U.S. Public Health Service's Centers for Disease Control and Prevention (CDC). Since 1980 there have been fewer than five cases a year in the United States.

Diphtheria is rare in this country because of vaccination. It has not disappeared from the rest of the world, however, and it could return to the United States on the next flight from abroad. Without continued vaccination, diphtheria could very well come back. And diphtheria still kills from 4 to 12 percent of the people who catch it, primarily young children and the elderly.

Indeed, diphtheria *has* come back in the former Soviet Union. Amid the turmoil of that country's breakup, vaccination rates slipped, and in the early 1990s diphtheria became epidemic throughout all fifteen of the New Independent States, as they are called, from the Baltic to the Pacific. More than 80,000 people have contracted the disease, and over 1,700 have died. At least twenty people from other parts of Europe and two Americans have caught it there. One was a twenty-two-year-old woman from New Jersey who got diphtheria in Ukraine.

One factor in diphtheria's return to the former Soviet Union is that many adults in these countries are not immune to diphtheria and thus can catch and spread the disease. And what worries public health officials here is that a similar situation exists in the United States. From 20 to 60 percent of American adults, the Public Health Service warns, are not immune to diphtheria.

## Cause

A bacterium called *Corynebacterium diphtheriae* causes diphtheria. The *Coryne-* part of its name comes from the Greek word for "club." The bacterium was given this name because when it grows in the lab, its cells sometimes take on a clubbed appearance.

*Corynebacterium diphtheriae* makes its home and grows and multiplies in the upper respiratory tract—the nose, mouth, and throat—of human beings.

## How It Spreads

A person who is infected with diphtheria bacteria sheds these organisms in secretions from the nose and throat. When the person coughs or sneezes or talks, droplets of moisture containing the bacteria are sprayed. These droplets can get into another person's nose or mouth. The bacteria settle down, usually in the throat, and grow and multiply there.

Your child can catch diphtheria from a person who does not know he has the bacteria. A person coming down with diphtheria sheds bacteria for several days before there are any symptoms, and people can carry diphtheria bacteria in their throats—and shed them—for weeks or months sometimes without ever getting sick.

## Incubation Period

If your child is infected with diphtheria bacteria, it usually takes from one day up to a week for symptoms to appear.

## Symptoms

Diphtheria is a frightening disease. As diphtheria bacteria grow and multiply in a person's throat, they produce a powerful toxin. A toxin is a poison made by a living organism. Diphtheria toxin is what causes most of the trouble, most of the symptoms of the disease.

The toxin gets inside the cells of the tissues lining the throat and destroys them. The patient usually has a severe sore throat first, with a fever. Then so many dead throat cells accumulate, along with white cells fighting the infection, that they can form a thick, leatherlike membrane stuck tightly to the throat. (This membrane gives the disease its name; the word *diphtheria* comes from the Greek word for "leather.") The person's neck may swell so much that its contours are no longer visible. Doctors call this bull-neck swelling.

The appearance of this thick, grayish membrane in the throat occurs in about half of diphtheria patients. It can grow downward into the person's larynx and windpipe and, in combination with the swelling, can block the airway, cutting off the air supply to the lungs. This is how diphtheria most commonly kills a person. Most such deaths occur in the first three or four days of illness.

During the first or second week of the disease, often as the swelling in the person's throat is going down, the diphtheria toxin can get into the bloodstream and circulate throughout the body. In up to 25 percent of patients, the toxin attacks the heart, causing inflammation of the heart muscle and killing muscle cells. This can interfere with the heart's rhythm and cause death from heart failure.

Diphtheria toxin can also damage a person's nerves, causing temporary muscle weakness or paralysis. It usually starts with the nearest nerves, the ones in the throat, and may paralyze the muscles used for swallowing. There is then the risk that one may swallow food or aspirate food, into the lungs. Weeks or even months later, the toxin may cause weakness of other, larger muscles in the body.

## CALL YOUR DOCTOR

- If your family is planning to travel outside the United States to countries where diphtheria is prevalent. You should make sure that your child has been vaccinated against this disease and that everyone's shots are up-to-date.

- If your child develops a sore throat while you are traveling in any country where diphtheria is prevalent, the Public Health Service advises, or during the two weeks after you return. The risk is minimal, but if you have a severe sore throat after traveling abroad, the prudent thing would be to consult your physician.

# Diagnosis

If the doctor suspects a person may have contracted diphtheria, she will use throat swabs to collect samples of his nose and throat secretions and also of the membrane, if he has one, in his throat. She will then ask a laboratory to culture (grow) and identify any microorganisms present.

# Treatment

A child who has diphtheria needs to be hospitalized and treated promptly. By the time she has a sore throat or other symptoms of diphtheria, the toxin is already at work doing its damage.

The main treatment for diphtheria is still diphtheria antitoxin like the one the sled-dog teams carried to Nome in the 1920s. Antitoxin is serum that contains antibodies against diphtheria toxin. Antitoxin binds with and neutralizes the toxin circulating in the patient's bloodstream. The sooner the patient gets antitoxin, the better because once the toxin gets into her cells, the antitoxin can no longer reach it to neutralize it. The patient gets antitoxin in a single dose, usually intravenously.

Antibiotics, usually penicillin or erythromycin, will be needed to eliminate the diphtheria bacteria in the throat, which are the source of the toxin. Antibiotics, however, are no substitute for antitoxin; antibiotics do nothing to neutralize diphtheria toxin.

People who recover from diphtheria do not necessarily develop immunity to the disease, and thus, as part of their treatment, patients are usually also vaccinated against the disease.

When someone does contract diphtheria, physicians usually also give prophylactic antibiotics, erythromycin or penicillin, to any other persons—adults and children—who may have been exposed, that is, those living in the same household or who have other close contact with the patient. Doctors also usually culture these other people's throats for diphtheria bacteria and make sure their diphtheria vaccinations are up-to-date.

# Prevention

*The U.S. Public Health Service and the American Academy of Pediatrics both recommend that children and adults routinely get vaccinated against diphtheria.*

Your baby needs a series of five shots against diphtheria, the first at two months old, the second shot at four months old, and the third at six months.

*All fifty states require that children attending day-care centers be immunized against diphtheria.*

At least six months later, when your child is between twelve and fifteen months old, a fourth, reinforcing shot is given.

When a child is between four and six years old, a fifth, booster shot is needed. *All fifty states also require that all children attending school be immunized against diphtheria.*

If for some reason you have missed this schedule, your pediatrician can advise you about a makeup schedule.

Babies usually get their diphtheria shots as part of a three-in-one shot called DTP: D for diphtheria, T for tetanus, and P for pertussis (a fancy name for whooping cough).

Diphtheria vaccine protects over 85 percent of children who receive all their shots, and if an immunized person does catch diphtheria, she is more likely to have a mild case of the disease. Vaccination also reduces the number of people who carry diphtheria bacteria in their throats and can spread the organisms to others.

This immunity to diphtheria, however, wears off in time. The Public Health Service thus recommends that everyone living in the United States get revaccinated against diphtheria at ten-year intervals at ages fifteen, twenty-five, thirty-five, and so forth. Physicians usually give diphtheria vaccine to adults in the same shot as tetanus vaccine, which we also need at ten-year intervals throughout our lives.

Diphtheria shots rarely cause any significant adverse reactions. Diphtheria vaccine is a toxoid: diphtheria toxin that has been inactivated chemically so that it can no longer cause disease yet can still stimulate our immune system to make protective antibodies (antitoxin). You cannot get diphtheria from diphtheria vaccine.

The most common side effects of diphtheria shots are tenderness and swelling at the site of the injection; 16 to 27 percent of those vaccinated experience this. About 2 percent have some redness around the injection site.

## *Resources*

You can get more information about diphtheria and diphtheria vaccine from the U.S. Public Health Service's Centers for Disease Control and Prevention (CDC) by calling 1-800-232-SHOT.

If your family is traveling abroad, you can find out whether diphtheria is a threat in any countries you plan to visit by calling the CDC's Travelers' Hotline at 1-888-232-3228. Or you can get information about diseases, vaccines, and travel from CDC's Web site at http://www.cdc.gov.

# EAR INFECTIONS

## *Ear Infections—Middle Ears*

Also called otitis media. *Oto-* means "ear"; the ending *-itis* means "inflammation," and *media* means "middle."

### SYMPTOMS

- Earache

- In a child too young to talk, irritability, scratching, or tugging at the ears

- Possible fever, which can be high, 102° to 104°F.

- Sometimes discharge from the ear

- Hearing loss

Infection of the middle ear is among the most common diseases of childhood, an illness your child probably will experience. Eighty percent of all children have at least one episode of middle-ear infection during their first three years of life. Most of us probably had middle-ear infections long before we were old enough to remember them.

If your child has a middle-ear infection caused by bacteria, she needs to take an antibiotic. Ear infections are one of the most common reasons that young children are given antibiotics.

Middle-ear infections are also the most common illness for which children visit physicians, causing 24.5 million visits a year, according to the National Center for Health Statistics. And middle-ear infections are the reason that hundreds of thousands of children each year undergo a surgical procedure to insert drainage tubes (see figure on page 92) through their eardrums.

The middle ear is a part of the ear entirely hidden inside the head. There are three parts to the ear: the outer ear, middle ear, and inner ear. (See below.)

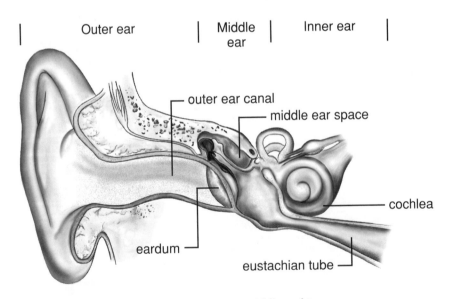

*Cross-section of ear showing outer, middle and inner ear.*

The outer ear is simply the familiar shell-shaped funnel that you see when you look at a person's ear, plus the ear canal leading inward. At the base of the ear canal is the eardrum, which is a thin, flexible membrane. The ear canal directs incoming sound waves—which are vibrating molecules of air—to the eardrum. When sound waves strike the eardrum, they cause it to vibrate in response. Infections of a child's outer ear are less common and less potentially serious than those of the middle ear. See *Ear Infections— Outer Ears*, page 93.

The middle ear is a narrow, slitlike space lying just beyond the eardrum. It contains three tiny bones in a row: a hammer-shaped bone called the malleus; an anvil-shaped bone, the incus; and a stirrup-shaped bone, the stapes. When incoming sound waves set the eardrum vibrating, it in turn sets these little bones vibrating. And the last little bone, the stapes, delivers the vibrations to the inner ear.

In the inner ear an organ called the cochlea contains hundreds of thousands of tiny hairs. These hairs bend in tune with incoming vibrations and convert them into electrical signals which travel along the auditory nerve to the brain. There we perceive them as sound: the song of a bird, the voice of a friend, a clap of thunder.

Middle-ear infections are a disease of babies and toddlers. Children most commonly get these ear infections between the ages of six months and three years, and they usually develop them following a cold.

Infections with respiratory viruses cause the tissues lining the nasal passages and throat to swell and become inflamed, and the infections actually damage these tissues. This allows germs to spread from a child's nose and throat into the middle-ear spaces—which are normally sterile. Children who go to day-care centers get more middle-ear infections than children cared for at home because they get more colds.

Germs travel into a child's middle-ear spaces along narrow channels—called the eustachian tubes—that connect these spaces to the back of the throat. We are most aware of our eustachian tubes when we pop them open by swallowing to equalize the pressure in our ears, most commonly when we ascend or descend in an airplane or high-speed elevator. The eustachian tubes also drain the middle-ear spaces. The membranes lining the middle ears, like those of the nose and throat, constantly secrete fluids. The eustachian tubes allow these fluids to flow down into the throat, where they are simply swallowed.

The reason very young children get so many middle-ear infections lies in the anatomy of their eustachian tubes. In older children and adults, the tubes slant downward at an angle of about 45°, allowing fluids to flow freely down into the throat. In babies and toddlers, however, the tubes are nearly horizontal. (See page 86.)

This means that in babies and toddlers, germs can more easily spread into their middle-ear spaces. It also means that the openings of their eustachian tubes become blocked more easily by inflammation from a cold. And as germs grow and produce pus in the middle ear, the fluid cannot drain out as well and becomes trapped in the spaces. Middle-ear infections are basically a drainage problem.

Because middle-ear infections usually follow on the heels of colds, children tend to get them more frequently during the respiratory-virus season, from December through March. During these months at Children's Hospital, we see scores of children every week with middle-ear infections.

About one-third of all young children are susceptible to developing middle-ear infections

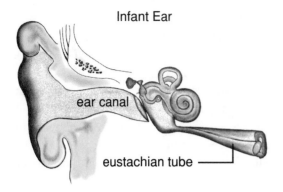

Infant Ear

ear canal

eustachian tube

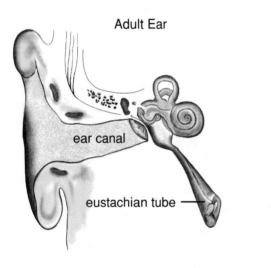

Adult Ear

ear canal

eustachian tube

*Eustachian tubes in babies and adults.*

over and over again. Doctors call these children otitis-prone. *Otitis*, remember, means "inflammation of the ear."

Some of these otitis-prone children probably have narrower eustachian tubes that are more easily blocked. Some have nasal allergies, so-called hay fever, which can also cause nose and throat tissues to swell and block the tubes. And some children have more ear infections because their parents are smokers. Smoke, even from someone else's cigarettes, may damage nose and throat tissues and allow germs to grow.

The vast majority of these children rapidly outgrow their susceptibility to otitis. It is unusual for a child over three to have a middle-ear infection.

## Causes

Many of the common viruses causing upper respiratory infections—colds—can spread into a child's middle-ear spaces and cause an infection there. Among them are the rhinoviruses (the most common causes of colds), adenoviruses (the most common causes of sore throats), influenza viruses, parainfluenza viruses, and the respiratory syncytial virus.

Among bacteria, the most common culprit is *Streptococcus pneumoniae*, also called pneumococcus and sometimes strep pneumo for short. Strep pneumo causes 30 to 50 percent of all acute middle-ear infections in children, 7 million cases a year, according to the U.S. Public Health Service. Strep pneumo also causes sinus infections, pneumonia, and meningitis. This is *not* the common strep bacterium that causes strep throats; that one is *Streptococcus pyogenes* (also called group A streptococcus).

In second place among bacteria as a cause of children's middle-ear infections is an organism called *Haemophilus influenzae*. This name may sound familiar because your baby should have been vaccinated against hemophilus bacteria with a series of shots starting at about two months of age; this is a vaccine both the U. S. Public Health Service and the American Academy of Pediatrics recommend that all infants receive. However, the vaccine does not protect your child against ear infections because it targets a different, more dangerous type of hemophilus (called type b) than the ones causing ear infections. The types involved in ear infections are also common causes of sinusitis. See *Hemophilus Infections,* page 130.

In recent years physicians have come to realize that a third bacterium, *Branhamella catarrhalis*, is also a significant cause of middle-ear disease in children. It also causes sinus infections. Another bacterium that cause ear infections, though less commonly, is *S. pyogenes* (group A strep, the strep that causes strep throat). In addition, viruses cause 10 to 15 percent of ear infections.

## How They Spread

Your child can catch any of the three bacteria that most commonly cause middle-ear infections from another child or adult who not only does not have a middle-ear infection but is not sick at all.

The bacteria that cause middle-ear infections are all ones that normally live in the nasal passages and throats without causing any symptoms. About 25 to 50 percent of healthy children carry strep pneumo bacteria without having any symptoms, and even among adults who have no contact with children, about 5 percent carry these bacteria. Even more children—60 to 90 percent—carry hemophilus bacteria in their noses.

## Incubation Period

Because the bacteria most commonly causing middle-ear infections often live harmlessly in people's nose and throat, their incubation periods are variable and not well known.

## Symptoms

When a child develops a middle-ear infection, she often appears to be getting over a cold, and then she gets worse in some way. She seems uncomfortable, or she gets a little more fussy.

As the virus or bacterium grows inside the middle ears, pus and other fluids accumulate and increase the pressure inside these spaces—which are normally filled with air. You can think of a middle-ear infection as a boil, an abscess, which is a pocket of pus within a closed space. This is a boil inside the ear. The buildup of pressure causes pain, and the child develops an earache, sometimes in both ears, sometimes just in one. This can range from a sense of fullness to extremely intense pain.

A child old enough to talk may tell you his ear hurts or feels funny or itchy, or he may complain about a throbbing or popping sensation. A baby may signal her discomfort or pain by tugging or scratching at her ears. She may become irritable and cry inconsolably. She may lose her appetite because she does not feel well, and sucking and swallowing may increase her pain. The earache may interfere with sleep.

When your child has an earache, he may or may not have a fever. The temperature can go up to 102° to 103°F. Sometimes ear infections start suddenly: a child with no previous symptoms may wake up with a high fever, screaming that his ear hurts.

The pus and fluid inside your child's ears usually cause him to lose temporarily some of his ability to hear well. The fluid restricts the movement of the eardrum and the three little bones, thus interfering with their ability to conduct sound waves to the inner ear. Hearing loss from an acute ear infection, however, is usually hard for parents to detect. You may notice a baby is not responding to sounds or an older child is turning up the volume on the TV, but children this young do not often tell you they cannot hear well.

Sometimes the pus inside a child's middle-ear space builds up so much pressure that it ruptures the eardrum, and yellowish or bloody pus drains out. Occasionally this is the first sign a child has an ear infection.

Parents are often alarmed when this happens, but it actually is therapeutic. It relieves the child's pain because the rupture releases the pressure inside the ear. Also, if a child does have a true bacterial infection, an abscess, the treatment for an abscess is to drain out the pus. And that is what the rupture does.

## Diagnosis

Your child can also develop an earache from an infection in her outer ear or a foreign object wedged in her ear canal. Even teething sometimes can cause a pain that a child feels in his ear.

Your pediatrician will examine your child's ears with a device called an otoscope. An otoscope is about the size and shape of a flashlight and has both a light source and a means of magnification. Your doctor gently inserts the otoscope's earpiece into your child's outer ear canal.

If your child's ears are healthy and not infected, the doctor sees a shiny, grayish eardrum that is translucent enough that he can see through it to the structures in the space beyond. He usually can see the handle of the first little hammer-shaped bone, which touches the eardrum, and also some of the second bone. If a child's ear is infected, however, your doctor may see an eardrum

that has become dull and also inflamed, sometimes even bright red. However, a child's eardrum can also turn red because she has a fever or has been crying in the waiting room. There are also many, more-subtle changes that doctors look for in addition to redness.

Your doctor may be able to see fluid trapped inside your child's middle-ear space; he may detect an air-fluid line or bubbles in the fluid. He may observe pus on your child's eardrum. Her eardrum may have become so thickened and opaque that the doctor cannot distinguish any of the bones beyond. Her eardrum may be bulging out into the ear canal because of the pressure of fluid behind it.

Your pediatrician can then use an otoscope to test how well your child's eardrums are able to move, that is, vibrate in response to incoming sound waves. He first increases and then decreases the air pressure on your child's eardrums. Doctors call this technique pneumatic otoscopy (*pneumatic* means "air"). This may hurt your child a little more if the ears are infected. A normal, healthy eardrum with no fluid behind it moves freely, but if your child's ears are infected, her eardrums may become stiff and lose their mobility.

(Parents sometimes wonder whether they should buy otoscopes so they can examine their children's ears themselves. We suggest not to. Ear exams require a great deal of experience to interpret correctly, and these are not diagnoses that parents can make.)

A clue to whether your child's ear infection is caused by a bacterium—in which case, as mentioned, she needs an antibiotic—or a virus is whether the infection affects both ears or just one. If your child has an earache and your pediatrician sees signs of infection, on just one side, it is more likely bacterial. Double-ear infections are more likely viral. Another clue is whether your child has a fever. Children with true bacterial infections almost always have a fever.

If your child has repeated middle-ear infections, your pediatrician may perform a more sophisticated test to measure the mobility of the eardrums, using an instrument called a tympanometer. A tympanometer is an electronic box outfitted with an earpiece, which your doctor places in your child's ear canal against the eardrum. The machine generates a tone and also varies the air pressure, then prints out a graph showing the responses of your child's ears. From the shapes of the curves, your doctor can gather more clues about the presence of fluid and the health of your child's ears.

Occasionally, if a doctor suspects there may be some complication of a middle-ear infection, he may have the child undergo some form of imaging—X-ray, CAT scan, or MRI (magnetic resonance imaging)—to investigate the problem.

## Treatment

If your child's middle-ear infection is caused by bacteria, he needs to take an antibiotic, as we have said, to kill the bacteria growing in his ear and prevent any complication.

If your child's ear infection is caused by a virus, however, he does *not* need to take an antibiotic. Antibiotics do not work against viruses; they do not kill viruses. And it is never a good idea for anyone to take an antibiotic or any medicine that is not needed. It is an unnecessary expense, and all medications can sometimes cause adverse reactions. Taking unnecessary antibiotics may also induce bacteria in your child's body to develop resistance to that antibiotic.

About 80 percent of children with abnormal-looking ears get better without any antibiotics. Presumably they had either a virus infection or a mechanical blockage of their eustachian tubes that resolved itself.

Do not be surprised, then, if your pediatrician does not immediately prescribe an antibiotic for your child. If his earache is not too uncomfortable and he has little fever, she may tell you that it is probably a virus infection and suggest observing him for twenty-four or forty-eight hours. If he is then getting better, that is good. If not and it now looks like a bacterial infection, your doctor will prescribe an antibiotic.

The standard treatment for children's middle-ear infections is amoxicillin, three times a day for five to seven days. This is taken by mouth, *not* put in the ears. Amoxicillin comes in several different forms: liquid for babies, chewable tablets for toddlers, pills for older children.

It is important that you have your child take all the doses of antibiotic to kill all the bacteria in his middle-ear spaces. Otherwise you run the risk of causing antibiotic-resistant bacteria to emerge.

### Other Medications

Whether or not your child is taking an antibiotic, you can give her acetaminophen, both to relieve the pain of her earache and reduce any fever she may have.

If your child's earache is more severe, your pediatrician may prescribe an anesthetic, which you drop into her outer-ear canals. Or if your child's ear pain is very severe, she may prescribe codeine, to be taken by mouth.

### Fluids

Make sure that your child takes in enough extra fluids to keep him from becoming dehydrated. Because he does not feel well, he may not drink as much as usual, and if he has a fever, he is losing fluid faster than usual. Babies particularly, because they are so tiny, can very quickly develop dangerous, even life-threatening, dehydration. With babies under a year, you need to give special fluids called oral rehydration solutions. See *Fluids*, page 290, in the Appendices for information about dehydration and these special fluids and also what fluids to offer older children.

While your child is taking the antibiotic, if he has a fever (101°F or above), you should keep him home from day-care. If he does not have a fever or once his fever is down, he can go to day-care if he feels well enough and his energy level is normal or near normal. You do not need to be concerned about your child spreading his ear infection to other children. These bacteria are so common that children are going to encounter them anyway.

Once your child starts taking the antibiotic, his earache should begin to disappear and his fever should be down within two or three days. If your child's ear infection does not clear with this course of antibiotic, your pediatrician may need to change the antibiotic. Your child may not be responding because he is infected with a strain of bacteria resistant to the first antibiotic. Your pediatrician may wish to see your child in three months to reexamine his ears to make sure the infection is clearing.

## Recurrent Middle-Ear Infections

The one-third of children who are otitis-prone (susceptible to getting middle-ear infections over and over again) fall into three different categories, depending on their response to antibiotics. These are three distinct problems with three different approaches to their treatment.

One group is children who get recurrent ear infections, sometimes six or more in a winter, but each time the infection is easily treated with antibiotics. The fluid completely disappears from their ears, and their hearing returns to normal.

For these children pediatricians sometimes suggest preventive antibiotics. The child takes a low dose, once a day, of an antibiotic throughout the winter months (no more than four to six months). Most children stop taking it over the summer, but if a child resumes getting ear infections again in the fall, she can start taking it again. A given child may need to take the antibiotic for several winters until she outgrows her susceptibility to ear infections.

It is questionable whether these children whose ears clear completely between episodes of infection ever need surgery to insert drainage tubes through their eardrums. (See the close-up illustration on page 92.)

A second group of otitis-prone children—the smallest of the groups—are those who have recurrent ear infections but their ears do *not* clear in between, even when antibiotics are changed repeatedly. They continue to have active, chronic ear infections with pus in their ears for prolonged periods. Some of these children do need tubes inserted in their eardrums, and a few need continuing care from an otolaryngologist, an ear, nose, and throat (ENT) specialist.

The largest group, however, is the 50 percent of children who still have fluid remaining in their middle-ear spaces following treatment for an acute ear infection. In many of them, the antibiotic kills all the bacteria, but their eustachian tubes remain swollen enough that fluid is still trapped in their middle ears. And sometimes children have fluid in their ears without ever having had an obvious ear infection. Children who just have fluid in their ears may or may not have any hearing loss.

Physicians call this condition otitis media with effusion. *Otitis media,* you recall, means "inflammation of the middle ear." *Effusion* is the medical term for fluid in a place where it does not belong, such a child's middle ear.

If these children with effusion do not take any more antibiotics, in most of them the fluid disappears from their ears within three months. If they do take another course of antibiotics, it does not hasten an improvement much.

Recently the U.S. Public Health Service's Agency for Health Care Policy and Research issued guidelines for treating children with otitis media with effusion. For otherwise healthy children, ages one through three, the agency recommends as initial therapy either observation or antibiotics—but not ear tubes.

Whether or not a child with just effusion ever needs ear tubes depends on whether she has a hearing loss, says the agency, and if so, how long she has had it. The years when children most commonly get middle-ear infections, up to three years, are the critical years when they are learning to talk and rapidly acquiring language. If a child is not hearing properly during these years, this could delay her acquisition of language and even her cognitive development.

You do not have to worry about the possibility of language delay, however, if your child has just one episode of middle-ear infection or even if she has recurrent infections that respond to antibiotics and clear each time.

The temporary decreases in hearing associated with ear infections that are rapidly treated do not appear to cause any long-term effects on language or speech. The fact that a child is having repeated ear infections does not mean that her language development will be delayed. But physicians are concerned about language development when a child has a chronic, active infection or fluid behind her eardrums with a hearing loss that persists continuously for six months or longer.

## Hearing Tests

The experts therefore recommend that a child have a hearing test well before that time. "A child who has had fluid in both middle ears for a total of three months should undergo hearing evaluation," recommends the Health Care Policy Agency; before three months a hearing test is optional. The American Academy of Pediatrics also advises, "When a child has frequently recurring acute otitis media and/or middle-ear effusion persisting for longer than three months, hearing should be assessed."

If a child with otitis media with effusion does turn out to have a hearing loss in both ears at three months, the Health Care Policy Agency recommends that he either take antibiotics or get ear tubes. If he has fluid and a hearing loss lasting four to six months, however, the Agency recommends that he should have ear tubes inserted through his eardrums.

Surgery for placement of ear tubes is not necessary, however, the agency stresses, unless otitis media with effusion is causing a child to have a hearing impairment in both ears.

## Ear Tubes

The insertion of ear tubes has become the most common surgical procedure that children in this country undergo. Hundreds of thousands of children, as mentioned, have this operation each year. And in one study children who attended day-care were seven times more likely to get ear tubes than were children cared for at home.

The tubes themselves look like miniature spools of thread. They are inserted in a child's ears by an ear, nose, and throat (ENT) specialist, usually in an outpatient procedure. At Children's Hospital we give these very young children a general anesthesia. The actual surgery takes only a few minutes. The ENT specialist,

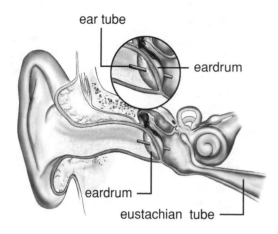

*Ear tube inserted into the eardrum.*

using a microscope, makes a small cut through each of the child's eardrums and then places a tube through each opening. The children recover from anesthesia and are ready to go home within a few hours.

Your doctor probably will call these tubes tympanostomy tubes. *Tympanic membrane* is another name for the eardrum, and the ending *-ostomy* means "artificial opening in a body part.

The tubes allow fluid to drain out of the child's middle-ear spaces, thus freeing the eardrum and the three little bones to vibrate normally. This usually restores the child's hearing to a normal level. The tubes prevent further accumulation of fluid and also equalize the air pressure across her eardrums and ventilate her middle-ear spaces. Ventilation of these spaces is also thought to decrease the severity and frequency of ear infections. Some children, however, may still need to take antibiotics for recurrent ear infections.

Like all procedures, ear-tube surgery has its down side. There is the cost, of course, and there is always some risk from any anesthesia. The surgery can produce scarring of an eardrum, or a child's ear may drain persistently. And the hole

in the eardrum can allow other germs to invade the middle ear from outside. To prevent this, it is necessary to keep water from getting into your child's middle-ear spaces. You need to be careful when you are bathing your child or washing her hair, and your doctor may suggest that she wear ear plugs when she is playing at the pool or swimming and avoid getting her head underwater.

As the incisions in the child's eardrums heal, the healing process gradually tends to push the tubes out of the eardrums. Most of the time, the tubes come out of the eardrums by themselves in six to eighteen months. Some children need to have ear tubes inserted more than once.

## Adenoidectomy

Some children who have repeated middle-ear infections or persistent middle-ear fluid are helped by having their adenoids removed. The adenoids are lymphoid tissue, part of the immune system, located at the back of the nose near the openings of the eustachian tubes. If a child's adenoids are enlarged, they can sometimes block the flow of fluid from a child's eustachian tubes. In children with recurrent ear infections, the adenoids may also be acting as a reservoir for bacteria that then can migrate up the eustachian tube to infect their ears. In such cases, removal could help.

This procedure is called an adenoidectomy; the ending *-ectomy* means "surgical removal of a structure." With the child under general anesthesia, an ENT specialist, using a mirror, reaches in through the child's mouth, behind the palate, to the back of the nose and cuts out the adenoid tissue. The whole operation, from the time anesthesia is administered until the child wakes up again, takes less than forty-five minutes. Older children can usually go home the same day, but at Children's Hospital we keep children who are two years old and younger in the hospital at least overnight. Children do have some discomfort afterward and usually take a pain medication (acetaminophen plus codeine). The wound heals in about a week to ten days.

## Complications

Rarely, middle-ear infections can lead to serious complications. Bacteria can spread out of a child's middle ear to the bone just behind the ear, the mastoid, and cause mastoiditis. This can cause permanent hearing loss by damaging the little bones that conduct sound vibrations to the inner ear. Bacteria can also spread to the inner ear itself and damage the cochlea. The infection can, very rarely, spread to a child's brain and cause an abscess or meningitis, inflammation of the membranes covering the brain.

Sometimes repeated ear infections lead to the development of a cystlike mass—called a cholesteatoma—within a person's middle-ear space. Cholesteatomas take long enough to develop that they are usually not detected until a person becomes an adult. The cyst can be removed surgically, but the person may be left with poor hearing.

Today, however, thanks to antibiotics, it is uncommon for a child to develop any of these complications. And with most people who have a permanent hearing loss, the problem is not the result of a middle-ear infection.

## Prevention

Since so many children and adults carry the strep pneumo and hemophilus bacteria that most commonly cause middle-ear infections in their nose and throat without being sick, you never know when you or your children might be shedding them in your nose and throat secretions.

Therefore, to reduce the chances of spreading these germs to others, cover your nose and mouth—and also teach your children to cover theirs—whenever you need to sneeze or cough. And encourage your children not to share cups or drinking glasses with other children or adults at day care or elsewhere or to eat from the same spoon or fork.

Another thing you can do to help keep your child from getting middle-ear infections is not smoke. "Keep your child away from tobacco smoke, especially in your home or car," advises the American Academy of Pediatrics. "Children who breathe in someone else's tobacco smoke have a higher risk of developing health problems, including ear infections."

Breastfeeding also protects infants against middle-ear infections. In a study of over 1,000 infants in Arizona, babies who were breastfed exclusively for four or more months had only half as many episodes of middle-ear infections as did babies who were not breastfed. Breast milk contains antibodies against strep pneumo, hemophilus, and the other organisms that cause middle-ear infections. These antibodies reduce the number of these germs, right there on the spot, at the back of a baby's throat.

## *Ear Infections—Outer Ears*

### *Outer-ear infections must be treated by a doctor.*

Also called external otitis or swimmer's ear. *Oto-* means "ear"; the ending *-itis* means "inflammation."

### SYMPTOMS

- Earache, itchy ear
- Pain when pulling on the ear
- Red, swollen ear canal
- Painful chewing

Outer-ear infections—also called swimmer's ear—are very common among children. They can be quite painful but are almost never serious. If your child is prone to these infections, you can take several steps to help prevent their recurrence.

The outer ear is simply the part of the ear that you can see plus the ear canal, which leads down to the eardrum. (See figure on page 84.) Outer-ear infections can occur at any age, but they most frequently affect preschoolers and school-age children.

Outer-ear infections are both less common and less potentially serious than are infections of the middle ear. See *Ear Infections—Middle Ears,* page 89.

## Causes

A number of bacteria cause most outer-ear infections. These include *Pseudomonas aeruginosa, Enterobacter aerogenes, Proteus mirabilis, Klebsiella pneumoniae,* and streptococci. Less commonly, some fungi can also infect the outer ear.

## How They Spread

The outer ear has an excellent self-defense system that protects it against infection. The earwax (doctors call it cerumen) that forms in the ear canal is naturally acidic and repels both water and germs. Tiny hairs near the opening of the ear canal push debris out of the ear. But if anything disrupts the ear's ways of protecting itself, germs can invade the canal, and your child can develop an outer-ear infection.

Sometimes the invaders come from the outside world: your child can get an outer-ear infection from playing in polluted water. But the great majority of these infections do not involve contaminated water. Sometimes the "invaders" are bacteria that live in your child's ear all the time without doing any harm.

The outer ear's defenses can be disrupted if a child's ear canal becomes too dry or if the skin inside there becomes traumatized. This can happen if you repeatedly try to clean out your child's earwax, even with something as benign as a cotton swab.

What often disrupts the ear's defenses, however, is repeated immersion in water. A warm, moist environment in the ear is the most hospitable setting for an outer-ear infection. That is why such infections are more common in the summer, when children tend to spend a lot of time in the water. But outer-ear infections can occur in any season, especially if you live in a climate that is warm all year round.

Nor does your child have to be a swimmer to develop swimmer's ear. Repeated immersion in water can also come from playing in the pool or from sitting in a hot tub or even the bathtub.

Several other factors can also predispose a child to outer-ear infections: earwax lodged in the ear, contact dermatitis (rash), or an ear canal that is especially narrow. Children who get recurrent middle-ear infections may also be more prone to these infections because any chronic draining associated with that condition can inflame the ear canal.

## Incubation Period

Symptoms may appear within a few hours or several days of becoming infected.

## Symptoms

In the earliest stage, your child's ear feels full and itchy. A young child may not tell you so, but you may see him rub his ear or put his finger in it. Scratching can irritate the skin further and make it susceptible to bacterial invasion. His ear starts to hurt. The opening of his ear canal may look red and swollen, and you may see some pus or flaking skin.

Your child's ear hurts even more if you push or pull on the outside of his ear. This differs from an infection in the middle ear. The pain caused by a middle-ear infection does not increase when you pull on the ear.

With more severe infections, the redness and swelling are worse, and the pain may increase enough to make your child cry. He may not want to eat because chewing hurts, and he may develop a low fever.

In the most severe infections, your child's ear canal may become so swollen that you cannot see into his ear at all. His pain may be constant, and it gets worse when he moves his mouth—even to speak or chew—or when you just touch his ear.

Your child may complain that he is having trouble hearing. This does not mean the infection has permanently damaged his hearing. Very likely the swelling and buildup of debris in the ear canal are blocking sound waves from reaching his eardrum.

### CALL YOUR DOCTOR

- If your child complains of ear pain.

## Diagnosis

Your pediatrician probably can make a diagnosis of an outer-ear infection simply by looking into your child's ear with an otoscope. (For information about this device and how doctors use it to examine the ear, see "Diagnosis," page 88, in *Ear Infections—Middle Ears*.) The single physical finding that clinches the diagnosis is exquisite pain when your doctor tugs on the external part of the ear.

## Treatment

Outer-ear infections do not go away on their own. Your child needs to be treated by a doctor.

To ease the pain until you get her there, you can give her acetaminophen.

You can also apply a heating pad, set on low, or a hot-water bottle to the affected ear. Do *not* try to relieve your child's pain or itching by putting a cotton swab (or anything else) into her ear. It will only make things worse.

Your doctor will begin by cleaning out the pus and debris from your child's ear canal. The doctor may use a very small tube to gently irrigate her ear with water or saline solution.

In most cases physicians prescribe eardrops containing an antibiotic for five to seven days to kill the bacteria causing the infection. This will also decrease the swelling, and as the swelling decreases, so will the pain. You should see an improvement in your child's symptoms within three or four days.

Using the eardrops as prescribed is the key to successful treatment, but it can be a struggle to get drops into the ears of a squirming child who is in pain. You probably will want to hold an infant or young child on your lap; have an older child lie down on the bed. Turn your child's head to one side and drop in the prescribed number of drops. Medicine at room temperature will feel better to your child than drops that are cold.

To make sure the drops go where they should, gently pull on your child's ear. If your child is under three, her ear canal curves upward, so you should pull *down and back* on the ear to straighten out the canal and help the drops move through it. In children older than three, the ear canal curves downward, so pull *up and back* on the ear.

Try to keep your child lying on her side for a few minutes afterward so that the eardrops do not drip out. But unless your doctor tells you to, do not put cotton in her ears to keep the drops in. Your child may push the cotton in too far or take it out and put it in her mouth.

If the ear canal is quite swollen and your doctor thinks that getting eardrops directly into your child's ear will be difficult, he may insert a special piece of cotton "wick" deep into your child's ear after saturating the cotton with an antibiotic preparation. The wick soaks up the medication and delivers it to the deeper recesses of the ear canal. Usually the wick falls out on its own within a day or two. That means the ear canal has opened up enough for that little wick to wiggle out, so the swelling has obviously diminished. You continue giving your child eardrops for a few more days.

In a small number of cases, depending on the particular bacterium causing the outer-ear infection, the doctor may also prescribe an oral antibiotic.

Your child's outer-ear infection is not contagious. So there is no reason to keep her out of day-care, school, or camp or limit her usual routine, as long as someone is available to give her the eardrops or oral medication.

Your child should stay out of the water, however, as much as possible until the infection has run its course, in about a week. Baths or showers should be as brief as possible, and afterward you should gently dry her ears with the corner of a towel. You can also use a hair dryer to dry her ears—but be sure to use the lowest possible heat setting and keep the dryer about two feet away from her ear.

If your child's hearing was affected, it will return to normal after the infection goes away. Only in rare cases, if an infection moves farther into the ear, is hearing at risk. In cases of an extremely severe infection, a child might be hospitalized to receive intravenous antibiotics, but this is very unusual.

## Prevention

Remember the old saying "Don't put anything in your ear except your elbow"? This is very true when it comes to preventing outer-ear infections. One way to traumatize the ear canal is by sticking something sharp into it and scraping the skin, so that you get an abrasion in the skin.

Earwax protects the ear canal, so if you routinely remove your child's earwax with cotton swabs, you are increasing his likelihood of developing an outer-ear infection. If your child is troubled by excess earwax, ask your doctor about using an ear bulb-syringe or earwax softener.

If your child has had a recent outer-ear infection or tends to get them often, try to limit his stay in the water to less than an hour at a time. When he comes out, use the corner of a towel to remove any excess water from his ear, or teach him to shake his head vigorously or hop on one foot, with his head bent to one side, to get the water out. Have your child wait about twenty minutes before reentering the water, to give his ears time to dry out completely.

As a further measure, if your child has recurring outer-ear infections, your doctor may suggest that you apply an acetic acid preparation or eardrops to his ears after each day's swimming or in the morning and at bedtime. These are available at the drugstore (some by prescription). Some types are applied with a tuft of cotton—not a cotton swab—that you keep in your child's ear canals for five minutes. Having your child wear earplugs in the water may also help prevent infection.

# E. COLI DISEASE

Sometimes called the "hamburger disease."

The possibility of getting *E. coli* disease is the reason public health experts are now recommending that you should always cook hamburgers until they are well done.

The lowly bacterium *E. coli* zoomed to national attention in 1993 when it caused a serious outbreak of food poisoning in the Northwest. Nearly 600 people in four states (Washington, Idaho, Nevada, and California) developed bloody diarrhea or severe kidney disease after eating contaminated hamburgers from a chain of fast-food restaurants. More than 170 people were sick enough that they needed to be hospitalized, and four young children died.

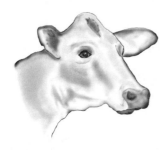

E. coli *normally lives in the intestines of healthy humans and cattle.*

Then, in 1997, *E. coli* was responsible for the largest meat recall in the nation's history, 25 million pounds of hamburger, after 17 people in Colorado became ill. *E. coli* has now become almost a household term, appearing regularly in newspaper headlines and on TV news, as Americans have been become increasingly concerned about the safety of our meat supply.

## Cause

*E. coli* disease is caused by a very common bacterium, well known for over a century. Its full name is *Escherichia coli*. Escher is the name of the German scientist who discovered the bacterium. The *coli* part of its name comes from where it lives: it is one of the many microbes that normally inhabit the colon (the lower part of the intestines) of humans and other animals.

There are hundreds of different strains of *E. coli,* most of them quite harmless; we all have *E. coli* living in our intestines. Some *E. coli* strains, however, cause diarrhea by attacking the tissues lining the intestines. Other strains produce powerful toxins. Toxins are poisons produced by living organisms. These toxins can circulate throughout the body in the bloodstream and damage distant organs. The strain that caused all the trouble in the Northwest—called O157:H7—produces a particularly potent toxin.

The *E. coli* O157:H7 strain was first identified as a cause of human disease in 1982, more than a decade before the big outbreak in the Northwest, when it caused similar outbreaks of food poisoning in Michigan and Oregon. A number of people in those states developed severe bloody diarrhea after eating contaminated hamburgers from another fast-food restaurant chain.

Since then, more and more episodes of *E. coli* O157:H7 disease have been reported. This is both because testing labs are now looking for the bacterium more and also, experts believe, because O157:H7 disease is, in fact, truly increasing. *E. coli* O157:H7 was the strain that prompted the big meat recall in 1997. The U.S. Public Health Service's Centers for Disease Control and Prevention now estimate that at least 20,000 people in this country get sick from *E. coli* O157:H7 each year and that it causes 250 deaths a year.

Recently, still other *E. coli* strains (among them, O104:H21 and O111:NM) have been identified that produce similar, potent toxins and can also cause severe disease.

## How It Spreads

Hamburger continues to be the most common source of the dangerous *E. coli* O157:H7 strain.

*E. coli* O157:H7 normally lives in the intestines of healthy cattle, and it can contaminate beef when cattle are slaughtered. When the beef is ground into hamburger, the bacteria can become mixed throughout the meat. If hamburger is not thoroughly cooked, *E. coli* can survive, and people can become infected when they eat it. *E. coli* O157:H7 is not just a problem in fast-food restaurants. People have also gotten sick from *E. coli* O157:H7 in hamburger they bought in local markets and cooked at home.

While the O157:H7 strain is less likely to survive on beef that is not ground, people have also caught *E. coli* disease from other cuts of meat. In North Dakota in 1990, seventy people became ill after eating rare roast beef at a buffet dinner. Sixteen people, including two children, had to be hospitalized. *E. coli* O157:H7 has also turned up in raw (unpasteurized) milk; in yogurt; in alfalfa sprouts; in fresh, unpasteurized apple cider; and in dry-cured salami in California and Washington state.

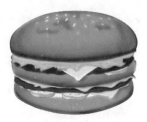

*Contaminated beef, ground into hamburger, has caused some people to become ill.*

The O157:H7 strain and other disease-causing *E. coli* can also get into food from the hands of infected people. An infected person sheds the bacteria in his stools and can get them on his hands when he goes to the toilet. If he does not wash his hands thoroughly afterward and then fixes food, he can contaminate the food.

*E. coli* bacteria spread particularly easily in day-care centers. Babies and toddlers who are not toilet trained can get *E. coli* on their fingers, and they then can leave the bacteria on anything they touch, such as a toy. Another child touches the toy and puts her hand to her mouth, and she becomes infected.

E. coli can also spread in water that has been contaminated with sewage. People can get *E. coli* disease from drinking impure water or swimming in lakes or streams polluted with the bacteria. Recently, there was an outbreak in a water park traced to a child with diarrhea who was swimming in the pool.

## Incubation Period

With most strains of disease-causing *E. coli*, it takes from less than half a day to up to six days for a person to get sick after ingesting the bacteria. With the *E. coli* O157:H7 strain, the incubation period is usually three to four days, but it can be as long as eight days.

## *Symptoms*

If your child does become infected with a disease-causing strain of *E. coli,* it most commonly causes him to have diarrhea—that is, loose stools. Various strains of *E. coli* cause different types of diarrhea. Some cause a child to have watery diarrhea, sometimes profusely watery diarrhea. Other strains can cause him to have blood in his stools. Bloody diarrhea is also called dysentery.

Along with diarrhea, your child may—or may not—also have abdominal cramps (which can sometimes be severe) and a fever or a headache, and he may be vomiting too. These symptoms can last, depending on the strain of *E. coli,* from a few days to several weeks.

Certain strains of *E. coli* are a leading cause of the so-called traveler's diarrhea that a person may catch while traveling in Mexico or other developing countries.

Any kind of diarrhea can be serious, even life-threatening, particularly in infants. A baby can lose so much fluid in his frequent or watery stools, and also through vomiting, that he very quickly can become dangerously dehydrated. See *Fluids,* page 290, in the Appendices for more about dehydration.

*E. coli* bacteria are also the most common cause of urinary infections in children. The bacteria can travel up into a child's urinary tract and infect his bladder or his kidneys. (See *Urinary Tract Infections,* page 278.) In newborn babies, *E. coli* occasionally causes meningitis (infection of the membranes covering the brain) or sepsis (infection of the blood).

With the dangerous *E. coli* O157:H7 strain, a person usually has blood in the stools; this strain is a leading cause of bloody diarrhea. The person usually also has severe cramping in his abdomen, but he usually does not have any or

---

### CALL YOUR DOCTOR

- If your child has any blood in her stools or has diarrhea with abdominal pain for more than an hour or two.

- If your child is having watery bowel movements more than ten times a day.

- If your child has diarrhea and is under a year old.

- If your child shows any signs of dehydration: if he is not urinating as much as usual, if his mouth is dry, and if he is less active than usual.

---

much fever. The diarrhea typically runs its course and is over in five to ten days.

The life-threatening kidney disease that the O157:H7 strain causes is called hemolytic uremic syndrome (HUS). HUS particularly strikes children under five and the elderly. It usually develops a week or so after a child starts having bloody diarrhea. *E. coli* O157:H7's powerful toxin has presumably spread in the child's bloodstream and done damage elsewhere in his body. The disease destroys his red blood cells, causing him to become anemic; he may look paler than usual, and his energy level may be down. The disease also damages cells in his kidneys, causing his kidneys to fail and urea to build up in his blood instead of leaving his body in his urine.

It is now realized that *E. coli* O157:H7 and its relatives are the major cause of this hemolytic uremic syndrome, which in turn is the leading cause of acute kidney failure in children. The syndrome, however, is not common. The Public Health Service estimates that only about 6 percent of people infected with *E. coli* O157:H7 develop this syndrome.

# Diagnosis

Physicians can find out what microorganism is causing a child's diarrhea by taking a sample of her stool and having a laboratory try to culture (grow) and identify the offending organism. Most of the time, however, it is not necessary for your pediatrician to do this. If your child has mild diarrhea that is not bloody and she has had the diarrhea for only a few days, your physician probably will not attempt to identify the germ.

If you and your child have recently been traveling in a developing country, the doctor may test your child's stool for the strains of *E. coli* that most commonly cause traveler's diarrhea. Or, more likely, the doctor may assume your child has this type of diarrhea and treat her for it.

If your child has more severe diarrhea, particularly if it is bloody or has lasted more than a few days, your pediatrician may have a lab test a sample of her stool for *E. coli* O157:H7 and its relatives.

# Treatment

When your child has diarrhea due to any cause, the most important treatment is to make sure that he takes in enough liquid to replace the fluids he is losing through his frequent and loose stools and also through vomiting. If your baby is under a year, pediatricians advise that you give him special fluids called oral rehydration solutions.

See *Fluids*, page 290, in the Appendices for more about these fluids, how to give them and what fluids to offer and not offer older children. See also "Treatment," page 57, in *Diarrhea* for information about what else to do and not do when your child has diarrhea.

Most diarrhea due to *E. coli* is mild enough and goes away soon enough on its own that your child does not need to take any antibiotics. If he

has more severe *E. coli* diarrhea, your pediatrician may need to prescribe an antibiotic such as neomycin or trimethoprim-sulfamethoxazole.

# Hospitalization

If a child does develop hemolytic uremic syndrome as a result of *E. coli* O157:H7, she usually must be hospitalized. She does not need an antibiotic. Antibiotics do not make any difference in the outcome of this disease. She may need to undergo dialysis until her kidneys repair themselves and are working normally again. This usually takes a week or so, but some people with hemolytic uremic syndrome have so much kidney damage that they need long-term dialysis or a kidney transplant. The syndrome kills about 3 to 5 percent of the people who develop it.

# Prevention

You can keep your child and others in your family from getting bloody diarrhea or hemolytic uremic syndrome from *E. coli* O157:H7 by thoroughly cooking beef. The U.S. Department of Agriculture recommends that you cook hamburger and meat loaf until the center reaches a temperature of 160°F. The juices should run clear, and the center of the meat should no longer be pink but gray or brown throughout. To be sure, you can measure the interior with an instant meat thermometer.

This is particularly important for young children, older people, and people whose immune systems are not normal, who are more susceptible to *E. coli* O157:H7 disease. It is not a good idea to feed rare hamburger or steak tartare to your baby.

*E. coli* O157:H7 contamination may be less of a problem with steaks and roasts because any bacteria would be on the surface of the meat and more readily killed when you cook it. Yet, as mentioned, there have been several outbreaks of *E. coli* O157:H7 disease from rare roast beef. It is also not a good idea to feed your child rare steak or roast.

You should also take care not to spread any possible *E. coli* or other germs around your own kitchen. After you shape ground beef into patties or a meat loaf, wash your hands thoroughly with soap and hot water before you touch any other food or anything else. If you get *E. coli* on your hands and then tear up lettuce, for instance, you could contaminate your salad. And remember that *E. coli* could remain on any surface or utensils that touched the raw meat. Do not put the cooked hamburgers back on the same platter that held the raw patties without first scrubbing it thoroughly with soap and hot water. For other tips on how to handle and prepare meat and other foods safely, see *Preventing Food Poisoning*, page 125.

And remember that *E. coli* O157:H7—as well as many other disease-causing germs—can also occur in raw (unpasteurized) milk. The U. S. Public Health Service and the American Academy of Pediatrics both advise that your child never drink unpasteurized or raw milk.

Since the O157:H7 strain and other *E. coli* bacteria—like many other diarrhea-causing germs—also spread directly from person to person via the feces-to-mouth route, you can help keep your family from catching these germs by washing your hands—and teaching your children, as soon as they are old enough, to wash their hands—after going to the toilet and before preparing or eating any food.

Day-care centers need to take particular care to keep from spreading *E. coli* and other germs from child to child. See *Recommendations for Day-Care Providers*, page 297, in the Appendices for advice about how day-care centers can help prevent the spread of disease-causing organisms.

# ENCEPHALITIS

*Encephalitis must be treated by a doctor.*

## SYMPTOMS

- Fever
- Neck pain
- Headache
- Abdominal complaints (nausea, vomiting)
- Rapid breathing
- Increasing sleepiness
- Hallucinations or confusion
- Weakness
- Dizziness
- Speech difficulties
- Seizures or tremors

Encephalitis is an infection or inflammation of the brain tissue that causes changes in the function of various portions of the brain and spinal cord. Acute infectious encephalitis is caused mainly by viruses, but other microorganisms and noninfectious diseases and even certain kinds of injuries are also responsible for encephalitis. Many of the same viruses that cause meningitis (see page 183) also produce encephalitis. The symptoms usually last anywhere from several days to two or three weeks. At The Children's Hospital of Philadelphia we are unable to find the cause in about one-third of patients, but it is important to try to determine a specific diagnosis because certain kinds of encephalitis can cause paralysis or even death.

While encephalitis can be serious, most of the time it is a mild condition and your child will make a complete recovery. Some very young children experience developmental delays as a result of encephalitis. That is why your physician may recommend a formal cognitive evaluation by a psychologist when your child recovers. However, encephalitis is seen more frequently in older children and adolescents.

We do not completely understand why encephalitis develops in one person and not in another, since most affected children are otherwise healthy. It is suspected that the immune system may be a factor. Also, where you live and how you spend your recreational time may also be a factor because some rodents, ticks, and mosquitoes carry encephalitis.

The names of some varieties of encephalitis are deceiving and reflect where we find the carrier mosquitoes, ticks, or other animals. For instance, Rocky Mountain spotted fever, which can cause encephalitis, is now commonly reported along the eastern seaboard rather than in the Rocky Mountain states. California encephalitis is found throughout the United States and is most common in the Midwest.

Certain forms of encephalitis seem to occur seasonally, and epidemics result from conditions that favor the breeding of mosquitoes, such as excessive rainfall and irrigation. However, with herpes simplex virus encephalitis, the most common cause of a nonepidemic form of the disease, there is no specific seasonal pattern. This is one of the kinds of encephalitis that responds to drugs. It occurs at any age in otherwise healthy people.

At one time in the United States, mumps and measles were a common cause of encephalitis, but thanks to vaccines, these diseases are no longer problems. On the other hand, some diseases—cat-scratch disease, for example—are recognized more frequently as testing makes diagnoses easier. In North America the most common strains of encephalitis are St. Louis encephalitis (SLE), eastern equine (EEE), and California (CE). Japanese encephalitis (JE) does not occur in North America, but it is found throughout rural Asia and can be deadly. Speak to your doctor if you plan to travel to that area of the world, because there is a vaccine available.

## Causes

Many kinds of viruses can cause encephalitis. Acute infectious encephalitis is caused primarily by viruses, but a wide variety of other microorganisms as well as a number of noninfectious diseases also cause the disease. In the United States the most common viral causes of encephalitis are the enteroviruses, herpes viruses, and arboviruses (bug-transmitted diseases).

Among the arboviruses, there are more than sixty different species of tick and mosquito-borne viruses carried by wild birds, rodents, and other small animals. The arboviral and enteroviral types of encephalitis tend to occur in clusters or epidemics from midsummer to early fall. The herpes viruses (which generally infect directly, in contrast to animal-borne infection) and other infectious agents account for sporadic cases year-round. Sometimes encephalitis is caused by infectious agents other than viruses.

The viruses and other organisms that cause encephalitis can reach the brain in several ways. Most commonly they multiply in other organs, such as the liver, spleen, or lymph nodes, and are carried by the bloodstream to the brain, where they reproduce. Some, like herpes simplex virus, may exist in a latent state within the brain tissue and reactivate spontaneously.

The rabies virus that causes encephalitis invades the skin from the saliva of the infected animal and enters a nerve, which gradually transmits the virus to the brain and spinal cord. Tick or mosquito-borne arboviruses are inoculated into the skin or muscle, where they multiply before entering the bloodstream.

## How It Spreads

Encephalitis, caused by arboviruses, is not contagious from person-to-person. It is spread to humans only by infected mosquitoes or certain ticks. However, your doctor may want to isolate your child at first until the cause of the illness can be determined and a communicable disease is ruled out. Enteroviruses are spread human-to-human. Herpes virus encephalitis can occur by person-to-person contact or reactivation of the dormant virus.

## Incubation Period

The incubation period depends on the particular virus or bacterium that causes the disease.

## Symptoms

The symptoms of encephalitis are similar regardless of which organism causes the infection. Although the onset of encephalitis may be sudden or gradual, a typical case is preceded by several days of nonspecific symptoms, such as fever, cough, sore throat, headache, or abdominal distress. Therefore, you may not realize that your child has anything more serious than a cold. Generally, children with encephalitis often begin to breathe rapidly. Your child will probably be increasingly sleepy. You will notice some kind of behavioral changes that may include confusion, hallucinations, weakness, and dizziness. With older children you may notice speech difficulties. In severe cases there might be a high fever, seizures, tremors, and coma that could proceed to death.

## Diagnosis

To diagnose encephalitis, your physician may look for the antibodies to the specific encephalitis germ in the blood, although the germ itself will not be in the blood. She may also perform a spinal tap (lumbar puncture) to examine the cerebrospinal fluid (CSF). Your child will most likely have an EEG (electroencephalogram) to measure brain-wave activity and a brain (CAT or MRI) scan to look for swelling or focal abnormalities. In rare instances a biopsy of brain tissue (a delicate but generally safe procedure) is the only sure way to identify the germ.

Your doctor will ask many questions to try to determine how your child may have contracted encephalitis. She will inquire about your child's travel history or exposure to illness in other people, exposure to ticks or mosquitoes or animals (especially sick ones such as horses), recent injections, and exposure to environmental poisons. This information is invaluable in helping to identify the specific germ and pinpoint a diagnosis.

## Treatment

Fortunately, for encephalitis from herpes simplex virus, antiviral medicine is available and helpful. For other types, like enteroviral encephatis, recovery depends on the development of antibodies to destroy the virus. Encephalitis patients are admitted to the hospital, where treatment can control fever and headache pain. Your child will stay in a darkened room to reduce external stimuli and will be observed closely for neurologic change. Conventional antibiotics may be used for certain cases of encephalitis not caused by viruses.

The prognosis for children with encephalitis depends upon a number of variables, including the agent that caused the disease, the child's age (children under one year of age are most vulnerable), and the severity of the illness. For example, encephalitis that is caused by the mumps virus and the enteroviruses is generally mild. Newborns who survive encephalitis caused by the herpes simplex virus may have serious, long-term handicaps. In older children prompt diagnosis and antiviral treatment for herpes simplex encephalitis will limit long-term complications such as seizures or developmental delay.

## Prevention

At present there are no medications to prevent encephalitis. Since mosquitoes feed from dusk to dawn during the hot summer months, humans are more likely to be bitten by infected mosquitoes at night. It's best to keep your children indoors or in screened-in areas when mosquitoes are actively biting. Mosquitoes are attracted to dark clothing, so dress your child in light-colored clothing that covers the skin. Use repellent containing 6 to 10 percent DEET on clothing as well as on the skin. If you have stagnant water around, get rid of it or anything else that acts as a breeding ground for mosquitoes.

Vaccination programs have greatly reduced the incidence of encephalitis in children, particularly the majority of cases associated with childhood diseases like measles, mumps, and rubella.

# EPIGLOTTITIS

*Epiglottitis is an emergency and must be treated by doctors in a hospital.*

The ending *-itis* means "inflammation."

## SYMPTOMS

- Difficulty breathing
- Extremely sore throat
- Drooling
- High fever (102° to 104°F)
- Insists on sitting up

*Epiglottitis is increasingly rare, but you should know about it because it is a medical emergency. If your child develops epiglottitis, you need to call 911 or rush your child to your local hospital emergency room.*

Epiglottitis is an inflammation of a child's epiglottis. The epiglottis is a very useful flap of tissue in the throat. Two tubes in the throat run downward into the chest. The one in back is the esophagus (gullet); this tube conveys food to the stomach. The other one, in front, is the trachea (windpipe); this tube directs air to the lungs.

The epiglottis sits atop the windpipe. When we swallow, the epiglottis automatically flops down over the top of the windpipe, closing it off and keeping food and liquids from going down into the lungs. When we finish swallowing, the epiglottis opens up again to allow air to flow to the lungs.

We are most aware of the epiglottis when it occasionally gets stuck in its up position as we swallow. We choke a little and say our food has gone down the wrong way.

When a child has epiglottitis, an infection has caused her epiglottis to become so swollen that it may block her windpipe, threatening her life by making it difficult or impossible for her to get enough air into her lungs.

Epiglottitis can affect people of any age, but it is rare in babies under a year. A child can develop epiglottitis at any time of year, but it is more common in winter and spring.

## Causes

Until recently 95 percent of episodes of epiglottitis in children were caused by a bacterium named *Haemophilus influenzae* type b. This type of hemophilus also causes meningitis and pneumonia in young children.

Today your child is much less likely to develop epiglottitis, thanks to a vaccine against this hemophilus bacterium introduced in 1985. See *Hemophilus Infections*, page 130, for more about this vaccine and the other diseases it prevents.

Epiglottitis, however, has not completely disappeared. There are still other bacteria around that occasionally cause a child to develop the disease.

## How It Spreads

*Haemophilus influenzae* type b is one of the many common germs that normally live in our respiratory tract. Before the introduction of hemophilus vaccine, about 5 percent of children carried these bacteria in their noses without having any symptoms. A child could get epiglottitis from a person who not only did not have epiglottitis but was not sick at all.

Such hemophilus carriers and people with active infections shed these bacteria in their nasal secretions. If they sneeze or cough without covering their nose or mouth, they can spread droplets containing the bacteria to another person and infect him with hemophilus. Or as they talk, they can inadvertently spray a person with the bacteria.

It is hard to know what tips the scale from a child simply carrying this bacteria in his nasal passages to having it cause epiglottitis. The child may have had a prior upper respiratory tract infection that has caused tiny breaks in the membranes lining his nose and throat. These breaks could allow the bacteria to circulate into the blood stream eventually settling in the tissues of the epiglottis.

## *Incubation Period*

The length of time it takes for a child to develop epiglottitis after being infected with Hemophilus type b bacteria is not known. It probably varies considerably.

## *Symptoms*

A child with epiglottitis becomes very ill very abruptly. Epiglottitis moves along at a rapid clip.

It usually starts with the child showing symptoms of an upper respiratory infection: a runny nose, maybe a cough, some fever. Then, as the bacteria multiply in his epiglottis, it becomes inflamed and begins to swell. His throat quickly becomes extremely sore and painful. His temperature may reach 102° to 104°F, and he may have so much trouble swallowing his saliva that he starts to drool.

Within hours the child's epiglottis can become so enlarged that it threatens to block the airway to his lungs. He may have so much difficulty breathing that he develops what is called respiratory distress.

As he takes each breath, you may hear him making a harsh, sometimes high-pitched,

sometimes loud sound called stridor. This sound is a sign that he has an obstruction in his airway in the region of his throat.

As the child tries to get more air, his nostrils may flare out at the sides. He may use extra muscles, ones he does not usually use for respiration, to help him breathe, developing what are called retractions. Each time he takes a breath, you may see the muscles in the spaces between his ribs and also those in the spaces at the base of his neck, above his collarbone, pulling in (retracting). He may also use his abdominal muscles to help breathe, causing his breastbone to sink down with each breath.

With less air flowing to his lungs, less oxygen may be getting into his bloodstream and reaching his brain and other tissues. He may start turning grayish or bluish around his mouth and at the tips of his fingers.

Children with epiglottitis are also very apprehensive, very concerned, obviously anxious. Typically, they refuse to lie down. As young as the child is, he somehow instinctively knows how to position himself to keep his airway open as much as possible. He insists on sitting up, leaning forward, with his neck outstretched and his chin thrust forward, sometimes propping himself forward on his arms. Some refer to this as the "sniffing position."

Whatever you do, do not make your child lie down or try to change his position. If you move or reposition a child with epiglottitis, he sometimes loses that instinctive ability to keep his airway open and you could abruptly block his airway. Nor should you ask him to open his mouth and say ahh! This, too, could block his airway.

These children can become so ill that it is very difficult to distract them from their illness, to engage them in conversation or get them to smile. They are just concentrating on breathing.

Any delay in getting a child with epiglottitis to an emergency room could be fatal. Children can go from having no symptoms at all to total obstruction of their airway within hours.

### CALL YOUR DOCTOR

**CALL 911 or take your child to your hospital emergency department:**

- If your child has a severe sore throat and is having so much trouble swallowing his saliva that he is drooling.

- If your child refuses to lie down but insists on sitting up, with his neck outstretched.

- If your child shows signs of respiratory distress: he is making a harsh sound as he breathes (stridor); his nostrils are flaring; he is retracting (pulling in) the muscles between his ribs and at the base of his neck as he breathes; he has a bluish or grayish tinge around his mouth or the tips of his fingers; or he becomes lethargic and unresponsive.

## Diagnosis

Often with a glance pediatricians can identify that a child may have epiglottitis based on the way she is holding herself and the way she is drooling.

If epiglottitis is suspected, the child is taken to the operating room whene an ear, nose, and throat (ENT) specialist and an anesthesiologist immediately inspect the child's throat and epiglottis with a lighted fiberoptic instrument called a laryngoscope to see if her epiglottis is indeed swollen. It can be so inflamed and red that it resembles a cherry or strawberry.

The physicians may have X-rays taken of the child's neck from the side. These could show whether a swollen epiglottis is the cause of her problem.

Identifying whether *Haemophilus influenzae* type b or some other bacterium is causing the child's epiglottitis can be done during the inspection in the operating room. Then the physicians may take a sample of her blood and ask the lab to culture (grow) and identify the responsible germ.

## Treatment

This may require inserting a breathing tube down past his swollen epiglottis into his windpipe to hold his airway open.

After the child is safely treated in the operating room, he is admitted to the hospital, to an intensive care unit, where he may be placed on a respirator to help him breathe. He gets an intravenous antibiotic to kill the bacteria that are causing his epiglottis to swell. His heart and respiratory rates are monitored continuously, and he may receive extra oxygen and intravenous fluids if he needs them.

Children who have epiglottitis usually need to stay in the hospital for five to seven days.

## Prevention

*The U.S. Public Health Service and the American Academy of Pediatrics both recommend that all infants routinely receive hemophilus type b vaccine, which prevents not only epiglottitis but also meningitis and pneumonia caused by hemophilus.*

Your baby should get her first shot of hemophilus vaccine when she is two months old. Then she needs one or two more shots—depending on the particular vaccine preparation your pediatrician uses—at the age of four months and (if needed) at six months. She should get a booster shot when she is twelve to fifteen months old.

See "Prevention," page 133, in *Hemophilus Infections* for more about this vaccine and its possible side effects. See also *Vaccines*, page 301, in the Appendices for the schedule of all the shots your child needs.

If a child does develop epiglottitis (or other invasive hemophilus type b disease), it means that other people living in the same household, adults or children, may also be carrying this bacterium in their noses, even if they are not sick. And any other child in the household younger than four who has not received all his hemophilus shots could catch the bacterium from these carriers and develop epiglottitis or another hemophilus disease.

The American Academy of Pediatrics therefore recommends that any such not fully vaccinated child and everyone else in the household (except pregnant women) should, as soon as possible, take a course of the antibiotic rifampin to eliminate any hemophilus bacteria from their noses.

If a child who develops epiglottitis has been attending a day-care center, his physician may recommend that all the children attending the center, as well as the staff, also take rifampin.

If your child has been fully vaccinated against hemophilus type b, however, epiglottitis is not something you need to spend much time worrying about.

Before the vaccine, during the late 1970s and early 1980s, at Children's Hospital we used to see about ten children each year who had epiglottitis. Today fewer people carry the bacterium in their noses, and the incidence of epiglottitis and other hemophilus type b diseases has decreased dramatically. We now usually see no more than one child a year with epiglottitis, and some years go by without our seeing any at all.

A few children and adolescents, nevertheless, will still develop epiglottitis. While hemophilus type b is now much less common, the other bacteria that occasionally cause epiglottitis (like group a streptococcus) are still around and do, from time to time, cause the disease.

# FEVERS

Children run fevers far more frequently than adults do. You will find that a fever in your child is one of the most common reasons for you to call the pediatrician.

Your child can have a fever for any one of many reasons. It can be a reaction to a vaccine or a medication or the response to an injury. Most of the time, however, it means that some disease-causing microorganism—a virus, bacterium, or some other germ—has invaded your child's body, and the immune system is mounting an attack on the organism.

Children have a lot of fevers because they are encountering for the first time many germs (usually viruses) that we adults met long ago and to which we have long since developed some immunity.

## *Normal Body Temperature*

Normal body temperature varies by several degrees. The familiar 98.6°F is just the *average* temperature, measured in the mouth, of an adult. Young children normally have a higher body temperature. It gradually drops throughout childhood until it reaches adult level in their teen years.

Body temperature also fluctuates throughout the day, tending to be highest in late afternoon and early evening and lowest in the early hours of the morning. This is also true when a child has a fever. This daily cycle, however, does not become established until a child is about two years old. Body temperature also increases during exercises.

A normal adult oral temperature ranges from about 96° to 99°F. The normal range for a child is 96° to 100°F, measured in the mouth; 97° to 100.4°F (38°C), measured in the rectum—which is the way you need to take it in small children. Parents sometimes say that their child has a "fever" of 99.5°F, not realizing that this is within the range of normal for a child.

Our body temperature is kept within this range by a temperature-control center, a thermostat of sorts, at the base of our brain. If we start to become too hot, our thermostat causes us to perspire, cooling us by evaporation, and our blood vessels to dilate, cooling us by radiation. If we start to become too cold, our thermostat causes our blood vessels to contract, conserving body heat, and our muscle activity to increase, warming us up. Sometimes our muscles contract so much that we shiver.

## *What Is a Fever?*

When a person's immune system detects that a germ has invaded the body, it sends white blood cells to the site of the invasion—to the nose and throat, for instance, if the invader is an influenza virus. These white cells release substances called pyrogens (literally, "heat producers"), which travel in the bloodstream to the thermostat in the brain. The pyrogens turn the thermostat up, so to speak, and allow the person's body temperature to rise. She may shiver and have chills in order to generate heat and cause the body temperature to rise. The resulting fever means that the immune system is fighting the infection.

The official, textbook definition of a fever is a temperature of 100.4°F or more, measured in the rectum. It is most practical to remember 101°F. Mouth temperatures run about one degree lower than rectal temperatures, so measured orally, a fever is a temperature of 100°F or more.

When your child has a fever, she also breathes faster and her heart beats faster. The activity of her stomach decreases; she digests food more slowly and thus tends to lose her appetite. Her skin may become flushed. Most children are not bothered much by a fever, but at other times they are uncomfortable and may become cranky and irritable, even listless and lethargic.

Children can develop quite high fevers as they meet many germs for the first time. It is not unusual for a child to have a temperature of 105°F, and it sometimes reaches 106°F. This, however, is about as high as a person's temperature will go as the result of an infection, and 106°F is unusual. Influenza, roseola, and meningitis are among the diseases that can cause fevers this high. At The Children's Hospital of Philadelphia, we see twenty or thirty children a year with fevers of 106°F. Weeks can go by when we see none, and then in February, during influenza season, we may see one a day.

There is little correlation, however, between the height of your child's fever and how sick she is. She can have a high fever and not be seriously ill—with roseola, for instance. What does correlate with how sick she is is how she is behaving and how she looks and feels. If she is lethargic and irritable, she is more likely to be more ill. However, if she is eating and sleeping well despite her fever, smiling and running around the house, you probably do not have much to worry about.

You *do* have to be concerned about *any* fever, however, in a baby under the age of about three months. Babies this young usually do not get a fever, and although most babies with fever probably have a virus, it could be a sign of something more serious.

Many parents fear that fever can harm their child, that a high fever can cause brain damage

or even death. This is a common misconception. Fever alone does not cause brain damage. There are a few infectious diseases, fortunately uncommon, that sometimes cause high fevers and brain damage, but it is the infection that causes the damage, not the fever.

About 3 out of every 100 children, when they have a high fever—particularly if it rises rapidly—may have a seizure: the child becomes unresponsive for a few seconds or minutes; her arms and legs usually flail rhythmically; and she may fall to the floor. This occurs most often in children between three months and five years of age. While frightening, these febrile seizures, as doctors call them, usually do no lasting harm. About half of these children never have a second seizure. Children outgrow any susceptibility to febrile seizures by the time they are five.

## Taking Your Child's Temperature
### Fever Thermometers

Traditional glass mercury thermometers are inexpensive but a little tricky to learn to use. Before taking a temperature, you need to make sure the thermometer is reading well below normal. If not, you need to shake it down: you hold it like a pencil, and snap your wrist several times. A mercury fever thermometer can be hard to read; you need to rotate it back and forth until you can see the mercury line. Once you learn to use one, mercury thermometers are reliable.

Many parents these days buy an electronic thermometer with a digital readout. These are easier to use and faster. They are the kind we employ in the emergency department at Children's Hospital. Their batteries, however, can run down just when you need them most. It is a good idea to keep a mercury thermometer on hand as a backup.

There are now also ear thermometers that measure a person's temperature by sensing infra-red radiation from his eardrum. These are more expensive and also take a little practice to learn how to get an accurate reading. Once you do learn, they are easy and fast.

Whatever type of thermometer you use, make sure your child is not overheated because he is wearing too many clothes. And make sure that the thermometer is clean. Mercury thermometers you can wash with warm water and soap. With electronic thermometers, follow the manufacturer's directions. And afterward, clean the thermometer again.

## Taking Rectal Temperature

As mentioned, with a baby or young child, you need to measure his temperature in his rectum simply because he is too young to hold a thermometer in his mouth. At Children's Hospital we measure temperatures rectally until children are three to five years old.

If you are using a mercury thermometer, you need to use one with a special short, rounded bulb so that you do not damage your child's rectum. Lubricate it with a tiny bit of petroleum jelly.

One way to take a rectal temperature with a small baby is to place him, tummy down, on your lap and hold him still with one hand (see top right). Another way is the diaper-changing position; he lies on his back and you hold his legs up. Some children squirm so much that taking a rectal temperature is a two-person job.

With your free hand, slide the tip of the thermometer into your child's anus and into his rectum. Be gentle; do not force it in. It should go in no more than one inch. Remain with your baby all the time the thermometer remains in his rectum, holding the thermometer between your first and second fingers.

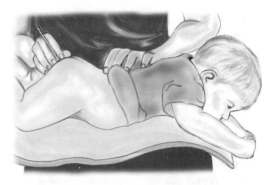

*Hold the tip of the thermometer between your first and second fingers, in your child's rectum.*

You need to leave a mercury thermometer in your child's rectum for two to three minutes. Electronic thermometers usually signal when they have finished a reading.

Again, your child has a fever if his rectal temperature is 101°F or above.

## Taking Oral Temperature

If you are using a mercury thermometer, you need one with a slender, elongated tip. Do not take an oral temperature right after your child has eaten or drunk hot or cold food or drinks; you will get an artificially high or low reading. Simply place the thermometer in your child's mouth, under her tongue, to the right or left. Make sure that she keeps her mouth closed. If you are using a mercury thermometer, also make sure that she does not bite down on the glass.

You need to leave a mercury thermometer in your child's mouth for two to three minutes. Her lips must remain closed around the thermometer throughout all this time. This is difficult for a child under three to five years to do; this is why you need to take rectal or armpit temperatures in such young children.

Your child has a fever, again, if her oral temperature is 100°F or above.

### Taking an Armpit Temperature

You can also measure your child's temperature in his armpit. We do not generally recommend this method because armpit temperatures are not as reliable at detecting fevers.

Armpit temperatures run about one degree lower than oral and two degrees lower than rectal temperatures. So if a child has an armpit temperature of 99°F or more, he does indeed have a fever. But a baby could have a normal reading in his armpit and still have a fever, and you would miss it.

There are some circumstances, however, when you might need to take an armpit temperature: if your baby has so much diarrhea or is fidgeting so much you cannot take a rectal; or with an older child, if you cannot take an oral because she is vomiting or cannot breathe through her nose. An armpit reading is better than nothing. We sometimes take armpit temperatures on babies in the hospital if they are stable and we do not want to wake them up.

To take an armpit temperature, you can use either a mercury or electronic thermometer with either a rectal or an oral tip. Place the tip of the thermometer under your child's armpit and hold—or have him hold—his arm firmly down against it, alongside his body. Make sure the thermometer is in contact with his skin and that no clothing is in the way. Hold a mercury thermometer there for three minutes.

## Treatment

Your pediatrician will try to determine the specific cause of your child's fever and treat the underlying disease that is causing it. If the fever

---

### CALL YOUR DOCTOR

- If your child is under three months of age and has a fever— a temperature of 101°F or higher measured in his rectum—call your doctor immediately.

- If your older child has a temperature of 101°F or higher and is also showing signs of lethargy, excessive tiredness or irritability. If your child is happy and playful despite his fever, continue to watch him carefully.

- If your child of any age has a temperature of 103°F or more.

**CALL 911 or immediately take your child to your hospital emergency room:**
- If your child has a seizure. See page 110.

---

is caused by a bacterial infection, for example, he may prescribe an antibiotic. However, whatever the cause, the following are some things you can or should do whenever your child has a fever.

## Home Care

With any fever, you should keep your child home from day-care or school. The American Academy of Pediatrics and the U.S. Public Health Service both advise that children be excluded from out-of-home child care whenever they have a fever.

## Fluids

Whenever your child has a fever, it is very important that you make sure she drinks plenty of extra fluids. She is losing fluid from her body more rapidly than usual, by evaporation from her warmer skin and, because she is breathing faster, from the tissues lining her respiratory tract. And she probably is not taking in as much fluid as usual because she does not feel well and her appetite is down. Babies particularly, because they are so small, can very quickly become dehydrated. See *Fluids*, page 290, in the Appendices for more information about dehydration and what fluids to offer children of various ages.

## Rest

Your child does not necessarily have to stay in bed. You can be guided by her energy level. If she wants to lie around on the couch or her bed and rest, let her. But if she wants to be more active and play quietly, that is all right too.

## Feeding

You do not need to worry if your child loses interest in solid food. He will lose a little weight, but when his fever goes down and he is well again, his appetite will return and he will gain the weight right back again.

In the meantime, do not withhold food from your child. If he is hungry, feed him. See *Feeding*, page 292, in the Appendices for information about what foods to offer and not offer your child when he sick.

## Clothing

Dress your child in light clothing; this allows her to lose body heat from her skin. Some parents believe that when a child has a fever, they should bundle her up and try to sweat it out of her. We sometimes see children with fevers who are swaddled in several layers of clothes and blankets, even on hot summer days. All this accomplishes is to make a child even more uncomfortable. So take off any excess clothing—but not to the point where she feels cold or is shivering.

## Room Temperature

Keep the air temperature in your child's room on the cool rather than the warm side, again, to allow him to lose body heat from his skin. A fan helps the air to circulate and might make him more comfortable—but again, not to the point that he feels cold.

## Medications

You do not necessarily need to give your child any medication to lower his temperature. Remember that the fever is a part of his body's normal response to an infection. If your child's temperature is below 103°F and he is happy and playful, he may not need any medicine. However, if his temperature is 103°F or above and he is uncomfortable or cranky or lethargic, a fever-reducing medicine can help him feel better.

The fever-lowering medication that doctors most often recommend for children is acetaminophen, which is available over the counter, without prescription. Acetaminophen works by literally lowering the point at which the thermostat in the brain is set. An alternative medicine is ibuprofen, which is also available over the counter.

You should not, however, give *any* fever-reducing medication to a baby under about three months old. Since a fever in a child that young could be a sign of something serious, your doctor needs to know whether or not he does indeed have a fever.

You should never give your child aspirin. In a child whose fever is caused by the influenza or chickenpox virus—and you never can be sure that it is not—taking aspirin is associated with a very rare but very serious, life-threatening, neurologic disease called Reye's syndrome. The Academy of Pediatrics "strongly advises" that you "not give your child or teenager aspirin or any medications containing aspirin when he has any viral illness." See *Reye's Syndrome*, page 217.

## Sponging

If your child's temperature is over 103°F and she is uncomfortable, you can also try sponging her to cool her off some. Have her sit in the bathtub in a few inches of lukewarm, or skin temperature—not cold—water. With a washcloth or sponge, drizzle water to wet her skin for 15 minutes or so. This cools her body by evaporation from her skin. Sponging should bring her temperature down about two degrees. Since sponging alone does not lower your child's thermostat, it is best combined with the use of acetaminophen.

* * *

Usually your child's fever decreases over a period of twenty-four to forty-eight hours. It is 105°F, then 103°F, 101°F, and then back to normal. It usually does not just suddenly drop down. If your child has a comfortable night and wakes up without a fever—and has not had any acetaminophen overnight—and his activity level seems normal or near normal, he can return to his day-care center or school.

# FIFTH DISEASE

Also called erythema infectiosum or slapped-cheek disease.

## SYMPTOMS

- Rash on cheeks
- Lacelike rash on arms, legs, and trunk, sometimes itchy

Fifth disease is a common rash disease of childhood that is so benign you rarely have to worry about it.

It typically causes a distinctive rash on your child's face. He looks as if he has been slapped, hard, on his cheeks with a spare rash around the mouth.

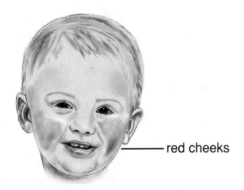
——— red cheeks

*Fifth disease.*

Your child is most likely to catch fifth disease between the ages of five and ten years. The disease is most often recognized in school outbreaks, which usually occur in the spring and may affect up to 60 percent of the children in a school.

Fifth disease acquired its name early in the twentieth century, when doctors were sorting out the various childhood illnesses that cause rashes. They called measles and scarlet fever first and second diseases respectively. Rubella (German measles) was third disease (what they thought was fourth disease is now lost in history). Fifth disease somehow kept its numeric name, probably because its formal, medical name—erythema infectiosum—is so complicated.

## Cause

It was not until the early 1980s that researchers realized fifth disease is caused by a virus named human parvovirus B19, often called B19 virus or just parvovirus.

## How It Spreads

While parvovirus is not primarily a respiratory virus, your child usually catches it via the respiratory route.

A child who is infected with parvovirus sheds virus particles in the secretions from the nose and throat. These secretions can be spread by coughing and sneezing.

What helps spread parvovirus is the fact that a child transmits the virus before he shows any signs of infection with fifth disease. By the time the rash appears he is no longer infectious; that is, he is no longer shedding virus particles and thus no longer able to infect others.

Once a person is infected, parvovirus settles down in the bone marrow, inside the cells that eventually turn into red blood cells. As the virus multiplies there, virus particles move into the bloodstream.

In pregnant women parvovirus particles can sometimes spread from the bloodstream across the placenta and infect an unborn baby. This, however, only rarely causes any problem.

## Incubation Period

If your child becomes infected with parvovirus, it usually takes from four days to two weeks for the first symptoms of fifth disease to appear, but it can take as long as three weeks.

## Symptoms

As virus particles flood into your child's blood, he at first has what seems to be an ordinary mild cold. He has a runny nose. His throat may be somewhat sore. He may have a slight headache, but he may have no fever at all. You have no reason to suspect he has anything other than a cold. In two or three days, he recovers from the "cold."

Then, a few days later, your child may break out in a very red rash. It typically starts on his face with the distinctive slapped-cheek rash; the area around his mouth often remains pale, accentuating the redness of his cheeks. A characteristic lacelike rash may erupt on his arms, legs, and stomach. The rash may itch a little, and it tends to come and go. Warmth sometimes brings it out. You may see it more when your child is out in the sun or has just taken a warm bath.

Adults who become infected with parvovirus are more likely to have pain and swelling in their joints, particularly in their hands and knees, on both sides, and they, too, may or may not also have a rash.

It is only when the rash appears that anyone usually recognizes that a child has fifth disease. Unfortunately, parvovirus is infectious and spreads only *before* he breaks out in the rash, when he seems to have just a cold. And if he never has the rash, you may never know he had parvovirus. After the rash appears, your child can no longer spread parvovirus.

About 50 percent of all of us have been infected by parvovirus by the time we reach adulthood—and probably most of us never had any idea that we caught it because we had no rash and were never sick.

## Complications

In some circumstances, however, parvovirus infections can be more serious. As the virus multiplies in a person's bone marrow, it cuts down on the body's daily production of red blood cells. In otherwise healthy children, this is no problem. But in children who have sickle cell disease or another chronic anemia, parvovirus infection can cause severe, even life-threatening anemia.

Parvovirus can also sometimes be a problem if a woman becomes infected while she is pregnant. If the virus crosses the placenta and infects her unborn baby during the first trimester of pregnancy, it may cause severe anemia in the baby. The baby usually recovers, but occasionally the virus can cause a woman to have a miscarriage.

The odds of this happening, however, are very low. The overall risk of losing a baby if a woman is exposed to parvovirus in early pregnancy, the U. S. Public Health Service calculates, is about 1 or 2 percent. Nevertheless, women who work in day-care centers or elementary schools, where parvovirus outbreaks most often occur, should be aware of the possibility.

Unlike some other viruses, which can cause serious birth defects if a woman catches them during pregnancy, parvovirus does not otherwise harm the baby. It does not cause any congenital malformations.

## Diagnosis

Your doctor can tell just by inspecting your child's rash that he does not have chickenpox or measles,

## CALL YOUR DOCTOR

- If your child has a rash and also has a fever or complains about feeling sick. With fifth disease she is unlikely either to have a fever or to feel sick.

- If your child has sickle cell or other chronic anemia and you learn about an outbreak of fifth disease at her school. Your doctor may want you to keep her home from school until the outbreak is over.

- If you are pregnant and discover you may have been exposed to parvovirus. Your obstetrician will want to monitor the situation.

**NOTE: If your child has fifth disease, you do not necessarily need to call your pediatrician. The rash, if she has it, is the only symptom that might prompt a call. If she is otherwise well and happy and has no fever, you may not need to call. What often happens, however, is that when the school nurse sees the rash, she sends your child home with a note saying you have to see a doctor and find out whether it is something contagious.**

which can be more troublesome than fifth disease.

If your child is grade-school age and has the classic slapped-cheek or lacelike rash, fifth disease is easy for your doctor to recognize, particularly if you tell her about the "cold" he had a few days earlier. Your doctor is also likely to know whether there is an outbreak of parvovirus in your area.

There are blood tests that can tell whether or not your child has been infected by parvovirus. If his blood has a high level of one kind of antibody (immunoglobulin G or IgG), it probably means he had a parvovirus infection at some time in the past and is now immune. If he has a high level of another kind of antibody (immunoglobulin M or IgM), it means he has a current or recent infection.

Since fifth disease is usually so innocuous, however, your pediatrician is not likely to have your child take these blood tests unless he has sickle cell or other chronic anemia. If you are pregnant and exposed to parvovirus, your obstetrician may want to test you to find out whether you are already immune.

## *Treatment*

Your child does not need to take any antibiotics when she has fifth disease. Antibiotics do not kill parvovirus—or any other virus.

There is no specific treatment for fifth disease. Your child's immune system will fight off and kill all the virus particles, and the disease is so mild there is really not much you need do for her except keep her comfortable. If she is bothered by a sore throat or headache, you can give her acetaminophen.

You do not need to keep your child home from day-care or school when she has fifth disease. By the time a child has the rash and you know she has a parvovirus infection, she is no longer shedding virus and able to infect others. Your doctor will probably give you a note for the school nurse saying it is okay for her to return to school.

The rash can last up to ten days or so. Over that time it may tend to intensify and then fade, particularly when your child is warm, out in the sun, or in a warm bath.

## Prevention

As with other viruses that spread from person to person by the respiratory route, you may be able to reduce the spread of parvovirus by teaching your children to wash their hands frequently. Hand washing cannot hurt.

# FOOD POISONING

## SYMPTOMS

**Most common:**

- Vomiting
- Diarrhea
- Abdominal cramps
- Possible fever

**Uncommon, depending on the particular germ involved:**

- Bone or joint infection
- Meningitis
- Seizure
- Kidney damage
- Paralysis
- Liver disease
- Swollen and painful muscles

Ever since nearly 600 people in the Northwest became ill—and several children died—after eating contaminated hamburgers from a fast-food chain in the mid-1990s, Americans have been increasingly concerned about the safety of our food supply. It seems as if almost every time we turn on the TV or pick up a newspaper, there is another headline about a food-poisoning episode: "Thousands of People Ill from Tainted Ice Cream," "Ailment Linked to Raspberries," "Tainted Alfalfa Sprouts Sicken 70 People." At Thanksgiving the food pages instruct us how to stuff our turkey—and at Christmas, how to make eggnog—safely.

Food poisoning causes some 6 million people in the United States to become sick every year, the Public Health Service's Centers for Disease Control and Prevention (CDC) estimates. Some other estimates put the number as high as 81 million people a year. CDC receives reports of 400 to 500 outbreaks—groups of people developing the same illness after eating the same food—every year. The majority of food-poisoning episodes, however, are never reported.

Most of these food-borne illnesses are mild, no more than a few passing twinges in the gut or a few loose stools. However, food poisoning can be far more serious for certain vulnerable people: babies and other young children, the elderly, and people who have chronic diseases or whose immune systems are not normal. The CDC estimates that food poisoning causes the deaths of 9,000 Americans every year.

The good news is that there is much you can do to help prevent your family from contracting food poisoning. According to the U.S. Department of Agriculture, "Some 85 percent of cases could be avoided if people just handled food properly."

## Causes

The most commonly identified culprits are bacteria, with salmonella and the less familiar campylobacter bacteria being the most common causes. Salmonella bacteria sicken 2 to 4 million Americans every year, the CDC estimates, and campylobacter infections may affect 2 to 4 million a year. Salmonella is the most commonly reported cause of food-poisoning outbreaks. Both salmonella and campylobacter infections most often target babies and children under the age of five. For more information, see *Salmonella Infections*, page 231, and *Campylobacter Diarrhea*, page 60.

Another common cause of food poisoning, particularly among preschool children, is a bacterium called *Yersinia enterocolitica*. See *Yersinia Diarrhea*, page 77.

Food poisoning is one of the ways that your child can become infected with shigella bacteria, which cause dysentery (bloody diarrhea). Hundreds of thousands of children and adults in the United States develop shigella infections every year. See *Shigella Diarrhea*, page 72.

The bacterium that contaminated the hamburgers in the Northwest was a particularly dangerous strain—called O157:H7—of a very common bacterium named *E. coli*. The O157:H7 strain was also responsible in 1997 for the largest recall of meat, 25 million pounds of potentially contaminated hamburgers. At least 20,000 people in the United States become sick from the O157:H7 strain each year. See *E. coli Disease*, page 97.

Other common bacteria that can produce food poisoning include *Staphylococcus aureus*, which also causes skin infections, pneumonia, and other diseases, and *Clostridium perfringens*, which causes 10,000 people to become sick each year. Among other bacteria occasionally causing food poisoning are *Bacillus cereus* (which usually causes several outbreaks a year, often related to improperly prepared fried rice), *Streptococcus pyogenes* (group A strep, the strep that causes strep throat), and two vibrios: *Vibrio parahaemolyticus* and *Vibrio vulnificus*.

Less frequently, listeria bacteria cause serious infections in about 1,850 people a year, most of them newborn babies or people whose immune systems are not normal. See *Listeria Infections*, page 166.

Botulism bacteria cause a particularly severe form of food poisoning. They used to cause more disease in the past, and 80 to 150 Americans still contract botulism every year, most of them babies under a year. See *Botulism*, page 16.

Viruses are less commonly identified as causes of food poisoning, but one of the ways your child can catch the hepatitis A virus is in food. (See *Hepatitis A*, page 136.) Other viruses that can spread in food or water include the Norwalk viruses (named for Norwalk, Ohio, where they were first identified) and a number of other gastrointestinal viruses.

Several protozoan parasites—microscopic, single-celled animals related to amebas—can spread in food: *Cryptosporidium parvum*, which most frequently affects children under two years (see *Cryptosporidium Diarrhea*, page 63); *Giardia lamblia*, which also most often infects young children (see *Giardia Diarrhea*, page 67); and *Cyclospora cayetanensus*. Cyclospora protozoans were first identified as a cause of human disease in 1979. Many people first heard of them in the mid-1990s when they turned up in raspberries imported from Guatemala and caused hundreds of people to become sick.

A tiny roundworm called *Trichinella spiralis* causes trichinosis, which a person can get from eating undercooked pork and other meats. Today only a few dozen people a year in the United States get trichinosis. See *Trichinosis*, page 271.

In most episodes of food poisoning, however, no one ever figures out what organism is responsible.

## How Germs Spread to Food

Many of these organisms are present in foods when you buy them at the store. Salmonella, campylobacter, *Y. enterocolitica*, *E. coli*, and listeria bacteria and cryptosporidium protozoans are among the many microbes that live in the intestines of animals, both domestic and wild. The animals are not necessarily sick but shed the organisms in their feces, and the germs can get onto meat when the animals are slaughtered. Germs can thus contaminate almost any raw food of animal origin: meat, poultry, and fish.

These organisms can infect dairy herds, again without making the cows sick, and the germs can spread into milk directly, or milk can become contaminated by cows' feces. Outbreaks of milk-borne food poisoning have occurred when schoolchildren visited dairy farms and were given raw, unpasteurized milk to drink. Listeria bacteria can also turn up in unpasteurized cheeses.

These same germs can contaminate the surfaces of fruits and vegetables if farm animals are kept in or near the fields or orchards where they are grown or if animal manure is used to fertilize these crops. People have caught food poisoning when they drank fresh, unpasteurized cider made from "drop" apples thus tainted with *E. coli* or salmonella bacteria or cryptosporidium protozoans.

Salmonella bacteria can contaminate eggs, not only the outside of an eggshell, from chicken feces, but also the inside of eggs. They can infect the ovaries of seemingly healthy hens, which then deposit the bacteria inside the shell before it hardens.

Pigs particularly and some wild animals (e.g., bears) can become infected with the trichinella worms that cause trichinosis when they eat the meat of other, infected animals. The larvae of the trichinella worms form cysts in the muscles—the meat—of animals they infect.

Some other food-poisoning germs—including shigella and *E. coli* bacteria, hepatitis A virus, and giardia protozoans—normally live in the intestines of human beings. Infected people shed these germs in their stools and can get them

on their hands when they go to the toilet. If they do not wash their hands afterward, they can then contaminate any food they are preparing or serving. And a person can shed these organisms without realizing it. You can be infected with shigella without having any symptoms, and with hepatitis A you shed the greatest number of virus particles while you are incubating the disease, the week before you discover you are sick.

*Staphylococcus aureus* bacteria also normally live on human beings. At any one time, about 30 percent of us carry Staph aureus, as it is called, on our skin or in our noses, throats, or hair. People can also shed Staph aureus from sores on their hands. Such carriers can contaminate any food they touch. Once in a food, Staph aureus multiplies rapidly at room temperature and produces a toxin (poison) that causes food-poisoning symptoms.

Flies can deposit salmonella and shigella bacteria onto foods if they first land on animal or human feces containing these germs. Flies can carry the bacteria on their legs, or they can get them in their gut and shed them in their own feces.

Some bacteria—*Clostridium botulinum* (which causes botulism), *C. perfringens,* and *Bacillus cereus*—are virtually everywhere around us because they form tough, dormant cells called spores. These spores are normal inhabitants of soil, and they float in the air and form part of our house dust. They thus may contaminate the surfaces of fruits, vegetables, and other produce. Cooking does not necessarily destroy these spores, which can also drift into foods after they are cooked. If you leave food out at room temperature, these spores can germinate and produce toxins in the food. Children in day-care centers became sick from *B. cereus* toxin when the bacteria grew in cooked rice that was held at room temperature and then only briefly stir-fried.

Botulinus spores germinate—and make a particularly potent toxin—only in places where there is little or no oxygen. People most commonly get food-borne botulism from inadequately processed home-canned foods. Or the spores can grow inside a baby's intestines and make their poison there.

When oysters and clams grow in water polluted with human sewage, they can become contaminated with hepatitis A, Norwalk, or other viruses. These mollusks feed by pumping great quantities of sea water through their bodies, filtering out the nutrients they need, a process that tends to concentrate in their bodies any germs that may be in the water. When we eat these mollusks raw or undercooked—and we often eat them whole, gut and all—we ingest whatever germs they may have in their digestive tracts.

You yourself can easily introduce germs into foods in your own kitchen if you do not wash your hands before you start to prepare or serve food. You can also spread germs by using the same knife or cutting board you used for meat or poultry to prepare other foods—to cut up vegetables for a salad, for instance—without first washing the knife and board. You can also contaminate cooked meat or other food if you serve it on the same platter you used for raw meat or poultry.

## Incubation Period

How long it takes for a person to become ill after ingesting a germ in food varies considerably. Staph aureus or *B. cereus* bacteria may cause symptoms within thirty to sixty minutes. Salmonella bacteria may cause a person to become sick in anywhere from six hours to ten days. Campylobacter bacteria usually take one

to seven days. With giardia protozoans, it can be one to four weeks; with listeria bacteria, it is usually three weeks; and with hepatitis A virus, it averages four weeks.

## Symptoms

Most people who contract food poisoning—as the bacteria or virus particles multiply in their intestinal tract—develop gastrointestinal symptoms: diarrhea or vomiting or both. Your child may also have a fever and painful cramps in the abdomen. The stools may be watery, or they may contain mucus or blood. Salmonella, campylobacter, shigella, and *Y. enterocolitica* bacteria are the most common causes of bloody diarrhea in children. Both staph aureus and *B. cereus* bacteria produce toxins that cause vomiting. See "Symptoms," page 52, in *Diarrhea*.

Some strains of *E. coli* are a leading cause of so-called traveler's diarrhea, which a person may catch by eating contaminated food or drinking polluted water while traveling in developing countries. Shigella, salmonella, and campylobacter bacteria and giardia protozoans are also among the germs that can cause traveler's diarrhea.

The danger of diarrhea and vomiting is that they may cause your child to become dangerously dehydrated. Body fluid is being lost through the diarrhea and vomiting. If she has a fever, she is also losing fluid through increased evaporation from her skin. Babies particularly can very quickly develop serious—even life-threatening—dehydration. See *Fluids*, page 290, in the Appendices for more about dehydration.

Less commonly, food poisoning can cause other severe or life-threatening symptoms. Occasionally salmonella or other bacteria spread out of a person's intestinal tract into other parts of the body and cause bone or joint infection or meningitis (inflammation of the membranes covering the brain). Such severe salmonella infections kill about 500 people a year in the United States, according to the CDC.

Some strains of shigella bacteria produce a toxin that rarely can cause a child to have a seizure. The dangerous O157:H7 strain of *E. coli* bacteria makes a toxin that can damage a person's kidneys, causing a life-threatening disease called hemolytic uremic syndrome (HUS). The CDC estimates that the O157:H7 strain kills 250 Americans a year.

Listeria bacteria cause little illness in most healthy people, but if a woman develops a listeria infection while she is pregnant, it can harm her baby. Listeria infections kill about one out of four people who develop them, 425 people a year, mostly newborn babies and people whose immune systems are not normal.

Botulism bacteria can cause a particularly severe form of food poisoning, which can kill a person by paralyzing his respiratory muscles; food-borne botulism causes two or three deaths a year in the United States.

The hepatitis A virus grows in a person's liver, and children may develop fever, nausea, and jaundice and lose several weeks or more from school.

In trichinosis the larvae of the trichinella worm migrate into a person's muscles and cause them to become swollen and painful. The person may have trouble breathing or his heart can fail. Today deaths from trichinosis are exceedingly rare.

For more about these other symptoms of food poisoning, see the "Symptoms" section in the chapters about each disease.

Infection with *V. vulnificus* bacteria from raw or undercooked oysters or other shellfish causes no harm to most healthy people, but for people with liver or other chronic diseases or whose immune systems are not normal, it can be one of the deadliest forms of food poisoning. It kills an average of seventeen or eighteen people a year in the Gulf Coast states.

## CALL YOUR DOCTOR

- If your child has diarrhea and is under twelve months old.

- If your child has any blood or mucus in her stools, is having watery bowel movements more than ten times a day, or has diarrhea with abdominal pain for more than an hour.

- If your child is showing any signs of dehydration: if she is not urinating as much as usual, if her mouth is dry, or if she is less active than usual.

NOTE: For when to call your physician for other food-borne diseases, see the "Call Your Doctor" box in the chapter about each disease.

## *Diagnosis*

If your child has diarrhea, your physician can find out what germ is responsible by having a laboratory try to culture (grow) the organism from a sample of his stool. If your child is vomiting excessively, the doctor may try to culture the germ from the material he is vomiting up.

Most of the time, however, this is not necessary. If your child has mild diarrhea that is not bloody and he has had diarrhea for only a few days, your physician probably will not attempt to identify the germ causing it.

At Children's Hospital we have our lab culture a child's stool sample if she has had diarrhea for more than five days or if her stools contain any blood or mucus. We routinely have our lab test for the four bacteria that most commonly cause bloody diarrhea in children: salmonella, campylobacter, shigella, and *Yersinia enterocolitica.*

If doctors suspect a child's diarrhea is caused by any of the protozoan parasites—cryptosporidium, giardia, or cyclospora—they have a lab inspect a sample of his stool under a microscope.

For more about how doctors diagnose each of the other food-borne diseases, see the "Diagnosis" section in the chapter about each illness.

When a significant outbreak of apparent food poisoning occurs, health-care workers interview the affected people to find out what food or foods they all ate in common. Then they have a lab test samples of the suspect foods, if they are still available, to try to identify the responsible germ. If an outbreak causes a potentially serious form of food poisoning, such as botulism, trichinosis, or *E. coli* infection, they also try to track down other people who may have eaten the contaminated food to make sure that they get any necessary treatment.

## Treatment

Gastrointestinal symptoms from food poisoning—diarrhea or vomiting—usually go away on their own as a person's immune system kills off all the bacteria or virus particles or the toxins are cleared from the system. Diarrhea due to salmonella, for instance, usually disappears in a few days or a week, although it sometimes can last longer. With the protozoan parasites cryptosporidium, giardia, or cyclospora, however, the diarrhea may last for a prolonged period, weeks or months.

Whenever your child has diarrhea, whatever the cause, the main treatment is to make sure he takes in enough extra fluids to replace the fluids he is losing through his frequent stools and through any vomiting or fever. If your baby is under a year, doctors advise that you give special fluids called oral rehydration solutions.

See *Fluids,* page 290, in the Appendices for more about these fluids, how to give them, and what fluids to offer and not offer older children.

See also "Treatment," page 57, in *Diarrhea* for information about what else to do and not do when your child has diarrhea.

For most types of diarrhea, your child usually does not need to take any antibiotics or other medications. There are no antiviral drugs that can kill the gastrointestinal viruses, and even for most food-borne bacteria, antibiotics usually do not help and may actually hurt. With most salmonella infections, for instance, antibiotics do not shorten the time that a child has diarrhea and may make him worse by prolonging the time he carries the bacteria in his intestines.

For some types of diarrhea, however, your child does need medication. If he has dysentery due to shigella bacteria, he needs an antibiotic. Shigella is among the few germs causing diarrhea in children in which antibiotics make a significant difference in promoting a speedy recovery. If a child has protracted diarrhea due to campylobacter or *Y. enterocolitica* bacteria, he may also need antibiotics. And, for diarrhea due to the protozoan parasites giardia and cyclospora, physicians also do prescribe medications. There are no known drugs, however, that kill cryptosporidium protozoans effectively.

If a child develops a severe salmonella infection outside his intestinal tract, in his blood or elsewhere, he needs antibiotics. And if a pregnant woman has a listeria infection, her physician can treat her with antibiotics. This may enable her baby to be born healthy.

People who have *V. vulnificus* infections from eating tainted raw oysters or other shellfish are treated with antibiotics. The disease can be fatal in those with cirrhosis, diabetes mellitus, or with a weakened immune system, causing death in more than 40 percent of those who develop it.

There are no antiviral drugs that can kill the hepatitis A virus. In time, a person's immune system destroys all the virus particles, but in the meantime he needs to rest and eat a nourishing diet. Most people recover completely.

The few people who get trichinosis these days take antiparasite agents to kill the trichinella worms. If a person has severe trichinosis, he may need to be hospitalized.

People who develop botulism from contaminated food must be hospitalized, often in an intensive care unit. If her throat muscles are affected, she may need to be fed by tube. If her respiratory muscles are weakened, she may need to be on a respirator.

Again, for more about the treatment of these food-borne illnesses, see the "Treatment" sections in the chapters about each disease.

## Prevention

Remember: disease-causing organisms may contaminate almost any raw food of animal origin: meat, poultry, seafood, eggs, and unpasteurized milk and other unpasteurized dairy products.

About one-third to one-half of raw chicken contains campylobacter bacteria, according to the U.S. Department of Agriculture (USDA), and 20 percent has salmonella bacteria. About 1 percent of raw beef and 5 to 7 percent of ground beef have salmonella. Hamburger is probably more likely to be contaminated than other cuts of beef because the process of grinding can mix any germs on the meat's surface throughout the interior. Raw pork is the most common source of *Y. enterocolitica* bacteria, and a small percentage of raw pork still contains the microscopic trichinella worms that cause trichinosis.

In some parts of the country, one out of every 10,000 eggs, according to the U.S. Public Health Service, may be contaminated with salmonella bacteria inside the shell.

Most food poisoning from seafood comes from eating raw oysters, clams, or mussels. One out of every 1,000 or 2,000 servings of these raw mollusks is likely to make someone sick, says the Food and Drug Administration (FDA), which regulates seafood. If these mollusks are illegally harvested from polluted waters, they may contain hepatitis A, Norwalk, or other gastrointestinal viruses or such bacteria as campylobacter, salmonella, or shigella. Oysters particularly can contain the deadly *V. vulnificus* bacteria, even if harvested legally from unpolluted waters.

Fruits and vegetables are less common sources of food poisoning, but they, too, can have germs on their surfaces from soil or from animal manure or human feces. In one study researchers found that 10 percent of honey samples they tested contained botulinus spores.

Here is a list of tips for preventing food poisoning:

- Remember that these germs can multiply rapidly in foods—to dangerous levels—when the food is held at temperatures between 40°F and 140°F, including at room temperatures. Therefore, plan your food-shopping expeditions so that you do other errands first and buy food last. In the store, select frozen foods and other foods that need to be refrigerated last. Avoid letting food sit in a hot car; drive home promptly.

• When you get home, promptly refrigerate meats, poultry, eggs, seafood, and other perishable foods. Raw juices from these foods often contain bacteria or other germs; make sure that you put the packages away so that they do not touch and their juices do not drip onto other foods. Keep eggs refrigerated at all times to prevent any salmonella from growing; do not buy eggs that are not refrigerated.

Your refrigerator should run at 40°F or below, advises the USDA. This temperature does not kill bacteria or other germs, but it does keep most of them from multiplying. Listeria and *Y. enterocolitica* bacteria, however, can grow in food even in the refrigerator.

If you are not going to use meat, poultry, or fish within a few days, freeze it immediately, advises the USDA. Your freezer should run at a temperature of 0°F or below. Again, freezing does not kill bacteria and other germs, but it does stop their growth.

With bottled and other processed foods, be sure to read their labels to find out whether you need to refrigerate them. Some are all right to keep on a shelf at room temperature before you use them, but once you open the jar or can, it may need to be refrigerated.

• Before you start preparing any food, always be sure to wash your hands with soap and warm water for at least 20

seconds, advise both the USDA and FDA, also making sure you do not have dirt under your fingernails. You may have all sorts of germs on your hands—from touching doorknobs, money, counters in stores, your children's toys, garden soil—and you do not want to introduce these germs into the foods you are fixing. Also wash your hands, adds the USDA, after you use the bathroom, before you start working with a new food or a new tool, when you finish food preparation, and before you serve food.

Dogs, cats, and other pets can get many germs on their paws and fur from soil outside and from their own feces. Cats, particularly, can pick up germs as they scratch in their litter boxes. Keep your pets away from your food and cooking equipment and off your kitchen countertops and dining tables. Wash your hands after you handle your pets before you touch any food.

Rinse fruits and vegetables thoroughly in water before you serve them, particularly those you are going to eat raw. When you are traveling abroad in developing countries, be particularly careful about raw fruits and vegetables. The general rule in these places, says the Public Health Service, is "Boil it, cook it, peel it, or forget it."

When you thaw frozen meat, poultry, or fish, do it in your refrigerator or microwave or in cold water, not out on your countertop at room temperature—which could allow bacteria and other germs to grow. Also, when you marinate food, do so in the refrigerator.

When you are preparing meat, poultry, or fish, be careful that you do not let any germs they may contain contaminate other foods in your kitchen. The USDA advises that you use a plastic rather than a wooden cutting board because the grooves in a wooden board could trap bacteria. Promptly wipe up any meat, poultry, or fish juices that spill on your countertop. After you have cut or trimmed these foods, scrub—with hot water and soap—your knife, cutting board, and any other utensils before you use them for any other food. And after handling raw meat, poultry, or fish, wash your hands again.

• To kill any bacteria or other germs that may be present in meat, poultry, or fish, you need to cook them thoroughly. "Thorough cooking . . . is the single most important step in preventing food-borne disease," the Public Health Service emphasizes.

The USDA recommends that you cook red meats—beef (including hamburger), lamb, veal, and pork—to an interior temperature of 160°F, measured with a meat thermometer. Red meat is done when it has turned gray or brown inside. Thorough cooking is particularly important for hamburgers because any germs could be mixed throughout the interior of the patties. CDC advises that you cook pork to a temperature of 170°F to destroy the trichinella worms that cause trichinosis.

Cook chicken and other poultry—turkey, duck, and goose—to 180° or 185°F, the USDA recommends, and until the juices run clear. At Thanksgiving—or anytime you stuff a turkey—stuff it just before you cook it. Do not stuff the turkey at home and then drive it for hours to grandmother's house. Use a meat thermometer, the USDA emphasizes, to make sure that the stuffing reaches a temperature of 165°F.

Fish is done when it flakes with a fork.

Eggs should also be cooked thoroughly, says the USDA. For information about how to cook eggs so they are safe, see "Prevention," page 235, in *Salmonella Infections.*

After cooking meat, poultry, or fish, do not put it back on the same platter or board you used when it was raw. Use a clean platter instead. When you are barbecuing outdoors, carry out a second platter to hold the grilled food.

If you marinate meat, poultry, or fish, remember that the marinade may pick up germs from the food in it. Heat it to boiling before you pour it back on cooked food.

Always cool foods in the refrigerator, not out at room temperature where germs could multiply. Cooking does not necessary kill all the germs in food; remember that some bacteria—including the one that causes botulism—form heat-resistant spores, and these spores can also drift into food after it is cooked. At room temperatures these bacteria can grow and make their poisons.

If you are serving a buffet, the USDA advises that you not leave the food out at room temperature for longer than two hours, while the FDA and Public Health Service both recommend that you not leave food out for more than four hours.

When you are reheating leftovers or takeout food, remember that some bacteria can grow even in the refrigerator. Bring sauces and soups to a boil, and heat other foods to a temperature of 165°F, that is, until they are hot and steaming.

Obviously, you should not serve or eat any food that looks, smells, or tastes bad. You should discard most moldy food because the mold you see on the surface is only the tip of an iceberg, so to speak; some molds can form poisons that may penetrate deeper down in a food. You should also toss—and not buy—any cans that are dented or swollen; when botulinus bacteria grow in a can, they produce a gas that may cause a can to bulge. "When in doubt," advises the USDA, "throw it out."

If you can foods at home, you need to use a pressure cooker when processing most foods in order to heat them to temperatures high enough to kill any botulinus spores. See "Prevention," page 19, in *Botulism*.

These precautions are particularly important for the people most at risk of developing serious disease from food poisoning: the very young and very old and people with chronic diseases or immune systems that are not normal. And certain people should avoid certain foods completely.

Babies under twelve months should not be given honey, both the U.S. Public Health Service and the American Academy of Pediatrics

recommend, to prevent the possibility of their developing botulism. See "Prevention," page 19, in *Botulism*.

Pregnant women, says the Academy of Pediatrics, "should avoid unpasteurized dairy products, soft cheeses and undercooked meats" to avoid infection with listeria bacteria, which could harm their unborn babies. See "Prevention," page 166, in *Listeria Infections*.

No one should drink raw, unpasteurized milk, advise both the Health Service and the Academy of Pediatrics, because there are so many germs that it may contain, including salmonella, campylobacter, and the dangerous O157:H7 strain of *E. coli*. Pasteurization, by heating milk, kills these germs and makes milk safe. Serve only pasteurized milk to your family.

You can protect your family and yourself against *E. coli* and other germs in apple cider by drinking only pasteurized or heat-treated cider.

To prevent food poisoning from spreading among children in day-care centers, the American Academy of Pediatrics recommends that centers have separate areas for fixing food and for changing children's diapers. If possible, different people should prepare food and change diapers or help toddlers go to the toilet. For more information, see *Recommendations for Day-Care Providers*, page 297, in the Appendices.

To prevent hepatitis A, a vaccine has been available since 1995. The Public Health Service recommends that you and your children receive this vaccine if you are traveling to countries where hepatitis A is more prevalent than it is here. If you know you have been exposed to hepatitis A, in food or elsewhere, and you have not been vaccinated against it, you can get temporary protection by taking a shot of immunoglobulin (IG) within two weeks after exposure. See "Prevention," page 138, in *Hepatitis A*.

## Resources

You can obtain additional information about handling and cooking food safely from the U.S. Department of Agriculture's toll-free Meat and Poultry Hotline at 1-800-535-4555 (1-202-720-3333 in the Washington, D.C., area). One of the most frequently asked questions on the hotline, says the USDA, is "I accidentally left food out overnight. Is it safe to eat?" The answer is "No. Throw it out." You can also connect to the USDA on the Internet at http://www.usda.gov.

For information about preparing fish and shellfish safely, you can call the Food and Drug Administration's Seafood Hotline, 1-800-FDA-4010 (1-202-205-4314 in the Washington area). The FDA also has a Consumer Information Line: 1-800-532-4440 (1-301-827-4420 in the Washington area). You can contact the FDA on the Internet at http://www.fda.gov.

If your child or you become involved in a significant episode of food poisoning, particularly if the suspect food comes from a restaurant or other commercial source, call your physician, or notify your local or state health department. Food poisoning that is mild for you could be more serious for someone else who is more vulnerable.

# HEMOPHILUS INFECTIONS

*A vaccine is available to protect your child against* Haemophilus influenzae *type b infections. See* Vaccines, *page 301, in the Appendices, for a list of all the vaccines your child needs.*

*A severe* Haemophilus influenzae *type b infection must be treated by a doctor and usually requires hospitalization.*

*Haem-* means "blood," and the ending *-philus* comes from the Greek word for "loving."

## SYMPTOMS

- Meningitis
- Epiglottitis
- Swollen, tender joints
- Pneumonia
- Skin infections (facial)

You may be familiar with the name *Haemophilus* because your baby probably started receiving a series of vaccine shots against this bacterium when she was about two months old.

The full name of this bacterium is a long one, *Haemophilus influenzae* type b, and it is a very dangerous germ. It causes severe, life-threatening diseases in children, most commonly meningitis, which is an infection of the membranes covering a child's brain and spinal cord.

Before the introduction of hemophilus vaccine, one out of every 200 children in the United States—12,000 to 18,000 children a

year—developed a serious hemophilus type b infection before he was five years old, according to the U.S. Public Health Service's Centers for Disease Control and Prevention. These infections killed about one out of every 20 infected children, 600 to 900 children each year.

Hemophilus type b bacteria particularly target infants and toddlers between the ages of three months and three years, at the age when their immune systems are not yet fully developed. About half of the infections are in babies under one year. And children who attend day-care centers are two or three times more likely to catch hemophilus infections than are children cared for at home.

Since the first hemophilus vaccine was introduced, in 1985, the vaccines have dramatically reduced the incidence of these severe hemophilus type b infections. At The Children's Hospital of Philadelphia, we used to see seventy to ninety children a year with severe diseases caused by this organism. Today we see fewer than three a year. This shows how important vaccines can be in preventing disease.

## Cause

The *Haemophilus influenzae* bacterium acquired the *haemophilus* part of its name because it has an affinity for blood. The bacterium got the *influenzae* part of its name because physicians at one time thought it was the cause of influenza. It does *not* cause influenza, but it was not until the 1930s that scientists discovered that the true cause of influenza is a virus, now just called influenza virus. For some reason, *H. influenzae* hung onto its misleading name.

There are several different types of *H. influenzae* bacteria, but "type b" was responsible for 95 percent of the serious hemophilus disease in children and is therefore the one that the vaccine protects your baby against. All types of hemophilus bacteria make their home only in human beings.

## How They Spread

Hemophilus bacteria are among the many common microorganisms that normally live in our nasal passages. Virtually every child carries hemophilus in his nose. Before the vaccine, about 5 percent of children at any one time carried type b—without having any symptoms. Your child could thus catch a serious hemophilus type b disease from another child who was not sick at all.

Such hemophilus carriers, as well as children with active hemophilus infections, shed the bacteria in their nasal secretions. When they sneeze or cough without covering their nose or throat—or even when they just talk—they can propel the bacteria several feet into the air, inside droplets of their secretions, and spray them directly on your child.

The classic situation is in day-care. One child sneezes, and ten other children may be exposed to hemophilus.

These other children can inhale the hemophilus bacteria inside the droplets of moisture into their nasal passages, where the bacteria grow and multiply. From a child's nose hemophilus bacteria can also sometimes spread into his bloodstream and from there into other tissues and organs of his body. This is how hemophilus type b can cause serious disease.

Because so many children have now been vaccinated against hemophilus type b, today it is unusual for a child to carry these bacteria. The vaccine not only reduced hemophilus disease, but it also reduced carriage, the amount of hemophilus type b bacteria in children's noses. So now there is less child-to-child transmission.

## Incubation Period

How long it takes for a child to become sick after being infected with hemophilus type b bacteria is not known. The time probably varies considerably.

## Symptoms

In unvaccinated children, *H. influenzae* type b bacteria can cause meningitis when they spread from a child's bloodstream into the membranes (meninges) covering the brain and spinal cord, causing these membranes to become infected and inflamed.

Before the vaccine, meningitis due to hemophilus type b bacteria used to take a terrible toll. Hemophilus type b was the most common cause of bacterial meningitis, the most serious kind of meningitis. Some 8,000 to 10,000 babies and toddlers in the United States developed hemophilus meningitis each year. It killed 400 to 500 children a year and left many of the survivors deaf or mentally retarded.

Since the introduction of the vaccine, the number of children developing meningitis due to hemophilus type b bacteria has declined dramatically, by more than 95 percent.

*See* Meningitis, *page 183, for more about this disease, the other germs that can also cause it, and the symptoms that should prompt you to call your doctor.*

Hemophilus type b infections also used to be the major cause of another potentially life-threatening disease—fortunately always rare—called epiglottitis.

The epiglottis is a flap of tissue in the throat. Hemophilus bacteria growing on a child's epiglottis can cause it to become so swollen that it blocks the windpipe, interrupting the flow of air to the lungs. Epiglottitis can develop so rapidly that it can totally obstruct a child's airway within hours.

Before the vaccine, hemophilus type b bacteria were responsible for 95 percent of episodes of epiglottitis. At Children's Hospital we saw about ten children each year who had epiglottitis. Today, thanks to the vaccine, it is rare to see a case of epiglottitis.

*See* Epiglottitis, *page 105, for more about this disease and the signs that should alert you to call 911 or take your child to your hospital emergency room.*

Hemophilus type b bacteria can also spread to a child's lungs and cause pneumonia. They can multiply in the blood itself, an infection called bacteremia. They can cause an inflammation of the membrane covering the heart (pericarditis). They can also invade a child's joints or grow in tissues under her skin, particularly around her eyes or cheeks, a condition known as cellulitis. Again, thanks to the vaccine, hemophilus type b bacteria today rarely cause these diseases.

Since hemophilus vaccine is effective only against type b strains of the bacteria, however, hemophilus bacteria that are *not* type b are still around. These other hemophilus bacteria commonly cause sinus and middle-ear infections in children. The vaccine has had no impact on the occurrence of these diseases.

## Diagnosis

If physicians suspect a child has meningitis, they find out what organism—whether hemophilus or some other germ—is causing his symptoms by obtaining a sample of the fluid surrounding the spinal cord and having a laboratory culture (grow) and identify the organism.

A physician obtains a sample of the child's spinal fluid by performing a procedure called a lumbar puncture (spinal tap). Using a local anesthetic, the doctor inserts a special needle through his back into the spinal canal and withdraws some of the fluid. For more about this lumbar-puncture procedure, see "Diagnosis," page 185, in *Meningitis*.

If emergency room doctors suspect a child has epiglottitis, an Ear, Nose and Throat doctor inspects the airway in a controlled way with anesthesia and a laryngoscope, to see if his epiglottis is indeed swollen. After the child receives emergency treatment to open his airway, they may draw a sample of his blood and have the lab culture and identify the responsible germ. See "Diagnosis," page 107, in *Epiglottitis*.

To diagnose whether haemophilus is the germ causing a child's other disease, physicians may have the lab try to culture the bacteria from his blood or from another body fluid.

## Treatment

Both meningitis and epiglottitis are medical emergencies.

If a child has hemophilus meningitis, she must be admitted to the hospital, sometimes to an intensive care unit, and promptly treated with doses of intravenous antibiotics to kill the bacteria. See "Treatment," page 186, in *Meningitis*.

If a child has epiglottitis, the emergency room physicians immediately make sure her airway is open enough that she can breathe. This may involve inserting a breathing tube down into her windpipe which is almost always performed in the Operating Room by an ENT physician. She must be admitted to an intensive care unit in the hospital, where her condition can be monitored closely and she can be treated with an intravenous antibiotic. See "Treatment," page 107, in *Epiglottitis*.

## Prevention

*Both the U.S. Public Health Service and the American Academy of Pediatrics recommend that children routinely be vaccinated against* Haemophilus influenzae *type b bacteria.*

Your baby needs an initial series of two or three doses of hemophilus vaccine, depending on the brand of vaccine your pediatrician chooses. Your baby gets his first shot when he is about two months old and his second shot at four months. If your doctor has chosen a vaccine brand that requires a third shot, your baby should get it when he is about six months old.

Your child then needs a booster shot of hemophilus type b vaccine when he is between the ages of twelve and fifteen months.

If your baby attends a day-care center, you should make particularly sure that he gets all these shots. Because children who go to day-care are at increased risk for hemophilus type b diseases, "efforts should be made," the Public Health Service emphasizes, "to ensure that all day-care attendees less than five years of age are fully vaccinated."

Hemophilus type b vaccines are among the safest of vaccines. All of the brands consist of pieces of the bacterium's outer coat, which can stimulate your baby's immune system to develop protective antibodies against the bacteria. Your child cannot get a hemophilus infection from any of these vaccines.

Your baby is also unlikely to have any significant adverse reactions to hemophilus vaccine.

About one baby in four has some mild redness, swelling or pain at the injection site. This usually disappears within twenty-four hours. About one child in a hundred has a fever over 101°F or diarrhea or vomiting or an episode of crying.

If a child does develop hemophilus meningitis or any other hemophilus type b disease, it means that other people living in the same household, adults or children, may also be carrying the bacteria in their nasal passages, even if they are not sick. Any other child in the household who is younger than four years and who has not received all his hemophilus shots could also catch the bacteria from these carriers and develop a serious hemophilus infection.

The U.S. Public Health Service and the American Academy of Pediatrics therefore recommend that any such unvaccinated child and everyone else in the household (except pregnant women) should—as soon as possible—take a course of the antibiotic rifampin to eliminate any hemophilus bacteria from their noses.

If a child who develops hemophilus disease has been attending a day-care center, his physician may recommend that all the children attending the center, as well as the staff, also take rifampin.

## Resources

You can get more information about hemophilus infections and hemophilus type b vaccine by calling the automated voice system of the Public Health Service's Centers for Disease Control and Prevention (CDC) at 1-800-232-SHOT or by connecting to their web site on the Internet at http://www.cdc.gov.

# HAND, FOOT, AND MOUTH DISEASE

Also called coxsackie virus.

## SYMPTOMS

- Achy feeling

- Sore throat

- Low-grade fever

- Loss of appetite

- Crankiness

- Lesions on hands, feet, and mouth and diaper area

This common childhood illness is aptly named, for it characteristically causes ulcers that appear on the hands, feet, and mouth. Many children who are infected do not get sick, and they may develop immunity without actually having the illness. Complications are rare.

Some children experience mild symptoms, while some experience no symptoms at all. For others the infection causes painful blisters in the mouth (in the back of the throat), on the palms and fingers of the hand, or on the soles of the feet. The blisters are filled with fluid that contains the virus.

Generally we see young children under the age of ten with hand, foot, and mouth disease because it spreads easily through hand-to-mouth contact. Young children tend to put their fingers in their mouths. For example, a child may touch his diaper area, get the virus on his hands, then suck his thumb or put his fingers in his mouth or in another child's mouth.

## Causes

The disease results from a virus called coxsackie virus A16, which belongs to the enterovirus family. Enteroviruses are common viruses that live only in humans. They are spread through the mouth and the feces. There are other coxsackie viruses besides A16 that sometimes cause hand, foot, and mouth disease. While it is possible to get hand, foot, and mouth disease again from a different coxsackie virus, it is unlikely.

## *How It Spreads*

When the virus in the blisters passes to another person, the disease spreads. The virus may be passed through the saliva from blisters in the mouth or through the fluid from blisters on the hands or feet. Another way the virus spreads is through the feces of an infected person. It does not really make sense to isolate a child with the disease because the virus can be excreted for weeks after the symptoms have disappeared.

## *Incubation Period*

The symptoms of hand, foot, and mouth disease usually develop after an incubation period of three to six days.

## *Symptoms*

Like many viral infections, hand, foot, and mouth disease often begins with symptoms of a common cold (achy feeling, sore throat, low-grade fever, and loss of appetite). Your child will be cranky, particularly when he begins to get the mouth ulcers. Generally there is a skin eruption on the hands before the ulcers erupt in the mouth. You might see anywhere from 30 to 100 lesions on the palms and soles and, on average, about 10 in the mouth, at the back of the throat. Initially the sores are very tiny (pinpoint sized), but within a couple of days, they get larger and become quite painful. The symptoms may last for seven to ten days.

## CALL YOUR DOCTOR

- If there are blisters on your child's hands, feet, and mouth, accompanied by a fever that does not go down after a couple of days.

- If the blisters bleed.

## Diagnosis

Your doctor will diagnose hand, foot, and mouth disease based on the course it follows and the symptoms. Ordinarily your physician will not need to do any tests to determine this disease. If your child is very ill, the disease can be confirmed by cultures of the throat or of the mouth lesions and from stool cultures.

## Treatment

There is no specific treatment for hand, foot, and mouth disease. The disease is self-limiting, which means that your child will recover without necessary medical intervention. Treatment is aimed at relieving your child's discomfort.

Because the lesions can be quite painful, your child may be very uncomfortable. Try giving her soothing mouthwashes, avoiding those that contain alcohol, phenol, or aromatic hydrocarbons. You can use a teaspoon of a mixture of one-half Maalox and one-half Benadryl as a mouth rinse mouth every two hours. If old enough, have your child rinse it around her mouth for two minutes and spit it out. Or for younger children, put the mixture on cotton tipped applicators. Or try stirring one teaspoon of baking soda in one quart of water. Have your child swish it around her mouth, then spit it out. Water or normal saline solution three times daily is also a good rinse-and-spit routine. Use nonaspirin pain relievers for fever and pain. Give your child small amounts of liquid frequently (she will welcome bland liquids and ice pops or fruit slushies). Avoid spicy food (no pepperoni pizza or buffalo wings, please).

Some doctors may recommend applying a topical anesthetic like lidocaine or benzocaine to the affected area with a cotton swab. Sometimes this is mixed with the Maalox and Benadryl mouthwash mentioned above. Ask your doctor whether this is necessary and advisable for your child's situation

## Prevention

Emphasize basic hand washing, especially after going to the bathroom, blowing the nose, and before or after eating. If you are going to change the diaper of an infected child, be certain to wash your hands thoroughly afterward. This is particularly important in nursery school or in a child-care center where the virus can infect the whole school. There is no point in isolating a child with this disease because the virus remains active after the symptoms are gone, so it can still spread. To prevent other family members from getting the disease, be vigilant about washing your sick child's towels and bedding.

# HEPATITIS A

*There is a vaccine against hepatitis A that is recommended for some children and adults. See* Vaccines, *page 301, in the Appendices for a list of all the vaccines your child needs.*

*Hepatitis A must be treated by a doctor.*

It gets its name from the latin roots *hepar* (liver) and *-itis* (inflammation); thus the word *hepatitis* refers to any inflammatory process involving the liver.

## SYMPTOMS

- Fatigue

- Jaundice (yellow skin or eyes)

- Foul breath and bitter taste in mouth

- Dark urine

- White or light-colored stools

- Vomiting and/or abdominal pain below either the right or left ribs

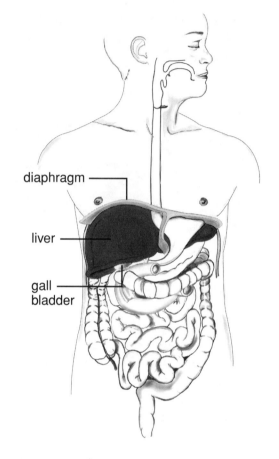

*The liver within the body.*

Hepatitis A is a highly contagious disease that affects the liver. The liver is the largest organ inside the body and one of the most vital, performing over 400 functions. An inflammation can adversely affect many of its functions. There are different, distinct types of hepatitis, of which hepatitis A is one.

The U.S. Public Health Service's Centers for Disease Control and Prevention (CDC) estimates that each year in the United States about 138,000 people of all ages get hepatitis A. This disease can be so benign that medical tests reveal that about 40 percent of urban Americans have had hepatitis A but only 5 percent remember being sick.

You may be completely unaware that you have had this disease.

In children, hepatitis A is the most common form of hepatitis. A person contracts hepatitis A by touching or eating anything that has been contaminated with the virus, which can pass through the mouth and into the body.

A person is at risk for acquiring hepatitis A if he has contact with someone who has the infection or with a worker who is handling infected animals. If a person travels to countries where hepatitis A is common, or shares a household or has sexual contact with an infected person, he is more likely to contract the virus. A person can also get this disease from a blood transfusion.

Hepatitis A infection generally doesn't last longer than two months. Once infected with the hepatitis A virus, a person has a lifelong immunity from future hepatitis A infections.

## Causes

Hepatitis A is caused by the hepatitis A virus (HAV), which can be found in the stools of infected individuals.

## How It Spreads

Hepatitis A is contagious and is spread through the oral-fecal route. The virus also spreads in contaminated water and foods, especially shellfish and milk, which is why it's easy for HAV to spread in overcrowded, unsanitary living conditions like residential institutions or day-care centers. Hepatitis A virus can live in the environment for long periods and will continue to thrive in water and ice, so freezing food does not kill the virus. Cooking food or boiling liquid at 185°F, however, will eradicate it.

If you eat food or beverages that have been handled by an infected individual and not subsequently cooked, you may get hepatitis A. Unsanitary conditions in institutions or day-care centers encourage the spread of this virus. We have seen outbreaks among children and employees in day-care centers since the 1970s. These outbreaks may be caused by careless hygiene among staff members whose jobs include changing diapers and also preparing food—a combination that requires stringent hygiene practices. In centers in which children are toilet trained and nobody is handling soiled diapers, we rarely see hepatitis A outbreaks.

Because young children often have no symptoms, hepatitis A is sometimes not recognized until an adult, frequently a parent of an infected child, gets sick.

## Incubation Period

Hepatitis A takes from two to six weeks to incubate, with an average incubation period of twenty-eight days. The symptoms usually begin abruptly. A person is most likely to infect others during the latter half of the incubation period (two or more weeks after exposure) and continuing for few days after symptoms appear.

## Symptoms

If your child is infected with hepatitis A, she may or may not have symptoms. You may notice that she seems more tired than usual. As the disease progresses, the chemicals normally secreted by the liver begin to build up, and your child will experience symptoms of a liver problem. She will develop jaundice (a yellowing of the skin and the whites of the eyes) and foul breath. She may complain of a bitter taste in her mouth. Her urine

### CALL YOUR DOCTOR

- If your child has symptoms or attends a school or program where someone has hepatitis A or has been exposed to anyone with the virus.

- If your child seems confused or drowsy, has skin or eyes that look yellow.

- If your child's appetite decreases and he is nauseated, vomiting, has diarrhea or caulk- or white-colored stools.

will be dark, and her stools will become white or light colored. There may be some vomiting with abdominal pain centered below either the right or left ribs.

Almost all children with hepatitis A who are otherwise healthy completely recover without any long-term complications. Some people or children with hepatitis A can be very sick for at least a month, and it can take up to six months for a complete recovery. Rarely, the hepatitis infection is so severe, liver failure is possible.

## Diagnosis

Your doctor will do a clinical examination and take a history of your child's recent contacts. If your doctor suspects a hepatitis infection, she will take a blood test to identify antibodies to the hepatitis A virus.

## Treatment

Mild hepatitis can be treated at home. Hepatitis A is a virus, and there is no medication to treat the disease. Instead, we treat the symptoms. Your child should rest in bed until his fever is gone and he regains his appetite. Be sure to offer him foods that are rich in protein and carbohydrates, and encourage him to drink plenty of water. You may want to try feeding him several small meals, and fluids that are high in calories, like milk shakes and chocolate milk. If your child is an older teen, make sure that he understands that alcohol is absolutely off-limits as long as he has this infection because it could worsen liver damage and inflammation.

## Hospitalization

If your child has a severe infection, she may have to be hospitalized. In the hospital she will be monitored closely and treated for symptoms accordingly, particularly if there is liver injury or damage.

## Prevention

One way to prevent hepatitis A is to practice good hygiene. Remind your child to wash his hands thoroughly after using the toilet and before eating. If anyone in your family develops hepatitis, frequent cleaning of any toilet or sink used by him is prudent.

If you travel to developing countries, be especially careful in areas where the water quality isn't known and sanitation is poor. Play it safe by using only bottled water, even to brush your teeth, and stay away from ice in beverages. Do not eat food or drinks (except those that are commercially bottled) from street vendors. Never eat shellfish that might have been taken from contaminated waters. Do not eat unpeeled fruits, salads, uncooked vegetables, or raw shellfish in developing countries, even in places that appear to be more modern or Western.

You can kill the virus by boiling food at 185°F for one minute. But should cooked food become contaminated after cooking, it can still spread the virus. Chlorination in water kills HAV.

Staff members of a day-care center, family members of infected persons, or sexual partners of someone with hepatitis A should get serum immune globulin (IG) if exposed. If an outbreak occurs, everyone in the child-care setting or family should get serum immune globulin to limit the transmission of the virus. Any child with hepatitis A should be isolated from other children for one week after the onset of symptoms.

If your family is going to travel repeatedly or plan to live for long periods in questionably risky or high-risk countries, then everyone should get the age-appropriate dose of hepatitis A vaccine. This vaccine stimulates the body's immune system to make antibodies that help protect against the virus. There are some very mild side effects that disappear within a couple of days. These include some soreness at the infection site, a slight headache, fatigue, and loss of appetite, but these symptoms disappear quickly. For travelers under two years of age, immune globulin is recommended.

# HEPATITIS B

*This is a disease for which there is a vaccine to protect your child, see* **Vaccines, page 301,** *in the Appendices.*

*Hepatitis B must be treated by a doctor.*

It gets its name from the Latin roots *hepar* (liver) and *itis* (inflammation); thus the word *hepatitis* refers to any inflammatory process involving the liver.

## SYMPTOMS

- Loss of appetite

- Nausea

- Vomiting

- Fever

- Stomach or joint pain

- Extreme exhaustion

- Jaundice (yellow skin or eyes)

Hepatitis B is a serious disease involving the liver. The liver is the largest organ inside the body and one of the most vital, performing over 400 functions. An inflammation can adversely affect many of its functions. Infection from hepatitis B can cause lifelong infection, cirrhosis (scarring) of the liver, liver cancer, liver failure, and death.

In this country more than 200,000 people of all ages get hepatitis B each year. In fact, one out of twenty people in the United States will get hepatitis B some time in their life. Most become infected as adolescents or adults, and infection is generally associated with other sexually transmitted diseases, including syphilis. Each year some 5,000 people die of illnesses caused by HBV. Although there are other types of hepatitis, hepatitis B is one of the most serious types. A person who has had other forms of hepatitis can still get hepatitis B.

Children at risk include those born to infected mothers, those with clotting disorders and others receiving blood products, hemodialysis patients, those with household contacts with hepatitis B carriers, and residents in institutions for the developmentally disabled.

Children who have hepatitis B may not look or feel sick when they become infected. Some may develop a mild illness that appears to be a flu. Others become quite ill, develop jaundice (yellow skin and eyes), and experience abdominal and joint pain. Many of these children have to be hospitalized.

Most people fully recover from hepatitis infections, but some never fully recover and carry the virus in their blood for the rest of their lives. This is known as chronic hepatitis B infection, and those who have it are called hepatitis B carriers. Carriers are capable of spreading the disease to others throughout their lives. Children who are infected with the hepatitis B virus are more likely than adults to become carriers. The younger a child is when he is infected, the more probable it is that he will become a carrier. Chronic infection can also lead to cirrhosis and liver cancer.

## Causes

This disease is caused by hepatitis B virus (HBV), which attacks the liver and causes inflammation of the liver.

## How It Spreads

A person can get hepatitis B by direct contact with the blood or body fluids of an infected person, for example, by having sex with an infected person or sharing needles with an infected person. The virus can also be spread to mucosal surfaces (for example, if infected secretions are splashed into another person's mouth or eyes).

HBV is also transmitted, although less commonly, through indirect means such as cuts, burns, and abrasions. A baby born to an infected mother can get hepatitis B during childbirth. Although HBV is not spread through the fecal–oral route, food or water, or by casual contact, a person can get the disease if someone living in the same household is a chronic carrier.

## Incubation Period

The incubation period of acute infection is 45 to 160 days, with an average of 120 days.

## Symptoms

Your child may not have any symptoms at all or symptoms that are merely flulike. Telltale signs of hepatitis B include loss of appetite, nausea, vomiting, fever, stomach or joint pain, and extreme exhaustion. This first stage lasts for about five to seven days. The jaundice stage—marked by yellow skin and eyes—follows the first stage and typically lasts less than four weeks.

## Diagnosis

Only a blood test can detect whether a person has HBV. Your doctor may suspect hepatitis B on examination, particularly if the liver is tender.

## Treatment

There is no cure or specific therapy for acute HBV infection. A patient hospitalized with hepatitis B

### CALL YOUR DOCTOR

- If your child's eyes or skin turn yellow or if his stools are light-colored and urine darkens.

- If your child loses all appetite.

- If your child experiences nausea, vomiting, fever, stomach or joint pain.

- If your child feels extremely tired and is not able to work or play.

is monitored carefully. Children generally recover quickly, but it may take from one to three months for the liver function to return and for your child to fully recover.

## Prevention

Since there is no cure for hepatitis B, prevention is extremely important. The best protection against HBV is hepatitis B vaccine. Three doses are needed for complete protection. In 1991, it was recommended that all babies at birth should be vaccinated with three doses of hepatitis B vaccine. All children eleven to twelve years of age who have not been vaccinated should be. A small percentage of children will have mild side effects—pain at the injection site and elevated temperature.

If you are a mother with HBV in your blood, your child will need a shot called HBIG along with the first hepatitis B shot within twelve hours of birth.

Today blood, organ, and tissue donors are carefully screened for HBV before they can donate. This eliminates the risk of infecting another person unwittingly.

# HEPATITIS C

***Your child must be seen by a doctor
immediately to treat hepatitis C.***

## SYMPTOMS

- Extreme fatigue
- Itchiness
- Joint pain
- Jaundice

Hepatitis C (HCV) is a viral infection that
affects the liver. This disease is responsible for
some 8,000 to 10,000 deaths a year in the United
States, with nearly 4 million people infected with
the virus. Presently, most people with HCV live
a normal life span. Although the annual incidence of acute hepatitis C has fallen in this country to less than a third of what it was a decade
ago, experts estimate that U.S. deaths due to liver
complications from HCV infection are expected
to triple over the next two decades. This increase
is largely the result of illicit intravenous drug use
and needle sharing. Worldwide, HCV is a
major reason for liver transplants in adults.

Although infectious hepatitis was first
described more than two thousand years ago, it
was not until 1990 that the viral agent responsible for hepatitis C virus (HCV) was identified.
Before the specific hepatitis C virus was recognized, the illness was known as non-A, non-B
hepatitis. We refer to HCV as a chronic illness.
The word *chronic* means that the infected person has had the infection for at least six months.
About 20 percent of adults with this disease
develop cirrhosis (scarring) of the liver. Severe
cirrhosis is associated with liver cancer.

What is interesting about hepatitis C is that individuals do not experience the disease in the
same way. A person's symptoms do not necessarily relate to how long he has had the disease;
someone with a mild infection may be symptomatic, while another person with more
advanced illness may have no symptoms at all.
Children especially may have an active infection
yet not exhibit symptoms for many years.

## Causes

This illness is caused by the hepatitis C virus.

## How It Spreads

Hepatitis C spreads by blood-to-blood contact.
This means that any way a person's blood comes
in contact with an infected person's blood can
spread the hepatitis C virus. The most common
route of transmission is by intravenous drug use
or sharing of needles. Transfusion-related acute
hepatitis C is fairly rare now, thanks to the
improved screening of blood. Your teen should
understand that this virus can also be transmitted through body piercing and tattooing.

If your child has HCV, you should take certain precautions such as informing anyone who
comes in contact with her blood (dentists, nurses,
blood technicians) of her condition. Also, she
should avoid sharing toothbrushes or razors.

Another possible mode of transmission is
through sexual activity, although the likelihood
of spreading it to a sexual partner is low. Menstrual blood can contain the virus. If you suspect that your teen is sexually active, be sure to
stress the importance of practicing safe sex.

It is very unlikely that a pregnant woman
infected with hepatitis C can transmit the virus
to her baby in the womb or during childbirth; it
occurs in only 5 percent of mothers known to

have HCV. We do not know whether HCV can be spread through breast milk, but the likelihood is so small that infected mothers may breastfeed their babies if they desire.

## Incubation Period

The incubation period for a hepatitis C infection can be anywhere from two weeks to six months. The illness is often barely detectable during that time. The average incubation period is six to seven weeks.

## Symptoms

Many people with HCV do not experience symptoms or experience very mild symptoms. Your child may appear to have jaundice, the yellowish cast that is a sign of liver infection. You may notice that your child is extremely fatigued. He may complain of joint pain. In addition, his skin may be itchy, although you will not see a rash.

### CALL YOUR DOCTOR

- If your child seems extremely fatigued, complains of joint pain or an unexplained itch, and looks jaundiced (yellow).

- If your child has had direct exposure through blood contact with someone infected with hepatitis C.

## Diagnosis

Generally, HCV is detected when the results of a routine blood test reveal an elevated level of liver enzymes. Further tests will identify the virus. Potential blood donors who are HCV positive are often identified when they are screened. If your doctor suspects that your child is at risk for this illness, he will do blood tests to check the liver function and, if indicated, do further testing. In most cases, the patient with HCV should be monitored by a specialist.

## Treatment

At present there is no vaccine for HCV. Treatment for this illness varies according to the extent of a person's disease. For some infected individuals, certain lifestyle changes such as eating nutritiously and giving up alcohol may be sufficient treatment. For an individual eighteen or older with a more active disease, the doctor may prescribe interferon alpha, a medication that has been approved for treating HCV. Interferon drugs may improve liver function and rid the virus from the blood in as many as 30 percent of HCV patients. However, a definitive treatment for hepatitis C probably will not be available until the development of new antiviral drugs that act specifically against this virus.

It is not necessary to isolate a child who has HCV, but it is important to notify anyone who might come in contact with the child's blood.

# HERPES SIMPLEX TYPE I

## SYMPTOMS

- Blisters on mouth, lips, and gums
- Fever
- Swollen glands
- Irritability
- Loss of appetite
- Achiness

Herpes simplex infections generally cause either cold sores around the mouth or blisters in the genital area. Herpes simplex types 1 and 2 belong to the herpesvirus family. Other members of this family that you may be familiar with include Epstein-Barr virus and varicella zoster virus (the virus that causes chickenpox).

Herpes simplex infections are characterized by their ability to reoccur throughout life. In other words, once you have a herpes simplex infection, you may have it again and again. After the first episode, herpes simplex type 1 virus (HSV-1) lies dormant in nearby nerves. There is no known way to eradicate this virus permanently.

The mouth is the most common site of HSV-1 infection. Herpes simplex gingivostomatitis is a disease characterized by ulcers in the mouth and a fever. For children the first episode of a herpes simplex infection is generally the worst and can be uncomfortable, but some children do not seem too bothered. Others have high fevers, irritability, and refuse to drink because of pain.

Herpes labialis is the most common form of recurrent HSV-1 infection. It is also known as a

fever blister or cold sore. While cold sores are painful to the touch and unattractive, they are generally nothing more than an annoyance. It can take a week before the cold sores heal. (CAUTION: *Infants, or those not previously exposed to HSV-1, can be infected by an adult with a cold sore, so careful hand-washing is important.*)

A child with HSV-1 genital infection may have unwittingly transmitted the infection from his mouth. However, when we see a young child with genital herpes, we must consider the possibility of sexual abuse.

HSV-1 simplex infections are transmitted from person to person, which means that your child gets an HSV-1 infection primarily from touching the sores of someone who is already infected. The virus also lives in bodily secretions and can be transmitted from contact with these fluids.

Most of us have had an HSV-1 infection at some time, and more than likely we acquired HSV-1 during childhood. More than 90 percent of adults age thirty or older show evidence of having been infected at one time or another. HSV-1 is also the most common cause of viral encephalitis (see page 103) in the United States.

When HSV-1 is reactivated or becomes symptomatic again, it may begin with a tingling and numbness in the mouth area. A blister emerges, then breaks and forms a crust. These cold sores usually follow some type of stress, either to the mouth or the whole body. The stress can be emotional or physical—unusually long exposure to sunlight, menstrual period, tooth extraction, common cold, or other infection. The sores usually last up to a week.

We do not know why some people have recurrent cold sores and others do not.

Herpes simplex virus is shed in the saliva for a long time, seven weeks even after the cold sores have healed, but a person is most infectious when the cold sore first appears.

## Causes

There is a great deal of confusion about these infections because the viruses that cause them are divided into two types. The herpes simplex viruses that cause these infections are divided into two types—type 1 (HSV-1) and type 2 (HSV-2).

HSV-1 usually involves the face and skin above the waist, while HSV-2 generally involves the genitalia and skin below the waist. However, either type of virus can be found in either location, depending on the source of the infection. In addition, either virus can rarely be transmitted by an infected pregnant woman to her newborn. The infection in infants can be very serious and needs immediate treatment when discovered.

## How It Spreads

The only way that herpes simplex virus spreads is through person-to-person contact with an infected person's sores or secretions. The virus can also pass in the saliva or genital fluids of someone who is a herpes carrier (someone who has the virus but exhibits no symptoms at the time of contact). Among children, about 5 to 8 percent pass HSV-1 in their saliva without actually having cold sores.

## Incubation Period

The incubation period for herpes simplex I virus ranges from two to fourteen days but most commonly is from six to eight days.

## Symptoms

Initially your child may have fever and complain of feeling achy. She may be irritable and have swollen glands. She may not have much of an appetite because it hurts to eat. Blisters develop on the lips and inside the mouth. These soon turn to painful ulcers. The gums may become red and swollen, and the tongue may get a white coating. Symptoms may last from three to fourteen days, with the sores lasting up to one week.

---

### CALL YOUR DOCTOR

- If your child has a painful open blister around the mouth.

- If your child has fever, swollen glands in the neck, or if mouth sores are causing difficulty eating.

---

## Diagnosis

Your physician can culture this virus fairly easily. It usually takes from one to three days to detect the virus. Some newer techniques, including direct fluorescent antibody staining of scrapings of the sores, can lead to a more rapid diagnosis.

In newborns herpes simplex virus infections are more serious. They can manifest as an infection involving the liver and lungs, a disease of the central nervous system, or a localized infection that may involve the skin, eyes, and mouth.

## Treatment

Depending on your child's age and medical condition, your doctor may prescribe an antiviral medicine like acyclovir or may recommend only symptomatic care such as pain control and plenty of fluids.

Acetaminophen (nonaspirin pain reliever) in the recommended dosage is a good choice to relieve pain.

Because your child will be uncomfortable from the cold sores, give him cool liquids or frozen juice bars to soothe the pain. Certain juices like apple and grape are gentler than acidic juices like orange juice or lemonade, which may sting. Sometimes holding an ice cube on the cold sore for a short time will relieve the pain. Be sure you keep the infected child's eating utensils separate from those of the rest of the family and wash them thoroughly with hot soapy water after each use.

## *Prevention*

Avoid touching the sores or ulcers of anyone who has an active herpes infection. Frequent handwashing is the best way to prevent the spread of this disease.

# IMPETIGO

*Impetigo must be treated by a doctor.*

## SYMPTOM

• Crested lesions on skin

Impetigo is a bacterial skin infection that sometimes begins around the nose and mouth, but it may affect the skin anywhere. The condition generally affects school-aged children. There are two forms of impetigo—called bullous and nonbullous. The latter is the most common form.

We usually see impetigo in the humid summer months, but it occurs in all climates. Impetigo is more prevalent in the warm season because the bacteria that cause the infection prefers skin that has already been injured in some way. In the warm months, children are outdoors and more likely to have poison ivy, insect bites, or a skin allergy. Once there has been some trauma, the skin is more vulnerable to attack by bacteria

## Causes

Nonbullous impetigo is often caused by group A streptococci bacteria, (*Streptococcus pyogenes*), the type of bacteria responsible for strep throat and scarlet fever. Nonbullous impetigo begins as tiny blisters. These eventually burst, and small wet patches of red skin that may weep fluid are exposed. In time a yellowish brown crust covers the affected area. The skin looks like it is covered with either honey or brown sugar.

The bullous form of impetigo is caused by *Staphylococcus aureus,* the bacteria that also causes toxic shock syndrome and food poisoning. This type of impetigo can cause large blisters that

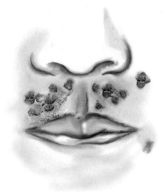

*Blisters on skin; a symptom of impetigo.*

contain fluid that is first clear and then cloudy or milky. These large blisters often break open leaving a "scab" or raw area of skin. Fortunately, impetigo infection does not leave scars.

## How It Spreads

Your child can spread impetigo on himself by scratching. Generally impetigo spreads along the edges of an affected area, but it can also spread to more distant parts of the body. Impetigo is contagious and can spread to others if someone touches the infected skin. It can also be spread to other family members through clothing, towels, and bed linens that have touched your infected child's skin. Because it is so contagious, impetigo spreads rapidly in group-living situations—child-care centers, schools, camps, and hospitals—which are breeding grounds for these bacteria.

Your child does not develop immunity after infection.

## Incubation Period

Impetigo has an incubation period of anywhere from a few days to several weeks. Usually it is around seven to ten days between the time of infection and the appearance of skin blisters. Impetigo is infectious as long as the lesions are draining and for forty-eight hours after starting either oral or topical antibiotics. Keep your child home as long as he is infectious.

## Symptoms

Generally there are no other symptoms except for the lesions. Your child will feel fine and may continue her regular activities. However, since impetigo most often affects school-aged children and frequently occurs on the face, your child may be somewhat self-conscious. Be sensitive to her emotional needs and assure her that this is a temporary condition.

### CALL YOUR DOCTOR

- If your child has signs of impetigo.
- If your child has impetigo and skin does not begin to heal after three days of topical treatment or if fever develops.

## Diagnosis

Your doctor may be able to diagnose impetigo from its distinctive amber color, although a culture of the infected skin lesions will confirm the diagnosis.

## Treatment

The physician may order antibiotics to be given orally for seven to ten days if a child has numerous lesions. You should see healing begin within three days of starting the medication.

An antibacterial ointment such as bacitracin ointment may be used if lesions are few, both to cure the infection and to help prevent the spread of impetigo on your child's body. Ask your pharmacist to help you choose a medication.

At home, use soap and warm water to wash the infected areas of the skin once or twice daily. Scrub the skin gently with a piece of gauze or clean washcloth. If an area is crusted, soak it first in warm soapy water to make it easier to remove the crust. Cover the infected areas with gauze and tape it down so that your child will not scratch the area and spread it or cause further infection. It is a good idea to cut your child's nails short.

You should keep your child home from school or child care until at least twenty-four hours after the appropriate treatment is started.

While impetigo is not a serious disorder, occasionally there are complications. Some group A strep can cause acute poststreptococcal glomerulonephritis, an inflammatory condition affecting the kidneys. While this is relatively uncommon, it does happen. Untreated impetigo can cause complications, especially if the bacteria reach the lymph glands, where it can make them swollen and very painful.

## Prevention

Teach your child good hygiene practices, particularly about handwashing. Pay attention to skin that has been injured, cleaning it after injury with warm, soapy water, and then keeping it clean and covered.

In extensive outbreaks, groups of children are sometimes given prophylactic antibiotics to prevent further spread, but generally health officials coordinate these efforts.

# INFLUENZA

*There is a yearly vaccine against influenza that is recommended for some children and adults. See* Vaccines, *page 301, in the Appendices for a listing and schedule of all the vaccines your child needs.*

Also called flu.

## SYMPTOMS

- Runny nose, nasal congestion, headache
- Possible sudden, high fever (105° to 106°F)
- Sore throat, cough
- Muscle aches and pains
- Fatigue
- Vomiting, nausea, abdominal pain

Influenza—familiarly known as the flu—is a common infection of the respiratory tract that we may catch more than once during our lives. And most of the time, we have the miseries of it for a few days and recover just fine.

But even in an average year, influenza causes the deaths of about 20,000 people in this country, according to the U.S. Public Health Service's Centers for Disease Control and Prevention. Most of these people are elderly adults.

And from time to time, influenza can be even more dangerous. Three times in the twentieth century, the disease has led to worldwide epidemics called pandemics. In 1918 and 1919, as World War I was ending, the so-called Spanish influenza swept around the globe in waves and left 20 million people dead. In the United States

alone, Spanish flu killed a half-million people, many of them young men and women in their twenties and thirties—more than ten times the number of those who died on the battlefields of Europe. In 1957–58 a pandemic of "Asian flu" caused the deaths of 70,000 people in the United States, and in 1968–69 the "Hong Kong flu" killed 34,000 Americans.

In this country influenza epidemics usually begin in November each year. Outbreaks often start among school-aged children, who carry the flu home and spread it to others. The disease usually hangs around all winter, reaching its peak from December through March. Then, in the spring, it disappears again until the following fall.

In the tropics, however, you can catch influenza at any time of the year, and in the Southern Hemisphere, influenza season occurs from April through September, during their winter.

Fortunately, as you are probably aware, there is a vaccine against influenza. Most children, however, do not need to take flu shots.

## Causes

Influenza is caused by a group of viruses called, succinctly enough, the influenza viruses. There are three types of influenza viruses, types A, B, and C. Influenza types A and B are the biggest troublemakers, type A much more so than B. Type A influenza viruses were responsible for all three twentieth-century influenza pandemics.

The reason we may catch influenza over and over again is that the influenza viruses constantly change their spots, so to speak. They are constantly evolving, undergoing genetic mutations that change their antigens, the protein molecules on their outer coats that our immune systems recognize and against which we develop protective antibodies.

Both influenza type A and type B gradually undergo small changes in their antigenic structure, called genetic drift. But from time to time, influenza A viruses abruptly undergo large changes in their structure, called genetic shifts. These major genetic shifts can create influenza strains to which few people in the world have any protective immunity. Such major genetic shifts produced the more dangerous type-A-virus strains that caused the three twentieth-century pandemics.

Such new strains of influenza A viruses often emerge out of China. Many people there live in close quarters with domestic animals such as ducks and swine, and when an animal or a person happens to become infected with an animal and a human flu virus at the same time, the genetic material of the two viruses can recombine and create a new strain.

New strains of flu viruses take their names from wherever in the world they are first identified. Thus in recent years we have had influenza strains named for, among many other places, Beijing, Shanghai, Wuhan, Guangdong, and Harbin, China; Taiwan; the Philippines; Panama; Johannesburg, South Africa; and Texas, Iowa, Alaska, Washington, New Jersey, and Pennsylvania.

In any given influenza season, how many people get sick—and how sick they get—depends on how much the flu viruses have changed or shifted since the previous season. If the viruses have not changed much, more people have some protective immunity to them, and fewer people will catch the flu, or if they do, more of them will have mild symptoms. If the viruses have changed substantially, fewer people will have much immunity, and more people will get more severely ill.

The very young and the very old are most likely to get severely ill from influenza. A young child encountering an influenza virus for the first time is likely to become sicker than an older child because the young one has no antibodies against any influenza antigens. Very elderly people whose immune systems are beginning to fail or who have other chronic diseases are likely to have more severe symptoms as well.

In addition to the influenza viruses, there are many other common respiratory viruses that sometimes cause flulike symptoms. If your child has flu symptoms during influenza season, November through March, the odds are that she is indeed infected with an influenza virus. But she could also have winter flu symptoms caused by adenoviruses or other viruses that may also cause colds and sore throats.

If your child has the "flu" during the late spring or summer, however—outside influenza season—it is more likely that she has been infected by one of the many enteroviruses, viruses that commonly cause summer illnesses. There are dozens of these enteroviruses.

## How It Spreads

During influenza season, your child can catch influenza from someone who does not yet know he is coming down with the flu. People who are infected with an influenza virus start shedding virus particles at least a day or more before they have any symptoms, and they are most infectious *before* they get sick. Young children, who have less immunity, tend to shed more virus particles and for longer periods of time.

An infected person sheds influenza virus in the secretions from his nose and throat. Whenever he coughs or sneezes, he releases millions of virus particles into the air and can spray them onto any person nearby or onto any surface, such as a table. When your child touches the table, she can get virus on her hands. Then she touches her nose or mouth and can infect herself with the virus. She can also catch the flu by sharing a drinking glass with an infected person or kissing someone who is infected.

Once the virus particles get into your child's respiratory tract, they settle down inside the cells of the membranes lining the nasal passages and throat, where they grow and multiply.

## Incubation Period

It usually takes about one to three days from the time your child is infected with a flu virus before there are symptoms.

## Symptoms

As flu-virus particles multiply in your child's respiratory tract, he usually becomes ill abruptly, with a sudden fever and severe, coldlike symptoms. With the flu he usually is sicker than with a cold because influenza affects the whole body.

With full-blown influenza, your child is more likely to have a fever than with a cold, but the temperature can vary considerably. Your child may have no fever at all, or it may range as high as 105° or 106°F, or it may fall somewhere in between. And if your child's fever rises quickly, he may shiver and have chills.

As with a cold, your child's nose runs, his nasal passages become congested with mucus, and he may find it difficult to breathe through his nose. Excess mucus may run down the back of his throat—this is called a postnasal drip—and cause his throat to become sore. Your child usually is coughing. And when he lies down to sleep at night,

mucus tends to pool in his throat and make his cough worse, and he may find it hard to sleep.

Influenza typically causes aches and pains in muscles throughout your child's body—in the arms, calves, thighs, and back. Sometimes children's leg muscles hurt so much they refuse to walk. But again, there can be a wide range of pain; your child may have only a few aches all over. He may also have a headache due to congestion in the sinuses.

Fatigue is usually more of a factor with influenza than with a cold. With a cold your child

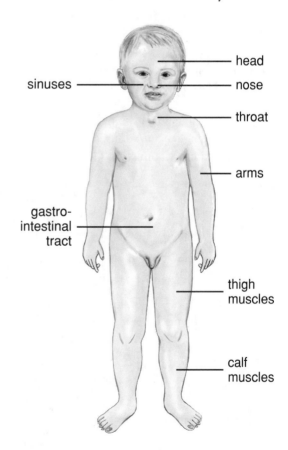

*The lines above indicate where influenza may affect children.*

can usually keep going. He has enough energy to function, to do whatever needs to be done, and to go to school. But when someone has the flu, there is little choice but to stop, stay home, crawl into bed, and go to sleep.

If your child is infected with one of the influenza type B viruses, he may also have some gastrointestinal symptoms: he may have diarrhea or be vomiting.

The influenza viruses can also cause diseases other than full-blown influenza. Babies or very young children may instead develop croup, an infection in their lower throat (see *Croup*, page 46). Older children may have just an ordinary cold.

## *Complications*

The most common, serious complication of influenza in both children and adults is pneumonia—an infection and inflammation in the air sacs of the lungs—or other lower respiratory tract disease. The influenza virus itself can spread downward into a person's lungs and cause pneumonia, or the virus infection can permit bacteria to invade the lungs and produce a bacterial pneumonia. For more about the different kinds of pneumonia and how they are treated, see *Pneumonia*, page 200.

The people who are most likely to become severely ill with influenza and develop pneumonia are, again, the very young and the very old and also those who have other, underlying diseases. These people include children who have a chronic lung disease, such as cystic fibrosis or severe asthma, or who were born prematurely, spent time on a respirator, and have some lingering lung damage, a condition called bronchopulmonary dysplasia. Also at risk are children who have sickle cell anemia, cancer, diabetes, chronic heart or kidney disease, or whose immune systems are not normal.

---

### CALL YOUR DOCTOR

- If your child has a fever of 103°F or more with cold/flu symptoms.

- If your child—particularly a baby under three months old—has a cough that is getting worse, or is not getting better, over a three- or four-day period.

- If your child is breathing faster than usual or you are concerned about the way she is breathing. Breathing rates increase with fever and will slow down when fever is controlled.

- If your child is working harder to breathe or showing signs of respiratory distress: her nostrils are flaring out and she is pulling in (retracting) the muscles between her ribs and at the base of her neck as she breathes.

- If your child feels so achy that he refuses to walk.

A persistent cough, fever, an increase in breathing rate, and respiratory distress are possible clues that a child may have developed pneumonia or other lung disease.
NOTE: When your child has a mild case of flu, she does not necessarily need to see her pediatrician.

## *Diagnosis*

When your child has a fever, stuffy nose, cough, and achy muscles and is very tired and feels terrible—and it is during flu season, November to April—he probably does indeed have influenza. You do not need to take your child to the doctor for diagnosis unless any of the signs of possible complications listed above set in. If you do go to the doctor, the following are some of the ways she might diagnose the illness.

Muscle aches and pains are a particularly important clue pointing toward a diagnosis of influenza. Your pediatrician may gently squeeze your child's arm or leg to find out whether his muscles are more tender or sensitive than usual.

Your doctor will examine your child to determine whether he has developed any complication such as pneumonia or other lung disease. She counts the number of breaths he takes per minute. With her stethoscope, she listens to the sounds he makes as he breathes in and out, and she observes whether he is having any trouble breathing. If she suspects your child has some pneumonia, she may request an X-ray of his chest.

Your doctor is unlikely to ask for any laboratory tests to confirm that your child is infected with a flu virus because, whatever the virus, treatment is usually the same. At Children's Hospital, we only test for influenza virus when a child is so sick that we are admitting him to the hospital. Then we need to know whether he has a flu virus because, if so, the hospital staff must isolate him so that he does not spread it to other patients.

To identify the virus, the doctors take a sample of the secretions from the child's nose, using either a swab or a suction device. Neither of these methods hurts a child; at most, they may make him slightly uncomfortable for a moment. The lab then runs a rapid test that can detect any influenza antigens that may be present in his infected nasal cells and also determine whether they are type A or type B.

## *Treatment*

When your child has flulike symptoms—whether they are caused by an influenza virus or another respiratory virus—she does not need to take any antibiotics. Antibiotics do not kill influenza viruses or any of the other viruses that can cause flu symptoms.

The treatment of most cases of flu is very similar to the treatment of colds. See "Treatment," page 38, in *Common Colds.*

### Medications

If your child is bothered by fever or by aches and pains in her muscles, you can give her acetaminophen. Acetaminophen will both lower her fever and also relieve her aches and pains.

You should never give your child aspirin, however, when she has flulike symptoms. If a child is indeed infected with an influenza virus, taking aspirin is associated with the development of a very rare but very serious, life-threatening neurologic disease called Reye's syndrome. The American Academy of Pediatrics "strongly advises" that you "not give your child or teenager aspirin or any medications containing aspirin when he has any viral illness." See *Reye's Syndrome,* page 217.

### Fluids

Whenever your child has a fever, whether caused by the flu or some other illness, it is very important that you make sure that she drinks plenty of extra fluids to prevent dehydration. Because of her fever, she is losing more fluid than usual by evaporation. If she has a very runny nose, she is also losing fluid in these secretions. Babies especially can very quickly become dangerously dehydrated because they are so small. With babies under a year, however, you should never give plain water; you need to give them special fluids called oral rehydration solutions. See *Fluids*, page 290, in the Appendices for more about dehydration and these special fluids and what other fluids to offer and not offer older children.

## Feeding

Whenever your child has a fever, she is likely to lose her appetite somewhat, and a young child may lose interest in eating solid foods. You do not need to worry about this. Your child may lose a little weight, but as soon as her fever goes down and she feels better, her appetite will return and she will gain the weight back. Encouraging fluids is far more important whenever your child is sick than worrying about whether she is eating solid food. See *Feeding*, page 292, in the Appendices for information about what foods to give and not give your child when she is sick.

## Sponging

Children are not always uncomfortable when they have a fever, but if your child has a high fever, over 103°F, and is very uncomfortable because of it, you can try to lower her temperature by sponging her with lukewarm water. See "Treatment," page 112, in *Fevers*.

## Humidity

Extra humidity in your child's room can help soothe the inflamed tissues inside her nose and loosen the excess mucus clogging her nose. See *Humidity*, page 293, in the Appendices for more information about humidity and humidifiers.

## Nose Drops

If your baby's nose becomes so congested and crusted that she has difficulty breathing, you can help clean her nasal passages with saline (saltwater) nose drops that you can make yourself. (See page 39.)

## Bed Rest

If your child has a fever (101°F or more), you should keep her home from day-care or school. Usually with the flu, as mentioned, your child feels so tired and miserable that she has no choice but to crawl into bed and rest. Some people seem to think there is some virtue in trying to keep on going when you feel terrible. However, resting more and sleeping more will help your child's body overcome the flu virus and also make it less likely that she will develop pneumonia or some other complication—and also less likely that she will spread the virus.

## Other Medications

If your child's nasal passages are congested, a nasal decongestant can help her breathe more easily. Nasal decongestants can reduce the inflammation in her nose and thus open up her nasal passages by constricting the tiny blood vessels in the membranes lining her nose. A nasal decongestant that pediatricians often recommend for children is pseudoephedrine, which is available without a prescription.

In babies less than twelve months, however, the possible side effects of nasal decongestants—notably, rapid heart rates—outweigh any benefits. For older children who are having trouble sleeping because of a congested nose, we often suggest they take a decongestant just at night, before bed, and just for the few days while they are getting over the worst of the flu.

If your child has a cough that is bothering her, you can give her a cough suppressant. The cough suppressant that pediatricians most often suggest for children is dextromethorphan, which is also available over the counter. If your child's cough is keeping her awake at night, you can give her a dose of cough suppressant just before she goes to bed. If her cough lasts for more than a few days, however, or is getting worse, it could be a sign that she has something more serious than the flu, which needs to be identified and treated.

However, you do not necessarily want to suppress your child's cough completely. She is coughing because excess mucus and pus are clogging and irritating the airways to her lungs. The cough is her body's way of trying to clear out these secretions.

The many nonprescription flu medicines that you see in your drugstore generally contain various combinations of the three categories of medications we have just discussed: a pain and fever reliever (such as acetaminophen), a nasal decongestant, and a cough suppressant. Some also contain an antihistamine.

Antihistamines are one of the types of medications used to treat allergies. (Allergies are not infectious diseases.) Antihistamines block a substance in the body called histamine, which is a main cause of allergic reactions. Antihistamines may help your child if she has nasal allergies that are contributing to her flu symptoms.

These four types of medications are the same ones usually found in over-the-counter (and prescription) cold medicines, which are often labeled "cold *and* flu" medicines. None of these ingredients, however, can cure influenza; they cannot kill influenza viruses or any of the other respiratory viruses that can cause flulike symptoms. Nor can these drugs shorten the duration of your child's flu symptoms.

Another consideration with these combination flu medicines is that your child may not have all the symptoms that a given combination targets. If your child's nose is not congested, she does not need a nasal decongestant. If your child is not coughing, she does not need a cough suppressant.

And it is not a good idea to give your child medicines she does not need. For one thing, it is an unnecessary expense. Also, all medications occasionally cause adverse side effects. You need to read the labels carefully to make sure that a flu medicine targets the symptoms your child actually has.

At Children's Hospital we usually do not give any of these combination flu medicines to babies under about ten to twelve months of age. These medicines usually do not help children that young, and some of the ingredients can actually harm them. In general, before giving any medication to your child, you might want to check with your doctor, especially during the first two years of your child's life.

* * *

It usually takes two or three days for influenza to run its course and for your child's immune system to make enough antibodies to overcome and kill off all the virus particles. But, again, how long influenza lasts can vary. Sometimes a child may have a fever that lasts a week or so, and the feeling of tiredness can sometimes drag on longer.

Once your child's fever is gone, however, and her energy level is nearly back to normal, you can send her back to day-care or school.

## Hospitalization

About one out of every 100 otherwise healthy children with influenza becomes sick enough that they need to be hospitalized. At Children's Hospital, during influenza season, we may admit two or three children each week because they have become dehydrated from their high fever or because they have developed pneumonia or another lung disease.

In the hospital the staff treats dehydrated children with intravenous fluids. If a child has pneumonia and is having trouble breathing, we measure the amount of oxygen reaching his bloodstream and give him extra oxygen if he needs it. If it is not clear whether a child's pneumonia is due to the virus or to bacteria, we may give him an antibiotic intravenously. The antibiotic will not kill any influenza virus, but it will kill the bacteria.

Occasionally physicians prescribe an antiviral drug called amantadine for children (and adults) who have influenza and are at particularly high risk of developing pneumonia or other complications of influenza, particularly those who have underlying lung disease (such as severe asthma and cystic fibrosis) or other chronic diseases. Children take amantadine by mouth once or twice a day, usually for several days.

Amantadine kills only influenza type A viruses; it does not work against influenza type B viruses. Therefore the lab first tests a sample of a child's nasal secretions to find out whether he is indeed infected with an influenza virus and, if so, whether it is type A or type B. Amantadine is approved only for children at least one year old, and for it to be effective, a child must start taking it within forty-eight hours of becoming ill. At Children's Hospital we prescribe amantadine rarely, only about five times each flu season.

## *Prevention*

Although it is difficult to prevent the spread of influenza, one of the most effective things you

can do is to teach your children to wash their hands frequently, especially before eating. During flu season they can easily pick up influenza virus on their hands as they go about their daily activities. And be particularly careful to wash your hands before you prepare food.

Since infected people shed flu virus *before* they get sick, it is also wise not to drink from the same glass or soda can or eat from the same spoon as another person.

To keep from spreading flu virus or any other germs to others, teach your children to cover their nose and mouth whenever they need to cough or sneeze. If they use a tissue, they should learn to discard it in a way that the virus on it cannot infect someone else.

When your child has the flu, she should stay away from others as much as possible until she is well again. It is particularly important not to infect very young children or very old people who might become severely ill if they caught influenza.

## Flu Shots

There is so much publicity about flu shots every fall, on the radio and TV and in the newspapers, that it is easy to get the idea that everyone should rush out and get vaccinated against influenza. Most healthy people, however, children or adults, do not need flu shots.

The U.S. Public Health Service and the American Academy of Pediatrics both recommend yearly flu shots for those children (and adults) who are at high risk of getting pneumonia or other serious complications if they do catch influenza. This includes people who have asthma or other chronic lung disease, chronic heart or kidney disease, diabetes or severe anemia; those whose immune systems are not normal; and also children and teenagers who have diseases (such as rheumatoid arthritis or rheumatic fever) that require them to take aspirin for long periods of time. These children and teenagers would be particularly at risk for developing Reye's syndrome if they did get influenza.

The Public Health Service and the Academy of Pediatrics also recommend yearly flu shots for healthy people, both children and adults, who live in same household as such high-risk children or who help take care of them. This is so that these family members do not catch influenza themselves and give it to the high-risk children.

Also, students who live in dormitories, advises the Health Service, "should be encouraged to receive vaccine to minimize the disruption of routine activities during epidemics."

If you are planning a trip abroad with your family, you might want to consider flu shots for everyone because you are more likely to catch influenza while traveling (just because you come in contact with so many more people) and you might not want to interrupt your trip. And remember: flu season in the Southern Hemisphere is April through September, and you can catch influenza in the tropics at any time of the year.

The U.S. Public Health Service also recommends annual flu shots for all adults age sixty-five and older, whatever the state of their health.

And it is okay for your child to get a flu shot even if she does not belong to any of the above groups. "Influenza vaccine may be administered," says the Health Service, "to any person who wishes to reduce his or her chances of acquiring influenza infection."

Adults need just one dose of flu vaccine. Children under the age of nine, however, who are being vaccinated against influenza for the first time, need two shots at least a month apart.

The vaccine is not recommended for babies under six months old, nor for people who are severely allergic to eggs because the viruses in the vaccine are grown in eggs.

If your child does need flu shots, she should get them some time between September and mid-November each year. This gives her immune system the time—a week or two—after the shot to develop enough protective antibodies before the flu season starts in November or December. If she gets her flu shot too early, her antibodies might not last throughout the entire flu season; her antibody levels may start to decline within a few months.

Your child needs to take a new flu shot, if she needs them, every year for two reasons. One is that her antibody levels do decline within a few months. (By contrast, when people are actually infected with an influenza virus, they develop antibodies that may last for many years.) The other reason is that the influenza viruses usually change so much from year to year that last season's vaccine will not protect your child against this season's viruses.

An international network of scientists, coordinated by the World Health Organization, monitors the strains of influenza viruses circulating around the globe. Early each year the Food and Drug Administration selects the three most prevalent strains to include in a new vaccine for the coming season for the United States. Thus, a flu shot protects you only against the three influenza strains in a given season's vaccine and only for the few months of that flu season.

The viruses in the vaccine are killed; you cannot get influenza from a flu shot. The most common side effect from the vaccine is some soreness at the site of the shot, which can last a day or two; less than a third of the people getting shots experience this soreness. About 5 to 10 percent of people have a mild headache or low fever for a day or so after their shot.

The effectiveness of flu shots depends in part on how closely the three virus strains in a given season's vaccine match the influenza strains that actually show up that season. When there is a good match, the vaccine usually prevents influenza in about 70 to 80 percent of the people who take it. However, your child can get a flu shot and still catch the flu for several reasons.

- The influenza viruses that do show up may indeed be very different from the ones in the vaccine.

- Your child may be one of the 20 to 30 percent of people who do not fully respond to the vaccine, who do not develop enough antibodies. If your child does get the flu, however, she is likely to have a milder case than if she had not gotten the shot.

- Your child may have flulike symptoms that are caused not by an influenza virus at all but by one of the dozens of other respiratory viruses that can cause similar symptoms.

Recently a new influenza vaccine has been developed that does not require a shot. This vaccine is given as a nasal spray. The testing in infants, children, and adults have been very promising. The vaccine is expected to be licensed in the United States in 1999.

Occasionally if a high-risk person does not get a flu shot in a given year because of a severe egg allergy or some other reason, his physician may try to keep him from catching influenza by having him take the antiviral drug amantadine or a related drug called rimantadine. The person needs to take the amantadine or rimantadine by mouth once or twice a day for the duration of the influenza season.

# JOCK ITCH

Also called tinea cruris.

## SYMPTOMS

- Rash that is red, tan, or brown, slightly scaly, with a fairly distinct margin

- Chafed, itchy, or irritated skin in the groin area, in the inner thighs, or the pubic or anal areas.

Jock itch is similar to athlete's foot (see page 14) but occurs in a different area of the body (as the name implies) and only in males. We rarely see this condition before puberty. It causes itchy, reddish, and scaly lesions in the groin area and on the thighs and may extend around onto the buttocks. It usually does not affect the scrotum or penis. Often obese males or males who perspire heavily get jock itch, especially while playing sports or during hot, humid weather.

For some reason teenagers are more susceptible to jock itch than adults, probably because children are more careless about hygiene. Keep in mind, however, that not every groin rash is caused by a fungal infection. Other conditions can look much like jock itch. If treatment for jock itch does not succeed, your doctor will look for another cause.

## Causes

Tinea infections are caused by one or more of the dermatophytes, which are fungi that live only on keratin, the dead body tissues of skin, hair, and nails. The tiny fungus that is responsible for jock itch grows best in dark, damp conditions. Other tinea infections include athlete's foot and ringworm.

## How It Spreads

Jock itch may be spread by direct contact. Males pass it to each other by sharing underwear or shorts, towels, benches, or shower stalls in locker rooms. It can also be spread through contaminated bedding, so infected children should avoid sharing beds or sleeping bags.

## Incubation Period

It takes three to five days for the infection to develop, but it may be anywhere from ten days to three weeks before symptoms appear.

## Symptoms

Jock itch brings a rash that is red to tan to brown color, is slightly scaly, and has a fairly distinct margin. Your child will have chafed, itchy, or irritated skin in the groin area, in the inner thighs, or in the pubic or anal areas.

## CALL YOUR DOCTOR

- If home treatment does not seem to be working and jock itch gets worse.

- If the rash begins to bleed.

## Diagnosis

Your physician will be able to diagnose jock itch by its appearance. You do not need to take your child to the doctor unless the itch gets worse and is not healing with over-the-counter treatment.

## Treatment

Generally over-the-counter antifungal creams are effective in treating jock itch, particularly if treatment begins immediately. Preparations containing miconozale are most effective. If these creams do not work, there are several prescription creams available. Your child should apply the cream once or twice a day, spreading it at least $1/2$ inch beyond the affected area. Treatment should continue for one week after the rash is gone.

If the rash is still present after a month of treatment, take your child to the doctor. He may need a different kind of medication. Some other topical medications include clotrimazole (Lotrimin), econazole (Spectazole), miconazole nitrate (Monistat-derm), and ketoconazole (Nizoral).

## Prevention

Instruct your child in good hygiene techniques. He should dry the groin area well after he showers. Be sure to instruct your child to dry his feet last—if he dries his feet first and then his groin, he may transfer a fungus. If your child perspires easily, he should use an absorbent powder.

Absorbent cotton underwear is advisable. Your child should stay away from tight clothing or synthetic fabrics. Remind him not to stay in a wet bathing suit too long. Discourage the use of anyone else's towels or clothes. Too much soap (which is alkaline and encourages fungal growth) can make jock itch worse, so make sure your child does not rub too much with soap and that he rinses off all soap, dries himself well, and keeps the groin area dry. Talcum powder reduces wetness and chafing.

# LICE

Also known as cooties or pediculosis. *Pediculus* is Latin for "louse," and the ending -*osis* means "disease."

You do not need to feel embarrassed if your child comes home with lice because lice infestations are very common among children. It is no reflection on how you bathe your child. An estimated 5 million people in the United States need to be treated for lice each year.

Lice are not a significant medical problem. They are totally curable and cause no long-term effects. Getting rid of them, however, can be a nuisance.

## Causes

Lice are tiny, wingless insects that feed by sucking blood. Three species feed on humans. Each of the three differs in the age group it targets and also where on the body it prefers to feed.

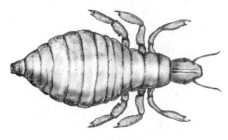

├─── Actual size: 2–3 mm ───┤

*Head louse (*Pediculus humanus*).*

The head louse (*Pediculus humanus capitis*), which is the most common, targets children of day-care and school age. Head lice, as befits their name, live and feed on the head. They glue their eggs—called nits—to a child's hair, close to the scalp. After the nits hatch, the adults feed on the skin of the scalp.

The pubic louse (*Pediculus pubis*) tends to infect teenagers and young adults between the ages of fifteen and twenty-five. Pubic lice are less fussy than head lice about where they live and feed. They attach their nits not only to pubic hair but also to other body hair—eyebrows, eyelashes, under the arms, a man's beard—and the adults feed on whatever skin is nearby. Pubic lice are also called crab lice because, under magnification, they look something like miniature crabs. Pubic lice infestations are sometimes called crabs.

The body louse (*Pediculus humanus corporis*) infests people of any age, but they are much less common in this country than head or pubic lice. Body lice lay their nits and live in a person's clothes and move onto his body only to feed, where they may suck blood almost anywhere.

## How They Spread

Head lice spread readily from child to child. Your child can easily pick them up at his day-care center or at school or camp. The insects can travel from an infected child to another when their heads come close while they are playing. Lice also can move from head to head when children try on each other's hats or other headgear; if they use each other's combs, brushes, or headphones; or if they sleep in the same bed.

Acquiring head lice has nothing to do with how clean you keep your child. You could bathe him and wash his hair every day, and he could still get head lice. The lice still have time to get in his hair and lay their eggs. Washing his hair does not remove the eggs, and then the eggs hatch.

Nor is hair length a factor. Boys with short hair are just as likely to catch head lice as are girls with long hair.

Pubic (crab) lice travel from one teenager to the next primarily through sexual contact, but they also can spread on such items as contaminated towels, bedding, toilet seats, and any loose hairs with nits attached that an infected person may have dropped.

Acquiring body lice, on the other hand, *does* have to do with how clean a person keeps herself. Body lice also spread from person to person via contaminated towels, bedding, and articles of clothing, and they are more common among people who live in shelters or on the street and do not wash their clothes regularly. Body lice, in turn, can spread several other diseases—typhus, trench fever, relapsing fever—that are uncommon in this country but prevalent in developing countries.

## Incubation Period

Once an adult louse lays her nits (eggs), it usually takes from six to ten days for the eggs to hatch and the lice to start feeding on the skin.

## Symptoms

The main symptom of a lice infestation is itching, sometimes intense itching, wherever on the body the insects are sucking their blood meal.

Head lice usually feed in a child's hair just behind his ears and at the back of his neck. Your child may complain that something is crawling in his hair, although children do not always notice anything if they have only a few lice. If your child scratches where it itches, he may damage his skin and produce small bloody or crusted sores, which can then become infected by bacteria.

If your teenager has pubic lice, he may also—in addition to itching in his pubic region and wherever else the lice are feeding—develop little blue spots on his skin. This is because the lice, as they are feeding, cause some bleeding in the skin. Body lice can also produce these little blue spots.

You do not necessarily need to call your physician if you are sure that what your child or teenager has is lice. What often happens is that the day-care center or school nurse sends home a note letting you know that a child or several children in your child's class are infested with lice. If your child is also clearly infested, you can just go ahead and treat her yourself.

If you do not get such a note but discover on your own that your child has head lice, let your child's day-care center or school know about it. The odds are that other children in the class, as well as other children she plays with outside school, also have them. And if your teenager has pubic lice, any person with whom he has sexual contact probably does too.

---

### CALL YOUR DOCTOR

- If your child complains of itching in her hair or she is scratching her head more than usual.

- If your teenager itches in his pubic region or other areas of his body, and you are not sure whether he has lice or something else.

NOTE: There is no need to call your doctor if you know your child has lice.

# Diagnosis

Lice is usually a fairly clear-cut diagnosis. Many parents can recognize the signs of lice infestations themselves. Look carefully on your child's scalp or skin wherever he says he itches or you see him scratching.

You may want to use a good light and a magnifying glass, but it probably is not necessary. For head lice, look most carefully behind his ears and at the nape of his neck. Adult head lice are very tiny, only 2 to 3 millimeters long (about $^1/_{10}$ inch). Pubic lice are even smaller, about 1 millimeter long ($^1/_{25}$ inch). They both look like little black dots on your child's scalp or your teenager's skin—but these little black dots are crawling about.

Or you may spot the nits. They look like little white specks glued to the hair near the base of the hair shafts and wrapped around the hairs like beads on strings. At first glance the nits may resemble dandruff, but you can easily blow or rub dandruff away, while nits are firmly attached to hairs. Lice are also itchier than dandruff.

If your teenager turns out to have pubic lice, her physician will probably check to find out whether she also has any other sexually transmitted disease for which she needs to be treated.

# Treatment

There are a number of medications in the form of shampoos and rinses that you can buy in a drugstore and use to kill the lice infesting your child.

With head lice, you need to do this before you send her back to her day-care center or school, to keep her from spreading the lice to other children. Also carefully inspect other members of your family. Some of them may also need treatment.

With a teenager who has pubic lice, his sexual partners need to be checked to find out whether they, too, need to be treated.

The medications generally contain one of the following lice-killing ingredients.

## Permethrin

Permethrin has "distinct advantages," says the American Academy of Pediatrics, over other lice-killing substances. It is available over the counter, without a prescription. It is unlikely to cause any adverse side effects, and it has a high cure rate. You first wash your child's hair with her regular shampoo and rinse and dry her hair with a towel. Then you apply enough of the permethrin rinse to saturate her hair and scalp. You leave the permethrin on her hair for ten minutes—but no longer—and then rinse it off with water. A single treatment is usually enough to kill all lice and nits.

## Pyrethrum

A number of pyrethrum-containing preparations are also available over the counter. You apply this type to your child's hair also for ten minutes only, but without shampooing her hair first. Some brands are intended for use against pubic as well as head lice. However, one treatment with these pyrethrum preparations does *not* kill all the nits. You need to give your child a second treatment seven to ten days later to kill any newly hatched lice.

## Lindane

Lindane-containing medications for both head and pubic lice are available by prescription only. Lindane preparations have the greatest risk of adverse side effects, the Academy of Pediatrics points out. If not used correctly, they can cause dizziness, convulsions, or seizures, particularly in young children. With lindane preparations you also wash your child's hair first with her regular shampoo. Then you put on different amounts of insecticide depending on the length of your child's hair and leave it on for four minutes only. A single treatment is usually enough.

Whichever type of medication you choose, be sure to read all the directions carefully before you use it on your child. You especially need to be careful not to get any insecticide near her eyes or on her mucous membranes, such as her mouth or inside her nose or vagina.

* * *

If your child has lice or nits on her eyebrows or eyelashes (usually these are pubic lice transmitted from an adult), you need to get rid of them some other way. You can coat her lashes and brows with petroleum jelly three to four times a day for eight to ten days. This will kill the lice and nits by smothering them.

People who have body lice do not need to use any of these insecticides because body lice spend most of their time in a person's clothes and move onto the skin only to feed. These people do, however, need to kill the lice on their clothing and in their surroundings. For how to do this, see below.

You can send your child back to her day-care center or school after you have given her the first treatment with an insecticide. Some schools, however, insist that you also remove all nits, dead or alive, from your child's hair before they will allow her to return. The insecticide will kill most of the nits, but there is always a chance it was not on long enough or part of the hair did not get well coated. It is better to remove as many nits as possible.

Removing nits can be a tedious task, the obvious origin of the term *nit-picking* to mean an excessive concern with details. You use a spe-

cial type of comb with extra-fine teeth. Such nit combs are often included in packages containing lice-killing medications.

You comb down through your child's hair with the nit comb, one section of hair at a time. The problem is that the nits are glued tightly around the hairs, right down at the very base of the hair shafts. You catch them with the comb, and then you need to pull them all the way off the end of the hair. This can be particularly difficult if your child has thick, curly hair.

How long this will take you depends a lot on your child, how old she is, and how long she can sit still. With a restless three-year-old, you might sit her in front of a video and do it ten minutes here and ten minutes there.

When you finish nit-picking, you may wish to decontaminate your child's clothing and surroundings. Remember that lice is usually spread person-to-person, so getting lice from the surrounding environment is less likely.

Nevertheless, you may wish to disinfect everything your child's head and hair—or in case of pubic lice, her pubic area and wherever else the lice were—touched for any length of time. To be safe, disinfect whatever she had prolonged contact with—that is, spent more than a couple of hours with—over the last month.

For head lice this means her hats, scarves, headbands and other hair ornaments, combs, brushes, coat collars, and also her towels, bedding (sheets, pillowcases, pillow, blankets, mattress), the upholstery of her favorite chairs, and also where she sits in the car. For pubic lice it also means her undergarments. If she slept in her sister's bed one night, you need to disinfect that bedding and mattress too. But you do not need to worry about a chair that she sat in just once.

In your washing machine, temperatures of 130°F for five minutes will kill both lice and nits, so anything washable—cotton and synthetic clothing, bedding, washable toys—you can wash on the hot cycle. Some articles you can just run through a hot dryer. Combs and brushes you can soak in hot water for ten minutes or wash with the insecticide shampoo.

Dry cleaning also kills nits and lice, but this, of course, can quickly become very expensive. A simple alternative for items your child does not need immediately is to store them away in plastic bags for about two weeks.

Use the vacuum cleaner or an upholstery cleaner on the couch and on any upholstered chair she may have contaminated and also on her pillow, mattress, and where she sits in the car. You do not have to worry so much about hard surfaces. Lice are more likely to hide in fabrics that have a pile to them, particularly in seams and piping.

Your child can catch lice over and over again. If the medication and these other measures do not work, the most likely reason is that your child is getting reinfested from someone, or from several someones, with whom she is in close contact or from her own clothing or other items that still have lice or nits on them.

## *Prevention*

To keep your child from getting lice and to keep you from having to go through all this again, teach your child not to share combs or brushes with other children or try on each other's hats.

# LISTERIA INFECTIONS

***Listeria must be treated by a doctor.***

Also called listeriosis. The ending *-osis* means "disease."

## SYMPTOMS

- Fever

- Headache

- Fatigue

- Muscle aches

- Vomiting or diarrhea

- If a woman is pregnant, possible miscarriage, stillbirth, or severely ill newborn

Listeria infections are a rare but potentially severe form of food poisoning. They are the reason the U.S. Public Health Service advises pregnant women to avoid eating soft cheeses such as Brie and Camembert.

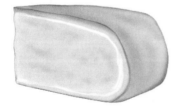

*Soft cheeses may harbor listeria bacteria.*

Most of us do not have to worry about getting listeria infections. However, if a woman does catch listeria disease while she is pregnant, she can lose her baby or the baby can be born with a life-threatening illness.

About 1,850 people in the United States develop serious listeria infections each year, estimates the Public Health Service's Centers for Disease Control and Prevention. Most of these people are either newborn babies or people whose immune systems for some reason are not normal.

## Cause

A bacterium called *Listeria monocytogenes* is the cause of listeria disease. The organism was named in honor of Joseph Lister, the nineteenth-century British physician who pioneered antiseptic techniques during surgery.

Although listeria infections are not common, listeria bacteria themselves are widespread in the world around us. They are found in soil and water, and they normally live in the intestinal tracts of many animals, both domestic and wild, including mammals, birds, and fish. These animals are not necessarily sick themselves; they can carry the bacteria in their intestines without being ill.

## How They Spread

Listeria bacteria have long been known, but it was not until the early 1980s that physicians discovered they can spread to humans in food.

Animals and people who are infected with listeria shed the bacteria in their feces. You can become infected if you get the bacteria in your mouth—most often from contaminated food—and then swallow them. If a pregnant woman becomes infected with listeria, she in turn can pass the bacteria to her unborn baby. A mother can also infect her baby with the bacteria at the time of delivery.

Listeria bacteria are so widely dispersed in nature that there are plenty of chances for them to get into food.

Dairy cows can be infected with listeria, and the bacteria are among the many germs that may get into raw, unpasteurized milk. At one plant in Los Angeles, over a period of months, unpasteurized milk repeatedly contaminated one brand of soft, Mexican-style cheese. Listeria bacteria subsequently infected ninety-three pregnant women who ate the cheese and also infected their babies. The bacteria have also been found in other dairy products, including Brie and Camembert cheeses.

Vegetables can become contaminated with listeria bacteria directly from soil or from animal manure. In an outbreak in Nova Scotia, manure from listeria-infected sheep contaminated cabbages growing in fields fertilized with the manure. The bacteria then made their way into coleslaw made from the cabbages, and forty-one people who ate the tainted coleslaw became sick.

People have developed listeria infections after eating contaminated meat and poultry that were not completely cooked and hot dogs that were not thoroughly heated. The bacteria have also turned up in cooked, ready-to-eat foods such as bologna and other cold cuts, ham and chicken salads, sliced turkey and roast beef, and in other foods purchased from delicatessen counters.

If such foods become contaminated with listeria after they are prepared, refrigeration is not sufficient to prevent the growth of these bacteria. Listeria is one of the few bacteria that are able to multiply at low temperatures.

## Incubation Period

From the time a person eats food contaminated with listeria bacteria, it usually takes about three weeks until the person develops symptoms, if there are any symptoms, but it can take anywhere from one to seventy days.

## Symptoms

Most healthy people who eat listeria bacteria in food never have any problem; they are never sick at all. Pregnant women, however, are about twenty times more likely than other healthy adults to develop listeria infections.

A woman may have flulike symptoms: fever, headache, fatigue, muscle aches, and sometimes vomiting or diarrhea. Even a pregnant woman, however, can be infected with listeria and have no symptoms—yet she still can spread the bacteria to her unborn baby.

Listeria bacteria can spread widely throughout the body of a developing fetus and infect many different organs, including the lungs, liver, spleen, and central nervous system. The infection may cause the woman to have a miscarriage or her baby to be born dead. Or the infection may cause the baby to be born prematurely with a life-threatening disease: he may have a listeria infection of his lungs (pneumonia), bloodstream (septicemia), or the membranes covering his brain and spinal cord (meningitis).

Less commonly a listeria-infected baby is born seemingly healthy, at full term and with a normal birth weight, and then when he is one to eight weeks old, he develops listeria meningitis. These babies with delayed listeriosis became infected at the time of delivery, and most of the time their mothers never realized they carried the bacteria.

Most other people who develop listeriosis—people who are neither newborn babies nor pregnant women—are, as mentioned, people whose immune systems are not normal. These include people who have cancer, were born with immunodeficiency diseases, are taking drugs (such as corticosteroids) that suppress their immune system, are infected with the human immunodeficiency virus (HIV), or have had an organ transplant. These people most commonly develop septicemia or meningitis.

---

### CALL YOUR DOCTOR

- If your newborn baby (up to twelve weeks of age) has any fever, that is, a temperature of 101°F or more.

- If your baby has signs of meningitis: irritability, lethargy, listlessness, poor feeding, a bulging soft spot. See *Meningitis*, page 183.

---

## Diagnosis

If physicians suspect that a pregnant woman, a newborn, or anyone else has listeriosis, they take specimens of tissues—such as blood, cerebrospinal fluid, amniotic fluid, or the placenta—for testing. The doctors have a laboratory try to isolate and culture (grow) the bacteria from the specimens in order to identify them.

## Treatment

If a pregnant woman has listeriosis recognized during her pregnancy, her physician can treat her with antibiotics, usually a combination of ampicillin and gentamicin. Prompt, early treatment with antibiotics may kill enough bacteria in her body and in that of her baby so that he can be born healthy.

Babies who are born with listeriosis or who develop the disease soon after birth are also treated with antibiotics.

Nevertheless, in the Los Angeles soft-cheese outbreak, thirty of the ninety-three pregnant women who were infected lost their babies. Altogether, listeriosis kills about one out of every four people who develop it. About 425 Americans die of the disease each year, according to the U.S. Public Health Service, again, mostly newborns and people with immune deficiencies.

## Prevention

Listeriosis "can be avoided by following a few simple recommendations," says the U.S. Public Health Service.

If you are pregnant or your immune system is not normal, the Health Service recommends that you "avoid soft cheeses (e.g., Mexican-style, feta, Brie, Camembert, and blue-veined cheese)." The American Academy of Pediatrics agrees that "pregnant women should avoid soft cheeses." There is no need, however, to avoid hard cheeses, processed cheeses, cream cheese, cottage cheese, or yogurt.

Because listeria and so many other germs can contaminate raw, unpasteurized milk, both the Health Service and the Academy of Pediatrics advise that people—especially pregnant women—not drink raw milk nor let children drink it. The Academy of Pediatrics advises pregnant women to avoid *any* unpasteurized dairy products.

Since listeria bacteria are able to multiply in food even in the refrigerator, the Health Service further advises pregnant women:

> *Leftover foods or ready-to-eat foods (e.g., such as hot dogs) should be reheated until steaming hot before eating. . . .Although the risk for listeriosis associated with foods from delicatessen counters is relatively low,*

*pregnant women and immunosuppressed persons may choose to avoid these foods or to thoroughly reheat cold cuts before eating.*

The Academy of Pediatrics also advises pregnant women to avoid eating undercooked meats. To kill any listeria or other germs that may contaminate meat or poultry, the U.S. Department of Agriculture recommends that everyone—pregnant or not—cook meat to an internal temperature of 160°F and poultry to a temperature of 180° to 185°F.

For more recommendations about how to protect your family from food-borne diseases, see "Prevention," page 125, in *Food Poisoning*.

# LYME DISEASE

*Lyme disease must be treated by a doctor.*

## SYMPTOMS

- Bull's-eye rash (red, circular, flat rash, more than 2 inches in diameter)

- Fever

- Muscle aches

- Sore throat

- Swollen lymph glands

- Facial palsy (drooping face)

- Headache

- Mild, stiff neck

- Arthritis (e.g. swollen knee)

Lyme disease has become the number-one illness that your child can catch from ticks in this country. It can cause a variety of symptoms, most commonly a rash and arthritis.

Fortunately, virtually all children who get Lyme disease can be cured by a single course of antibiotics. However, many people fear Lyme disease out of proportion to its frequency and usual severity. At The Children's Hospital of Philadelphia, we see many children with suspected Lyme disease—many of whom turn out not to have the disease at all.

Lyme disease was first identified in this country in 1975, thanks to two alert mothers in Old Lyme, Connecticut. The mothers were concerned because they knew so many people—children and adults—who were being diagnosed with arthritis. The women contacted physicians at Yale, who soon located several dozen more people with similar arthritis and realized the mothers had spotted a previously unrecognized disease.

However, Lyme disease turned out not to be so new. It has been known in Europe since the early twentieth century and also occurs in China, Japan, and Australia. Researchers have identified cases in this country dating back to the 1960s. Some experts suspect that Lyme disease has existed here at least since colonial times because early records contain so many references to annoying ticks. People from eastern Long Island, New York, have long talked about having "Montauk spider bite" (Montauk is the village at the eastern tip of the island), and some scientists think this may have been Lyme disease all along.

In recent years the number of people with Lyme disease reported each year to the U.S. Public Health Service's Centers for Disease Control and Prevention (CDC) in Atlanta has ranged from about 8,000 to over 16,000. However, "the actual incidence of Lyme disease in the United States is unknown," the CDC points out, because not all cases are reported and the disease is also often overdiagnosed and misclassified. At Children's Hospital we see some fifty or sixty children and teenagers a year with Lyme disease.

A person is most likely to catch Lyme disease in three geographic regions in the United States where infected ticks are most abundant. Most people who get Lyme disease catch it along the northeastern coast, from Maryland to Massachusetts. A second Lyme disease region is the upper Midwest, in Wisconsin, Minnesota, and Michigan, and the third region is northern California.

Within these three regions, infected ticks and Lyme disease tend to cluster in certain hot spots, among them, southeastern Connecticut;

Nantucket; Westchester County and eastern Long Island, New York; eastern Pennsylvania; southern New Jersey; and even particular roads, parks, and backyards. Near a nature preserve in Massachusetts, at one point, twenty-five of the thirty-eight nearest neighbors—66 percent—developed the disease.

## Cause

Lyme disease is caused by a bacterium called *Borrelia burgdorferi*. It gets the *Borrelia* part of its name from French bacteriologist Amédée Borrel. It gets the *burgdorferi* part of its name from Willy Burgdorfer of the National Institutes of Health, who first identified it, in 1982, in ticks collected on Shelter Island, off Long Island, New York.

Lyme disease bacteria live not only in the bodies of ticks but also in some birds and many small mammals, including chipmunks, voles, rabbits, rats, and mice.

## How It Spreads

Ticks are not insects but instead belong to a group called the arachnids, which also include spiders and mites. The most obvious difference between insects and arachnids is that insects have six legs, while adult ticks and spiders have eight.

The tick that most commonly spreads Lyme disease is the deer tick, also called the black-legged tick and *Ixodes scapularis* (formerly *Ixodes dammini*), which inhabits wooded, brushy, and grassy places in the Northeast and upper Midwest. In California the disease is spread by the western black-legged tick, *Ixodes pacificus*.

Deer ticks must drink a blood meal during each of three stages of their life cycle: as larvae, nymphs, and adults. The ticks initially become

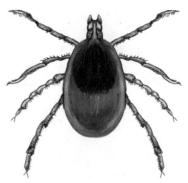

├─ Actual size (adult): 3 mm ─┤

*Deer ticks are often carriers of Lyme disease.*

infected with Lyme disease bacteria when, as larvae, they suck blood from small mammals that are infected, usually white-footed mice in the Northeast and wood rats in California.

The Lyme bacteria remain in the ticks' bodies as they molt into nymphs, and the nymphs are the stage that is most likely to infect a person. If one bites you, it may inject the bacteria into your body, along with its saliva, while it feeds.

In the Northeast, you are most likely to encounter deer-tick nymphs during the spring and early summer, from May through July, the very time of year your family is most likely to be out-of-doors. And nymphs are easy to miss if one does bite you because they are minute, only about a millimeter across, the size of a pinhead, a poppy seed, or a speck of dirt.

A person can get Lyme disease at other times of the year, however, from adult ticks, which usually are active during the fall, in October and November, but may also feed during mild spells in winter or early spring. Adult ticks are larger than the nymphs, 2 to 2¹/₂ millimeters across, so you are more likely to spot them and remove them before they can infect you.

Adult deer ticks prefer bigger game than mice and rats and may feed on raccoons, foxes, cattle, horses, and hogs, but their favorite food—as befits their name—is the blood of white-tailed deer. Deer are thus a marker for the possible presence of Lyme disease: wherever you see deer, there may also be ticks infected with Lyme bacteria.

The explosion of the deer population in recent decades is partly responsible for the emergence and spread of Lyme disease. Another factor is that so many people have now moved out into suburban and rural areas and are living closer to nature—and deer ticks. People have, however, caught Lyme disease in city backyards and parks. Infected deer ticks have been found, for instance, in New York City's Van Cortlandt Park.

Deer ticks may also feed on dogs and cats, and they, too, can contract Lyme disease. Or your dog or cat can carry a loose tick on its fur, which then could move to a family member and infect him.

People of all ages, children and adults alike, get Lyme disease. If your child is bitten by a deer tick, however, he will not necessarily become infected with the bacteria. Even in Lyme disease hot spots, less than half of the ticks may be infected. And an infected tick needs to stay attached to a person for twenty-four to forty-eight hours or more before it injects enough bacteria to cause infection.

## *Incubation Period*

It usually takes several days to several weeks from the time a person is infected with Lyme bacteria for him to start having early symptoms of Lyme disease—if he is going to get symptoms. However, some late symptoms may not appear for months. Thus, while infection usually occurs in the spring or summer, a person can develop symptoms of Lyme disease at any time of year.

## *Symptoms*

If your child becomes infected with Lyme bacteria, she may never have any symptoms. In Lyme disease areas many people become infected, but their immune system kills off all the bacteria, and they never realize they were infected.

If your child has symptoms, the earliest—and most common—is usually a distinctive rash, which may appear anywhere from several days to several weeks after she was bitten. This rash usually starts as a single large, flat, red spot, round or oval or triangular in shape and two or more inches in diameter. The rash is usually at or near the site of the tick bite. Your child may develop more than one spot from a single tick bite.

Most people who develop this distinctive rash, however, never noticed the tick because the nymphs are so tiny and the bites are usually painless. Most people thus do not know when they were infected.

Over the next few days or weeks, as the Lyme bacteria spread within your child's body, the red spot expands, sometimes reaching a diameter of a foot or more. The center of the spot typically clears, so that the rash takes on a bull's-eye appearance: a red ring surrounding a lighter center.

Your child could have Lyme disease, however, and never develop this distinctive rash. Some 20 to 30 percent of infected people never have—or never notice—the rash.

Your child may not have any symptoms other than the rash. Or as the bacteria spread into her bloodstream, she may have flulike symptoms along with the rash. She may have a low fever, or it may increase to 104°F, alternating with chills. Her muscles may ache, and her joints may feel sore or stiff. She may have a sore throat, swollen lymph glands, and nausea or vomiting. She may have a headache, sometimes severe, a mild stiff neck, and feel extremely fatigued. These symptoms may come and go over several weeks. Or these flulike symptoms can be so mild and fleeting that you may not notice them, particularly if she does not have the rash.

In later stages of Lyme disease, the bacteria can spread out of the bloodstream into other parts of the body, most commonly one of the joints, causing arthritis (inflammation of a joint). This was the symptom, remember, that led to the original identification of the disease; the Yale researchers called the illness Lyme arthritis at first until they realized it could also affect other parts of a person's body.

Arthritis is one manifestation of Lyme disease often seen in children. Arthritis can be the first and only symptom if your child missed or did not have the rash or flulike symptoms, and it can appear a few weeks to a few months after a tick bite. Or it can show up while your child still has the rash or flulike symptoms. At Children's Hospital we usually see several dozen children a year who have Lyme arthritis.

Lyme arthritis is usually not subtle. It usually affects just one side, one joint, often one close to the tick bite, most often the knee. (Long Islanders have long talked about having "Montauk knee.") The disease can cause a significant, incapacitating arthritis. The joint is obviously swollen and painful, hot, red, and difficult to walk on. Your child would be limping.

The bacteria also can cause inflammation in a person's nerves, most commonly the nerve that controls the muscles of the lower part of the face, partially or completely paralyzing them. This is called facial palsy or Bell's palsy. It usually affects just one side of the face; the person smiles with a lopsided smile because the muscles that pull up one side of the mouth are paralyzed. Lyme disease sometimes affects other nerves,

causing pain, tingling, numbness, or weakness in muscles of an arm or leg.

Rarely, Lyme bacteria can invade a person's heart, where they may interfere with the electrical signals that control the heart beat and cause a person's heart to beat more slowly or irregularly. Your child's pulse would be slow, but he would not necessarily complain of anything, and parents usually do not notice anything.

The bacteria can also invade a person's central nervous system and cause meningitis (inflammation of the tissues, or meninges, covering the brain and spinal cord) or encephalitis (inflammation of the brain). The person may have a fever, excruciating headaches, a very stiff neck, and overwhelming fatigue. Some people experience more subtle symptoms such as difficulty concentrating or loss of memory.

Late Lyme disease of the central nervous system, however, is very uncommon. And it is very, very unusual for fatigue or subtle symptoms to be a person's first or only sign of Lyme disease. Usually there are other, more obvious symptoms, such as the rash or arthritis.

Nevertheless, at Children's Hospital we see four to five teenagers a month who complain of headaches and fatigue and whose parents think they have Lyme disease. However, these symptoms have many, many possible causes and are much more commonly due to something else.

*You do not need to call your physician just because your child has been bitten by a tick.* Even in Lyme disease hot spots, remember, not all ticks are infected, and even if a tick is infected, it does not necessarily transmit the bacteria.

However, you should remove the tick promptly: it is virtually impossible to develop Lyme disease if the tick is attached for twenty-four hours or less. Then you should watch the place where your child was bitten for several weeks to see whether he develops the distinctive rash or any of the other possible symptoms of Lyme disease.

## CALL YOUR DOCTOR

- If your child develops a large, expanding rash. (See page 172 for a description of the distinctive Lyme disease rash.)

- If your child develops a swollen, painful joint.

- If your child has a weak muscle in his face or elsewhere or pain, tingling, or numbness in a muscle or nerve.

- If your child has a severe headache and stiff neck.

## *Diagnosis*

Diagnosing that a child has Lyme disease is most straightforward if she develops the distinctive rash. Each of the other possible symptoms of the disease—arthritis, palsy, slow pulse, or fatigue—has many other possible causes.

The Lyme rash is quite different from other rashes children usually get. The most common rashes are many tiny red dots that disappear in a few days. The Lyme rash, on the other hand, is usually solitary, flat, and large and lasts for days to weeks if left untreated. It is larger than most insect bites, and it does not appear right away; a rash that shows up in the first forty-eight hours after a bite is usually an allergic reaction, not Lyme disease. Nor is the Lyme rash streaky or intensely itchy, as poison ivy is.

In some cases, if your physician suspects your child may have Lyme disease, he may take a blood

sample and send it to a laboratory to be tested for Lyme antibodies—molecules that your immune system makes to kill the bacteria. It usually takes two or three days to get the results back. Unfortunately, the blood tests can yield both false-negative and false-positive results.

First, the lab tests the blood for antibodies using a technique called EIA (which stands for enzyme immunoassay). If the EIA test is negative, it generally means that your child does not have Lyme disease.

However, at the beginning of the infection, it usually takes the immune system several weeks after infection with Lyme bacteria to make enough anti-Lyme antibodies to be detected by the EIA test. If the EIA test is taken during these early weeks, the test could be falsely negative; your child could still have Lyme disease.

Also, if your child is taking antibiotics—for Lyme disease or another condition—during these early weeks, this could keep the immune system from making antibodies, and your child could have a false-negative EIA.

Even if the EIA test is positive, however, your child may not have Lyme disease. There are a number of other organisms that cause the immune system to make antibodies that also give positive results on an EIA test.

Therefore the lab performs a second blood test, using a different, more specific—but time-consuming—technique called Western blot. This can analyze whether the antibodies are truly against Lyme bacteria or against some other organism. Once your child is past those early weeks after a tick bite, if her Western blot is negative, she is very unlikely to have Lyme disease.

Even a positive Western-blot test, however, does not necessarily mean your child now has active Lyme disease. It just means that at some point, perhaps long in the past, your child had the bacteria in her body and mounted an immune response to them. Many people who live in Lyme-disease areas, you recall, become infected and never notice any symptoms. Your child's current symptoms could be caused by something else.

Therefore, to diagnose that a person has active Lyme disease, it is necessary not only that she have positive EIA and Western-blot tests but that she also have at least one of the typical symptoms of the disease: the rash, arthritis, or another symptom. Positive blood tests alone are often not enough.

Depending on your child's symptoms, your doctor may sometimes need to do other tests. If the doctor suspects your child has Lyme meningitis, he may perform a lumbar puncture (spinal tap) and have a lab examine the spinal fluid. (For a description of this procedure, see "Diagnosis," page 185, in *Meningitis*.) If she has arthritis, the doctor may have a lab examine fluid from the affected joint. If she has facial palsy or another nerve problem, he may do neurological testing. If he suspects your child has Lyme heart disease, he may perform an electrocardiogram and other cardiac tests.

## Treatment

If your child starts taking antibiotics within the first few weeks after he is infected with Lyme bacteria, he is less likely to develop any late or long-term complications and is more likely to recover completely.

However, your child does not need to take antibiotics if he was just bitten by tick but has not developed any symptoms of Lyme disease. Nor do most physicians prescribe antibiotics for people who have positive blood tests but no symptoms.

And your child should not take an antibiotic if he does not need it, since all antibiotics can sometimes cause adverse reactions. Or your child may develop an allergy to the antibiotic and then not be able to take it when he really needs it.

If a child does have the typical distinctive rash, most physicians start treatment without waiting for the test results to come back. In some circumstances, if a child is well except for the rash, no blood tests need to be performed.

There are a number of different antibiotics that your doctor may choose to prescribe, among them amoxicillin and doxycycline, depending on your child's age and specific symptoms. Your child will usually take the antibiotic by mouth two or three times a day for ten to thirty days, depending on his symptoms and how fast he responds.

If your child has more severe or late symptoms, your doctor may prescribe antibiotics intravenously, usually for a month. In one recent study, in Connecticut, of 201 children with Lyme disease, only seven children needed intravenous antibiotics. Three of these children had meningitis; two, facial-nerve palsy; one, both meningitis and facial palsy; and one, inflammation of the heart.

Your child can usually continue to go about his normal activities, including school, while taking oral or intravenous antibiotics for Lyme disease. For intravenous therapy the physician inserts a catheter in his arm. The catheter is connected to a tiny computerized device your child carries over his shoulder. The device automatically turns on the antibiotic infusion whenever he needs it, usually once or twice a day.

Sometimes a person needs other treatment for Lyme disease. If he has very severe arthritis, he may need to have fluid withdrawn from the affected joint. Rarely, a person with severe heart symptoms may need a temporary pacemaker and cardiac monitoring.

With antibiotic treatment, the rash usually disappears within a few days. Heart symptoms usually resolve on their own, even without treatment, leaving no long-term damage. Facial palsy usually goes away by itself within two to eight weeks—and your child can smile normally again.

However, even after the antibiotic has killed all the Lyme bacteria, the body still takes a while to return to normal. Your child may continue to have inflammation, swelling, and aching in his joints and flare-ups of arthritis for six months or more. He may need to take an antiinflammatory and pain-relieving medication such as ibuprofen or naproxen. And some people have persistent headaches, aching joints, and fatigue that last longer.

Of the 201 children in the Connecticut group, at the end of six months, all but one were completely well and back to normal. That one child still had mild, intermittent joint pain. Only one child needed retreatment with additional courses of antibiotics.

A common misconception sometimes leads people to take more antibiotic treatment for Lyme disease than they need. Some people believe, erroneously, that the antibiotic is going to turn their blood test negative again, so they keep taking more and more antibiotics, expecting the test to become normal. But it does not. Once you develop anti-Lyme antibodies, you generally continue to keep them in your blood and have a positive test forevermore. While the antibiotics kill the bacteria and cure the disease, they do not wipe out the antibodies.

The most common reason for antibiotic treatment for Lyme disease to fail is misdiagnosis. At Children's Hospital we often see this. A child or teenager has been treated for Lyme disease but still has headache or fatigue. It usually turns that she never had Lyme disease. So-called treatment failures are often diagnostic failures.

Lyme disease is not generally a life-threatening illness. However, there have been a handful of deaths due to Lyme disease reported in the medical literature. One Nantucket man who died had Lyme bacteria in his heart. But such deaths from Lyme disease are exceedingly rare.

Your child can get Lyme disease more than once. If he is treated early with antibiotics, he may not develop enough antibodies to fend off the bacteria if he is bitten again by an infected tick.

## Hospitalization

Occasionally a person needs to be hospitalized for Lyme disease. In the Connecticut group, only four of the 201 children were admitted to the hospital, three for meningitis and one for heart symptoms. They stayed an average of three days. At Children's Hospital we sometimes admit a child briefly to start his intravenous antibiotic therapy.

## *Prevention*

Obviously, the surest way of keeping your child from getting Lyme disease—or any other tick-borne disease—is to prevent her from getting bitten by a tick. This means staying away from places where there may be ticks infected with the bacteria. However, this may not be practical if you happen to live in a Lyme disease hot spot.

Your child is most likely to encounter infected ticks, remember, in grassy, brushy, or wooded areas. Where you see deer, ticks may be present, and also where there are mice or other rodents. And in the Northeast, a person is most likely to be bitten by the tiny nymphs during the spring and summer and by the larger adults at almost any time of year.

When walking in tick-infested areas, your child is less likely to be bitten if she keeps to the middle of trails or paths and avoids brushing against vegetation at the sides. Deer ticks are sedentary creatures: they have no wings, and they do not fly, jump, or drop down on a person from above. They mostly cling to grass and bushes, passively waiting for their next meal to walk by.

You can protect your child against tick bites by dressing her in a long-sleeved shirt, long pants, high socks, and high boots and tucking her pants legs into her socks or sealing her pants legs with tape. Also, if she wears light colors, it will be easier to see any ticks that may get on her clothes. Deer hunters in Lyme disease areas are warned to dress this way, but again, it is hardly practical if your backyard is a hot spot.

You can further protect your child by using a tick repellent. You can spray permethrin on her clothing, particularly on her pants, socks, and shoes—but not her skin. Or you can apply DEET (N, N-diethyl-m-toluamide) to her clothing or directly to her skin. For children, use repellents that contain no more than 6 to 10 percent DEET.

Read the labels carefully before applying either of these repellents and use them as directed. "If DEET is used, it should be used sparingly," warns the American Academy of Pediatrics, "because seizures have been reported coincident with its application in young children." It should be applied "only to exposed skin, not to a child's face, hands or irritated or abraded skin. These preparations should be removed by washing after the child comes indoors."

If you live in or visit tick country, it is a good idea to inspect your child's body for ticks every night during tick season. Once on her body, a tick may crawl almost anywhere; be sure to inspect hairy places, and remember that the nymphs are only the size of a poppy seed. You also need to check your dog and cat; people have caught Lyme disease from a tick the dog brought in. Deer ticks are much smaller than dog ticks.

If you do find a tick on your child or your pet or yourself, remove it promptly. Ticks are slow feeders: they must remain attached for several days to get their blood meal, and the longer one is attached, the more likely it is to infect the person. "If you remove a tick before it has attached for more than 24 hours," says the U.S. Public Health Service, "you greatly reduce your risk of infection." You can get some idea of how long a tick has been attached by its size. As it feeds, its body slowly enlarges.

To remove a tick, use tweezers. Grasp the tick as close as possible to the skin in order to get its mouth parts. Pull on the tweezers with a slow, steady pull. Try not to squeeze or crush the tick's body; its body fluids may contain the bacteria. Then wash the area with warm soapy water and also wash your hands. If you have to use your fingers to remove a tick, protect them with a tissue and wash your hands afterward.

Some people advocate suffocating the tick on the skin by coating it with a substance such as nail polish, nail polish remover, alcohol, or petroleum jelly. This is not advisable. If these methods work at all, they take too long. You need to get that tick off sooner rather than later.

Finally, a new vaccine against Lyme disease is being considered by the U.S. Food and Drug Administration. The vaccine has a three-dose schedule and is 79 percent effective. At this stage, the prevention measures mentioned above will still be very important—vaccine or not.

## Resources

You should be able to obtain information about whether infected ticks are prevalent in your area, the time of year they are most active, and also about possible methods of reducing tick populations from your local or state health or park department or your local office of the Cooperative Extension Service. You can find the Cooperative Extension Service in the phone book under the name of your state's land-grant university. In Pennsylvania the service is run by Penn State University; in New York, by Cornell University.

You can get more detailed information about Lyme disease from the U.S. Public Health Service's Centers for Disease Control and Prevention (CDC) in Atlanta by calling their toll-free Voice and Fax Information System at 1-888-232-3228. You can also connect to CDC on the Internet at http://www.cdc.gov. The material on this Web site includes color photographs of deer ticks.

The National Institute of Allergy and Infectious Diseases also has information about Lyme disease on the Internet (at http://www.niaid.nih.gov), including photographs of the tick as well as the distinctive rash.

# MEASLES

*A vaccine is available to protect your child against measles. See* **Vaccines***, page 301, in the Appendices.*

***Measles must be treated by a doctor.***

Also known as rubeola.

---

## SYMPTOMS

- High fever

- Runny nose

- Cough

- Red eyes, sensitive to light

- Rash (appears first on face and travels down body)

---

If you talk to an adult who had measles as a child, one striking memory is lying in bed in a darkened room. Most children today will not have that experience, thanks to an immunization schedule that has virtually eliminated measles from the list of common childhood illnesses. Yet before 1963, when the vaccine was first used, an average of 500,000 cases was reported in the United States each year.

Measles is best known for its distinctive skin rash. Initial symptoms include irritability, runny nose, eyes that are red and sensitive to light, hacking cough, and a fever that may be as high as 105°F. These early symptoms usually last for three or four days before the rash appears. Sometimes this early period, called the prodromal period, may last only one day or it may last as long as eight days.

Typically the rash begins on the nape of the neck and spreads downward over the face, neck, and body. It takes about three days for the rash to travel to the feet. It looks like large, flat, red to brown blotches that often meld into one another and appear to completely cover the skin, especially on the face and shoulders. It is curious that the rash fades in the same order that it appeared, forehead first and feet last.

One distinguishing characteristic that makes diagnosis of measles fairly easy for a doctor, is the

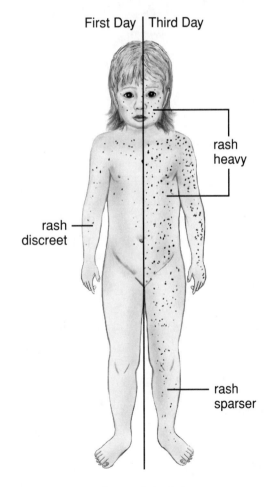

First Day | Third Day

rash heavy

rash discreet

rash sparser

*Measles rash on first and third days.*

appearance of Koplik's spots. These are small red, irregularly shaped spots with blue-white centers found inside the mouth. They usually appear one or two days before the rash and may be noticed by your doctor while examining your child.

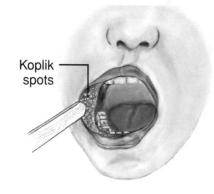

Koplik
spots

*Koplik's spots within the mouth.*

Measles is very contagious, and there is a high probability that anyone in your household who has not been immunized will develop the disease if someone else has it. Measles can cause a miscarriage or premature birth, so it is important if you are pregnant that you seek treatment if you have been exposed to measles.

Measles can lead to complications and can make the body more susceptible to ear infections or pneumonia caused by bacteria. Before the vaccine was available, measles occurred in springtime epidemics.

## Causes

Measles is a respiratory infection caused by the measles virus.

## How It Spreads

The disease spreads in fluid from the nose or mouth and in airborne droplets. That makes it easy to catch when someone with measles coughs or sneezes. Even if your child just talks to someone with measles, he may catch it because he can inhale the organism. He can even become infected simply by being in a room after an infected person has left because particles may remain suspended in the air.

People with measles are contagious from five days after exposure to five days after the rash appears.

Currently, outbreaks occur most often on college campuses among young persons who either have not been adequately immunized or whose immunity has decreased since childhood.

## Incubation Period

Generally there are eight to twelve days from exposure to onset of symptoms. In family studies, the average interval between the appearance of the rash in the first case and the appearance of the rash in other family members is fourteen days.

## Symptoms

Early symptoms include a runny nose, hacking cough, red eyes that are sensitive to light, and a high fever. Then the symptoms disappear except for the cough, which persists. A rash appears on the face and nape of the neck and travels down the body to the feet over the course of about three days.

## Diagnosis

The most definitive diagnosis is made from nose or throat cultures or by a blood test for antibodies. Generally, however, your doctor will diagnose measles by signs and symptoms, particularly if Koplik's spots are visible in your child's mouth.

## CALL YOUR DOCTOR

- Immediately if you suspect your child has measles.

- If your infant has been exposed to measles before being vaccinated.

- If your child has measles and his temperature goes above 103°F.

- If your child has measles and has an earache, breathing difficulties, severe headaches, stiff neck, seizures, severe drowsiness, difficulty waking up, or loss of consciousness.

- If your child has been exposed to measles and has tuberculosis, cancer, or is immunocompromised.

## Treatment

There are no antiviral drugs currently available for treatment of measles. Typically treatment of measles consists of managing the symptoms and keeping your child comfortable. If your child is otherwise healthy, keep her away from other children for four days after the onset of the rash.

Use acetaminophen to bring down fever. Do not use aspirin for a child who has a viral illness because the use of aspirin in such cases has been associated with the development of Reye's syndrome. (See *Reye's Syndrome,* page 217.) Children often have poor appetites in the early days of measles infection. Offer bland foods such as toast or crackers. Encourage your child to drink fluids—mostly clear liquids like soup broth, fruit juices, and popsicles to maintain and replace water lost in perspiration from fever. Using a cool-mist vaporizer reduces the chance of lung infections because it prevents lung secretions from thickening and clogging the breathing passages. Be sure to clean the vaporizer daily to prevent mold from growing. Avoid steam vaporizers that can scald or burn your child.

Your child may lose interest in watching TV, playing video games, or reading if the eyes become sensitive to light. Children often curtail their own activity when not feeling well. Encourage, but do not impose, bedrest. Your child should not return to school or a child-care center until five days after the rash appears. When there is an outbreak in a school or child-care center, any unimmunized child or adult should be immunized or excluded from the center until two weeks after the rash appears in the last case of measles in the facility.

Although vitamin A deficiency is generally not a recognized problem in the United States, it is evident in many children with more severe measles. The doctor will administer vitamin A to a child with measles under certain conditions, for instance, if the child is between six months to two years old and is hospitalized with measles and complications or if the child is older than six months and has an immunodeficiency.

## Prevention

All fifty states have laws requiring schoolchildren to be immunized against measles. The number of doses depends on your state. Measles vaccine is available in a single vaccine or in combination as measles, mumps, and rubella (MMR). MMR is the vaccine of choice for use in routine vaccination programs for children. MMR is an attenuated live virus vaccine, which means that after injection, the viruses grow and cause a very mild or asymptomatic infection in the vaccinated person. The person's immune system fights the infection caused by these weakened viruses, and immunity develops.

Most babies born in the United States receive some protection against measles (as well as mumps and rubella) from maternal antibodies. These antibodies can destroy the vaccine virus if they are present when the vaccine is administered. That is why MMR vaccine is not given until after a child's first birthday, when almost all infants have lost this passive protection. A small percentage of children may get a low-grade fever and slight rash following the MMR vaccine.

The first dose of vaccine should be given at twelve to fifteen months of age. MMR vaccine works well and will protect most children for the rest of their lives. But for about 5 percent of children, the first dose of MMR does not work. That is why a second dose is recommended—it gives these children another chance to become immune. This can be administered either when your child enters kindergarten or first grade, or else middle school.

This vaccine is usually not given to infants younger than thirteen months except when there are cases of measles in the community. Then a dose of measles vaccine alone is given, followed by the usual MMR immunization at fifteen months.

The measles vaccine should not be given to those with depressed immune systems or severe allergies to eggs or to the antibiotic neomycin—these children may risk life-threatening reactions to measles vaccine.

Measles vaccine is given to control measles outbreaks in schools. If this vaccine is given within seventy-two hours of exposure, it may provide protection to children who have no immunity to measles. If the exposure does not result in measles infection, the vaccine should protect against subsequent infection.

Immunoglobulin (IG) can be used to prevent or modify measles in an exposed, unvaccinated child but should be given within six days of exposure. IG is generally given to susceptible household members or contacts (particularly children younger than one), immunocompromised persons, and pregnant women (for whom the risk of complications is highest). If a mother is diagnosed with measles, her unimmunized children should receive IG because it is evidence that the mother did not have protective antibodies to transmit to her children before birth. These children should be given measles vaccine later (five to six months), provided they are at least twelve months old.

Children and adolescents with symptomatic HIV infection who are exposed to measles should receive IG preventive treatment regardless of vaccination status unless the child has been receiving IGIV at regular intervals and the last dose was within three weeks of exposure.

# MENINGITIS

*This is a disease for which there is a vaccine to protect your child. See* Vaccines, *page 301, in the Appendices.*

*Meningitis must be treated by a doctor.*

## SYMPTOMS

- Vomiting

- Fever

- Severe headache

- Stiff neck or back

- Sensitivity to light

- Extreme irritability

- Rash or bruise marks

- Seizure

- Bulging fontanel (soft spot) in infant

- Hallucinations or delirium

- Drowsiness

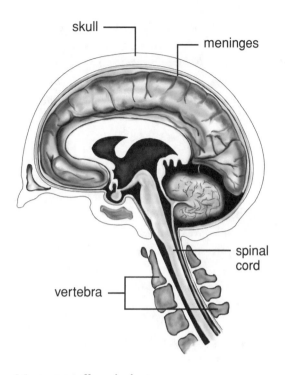

*Meningitis affects the brain.*

Meningitis is an inflammation of the meninges, which is the membrane covering the brain and spinal cord. It is the most common infection of the central nervous system, and because it affects the brain, meningitis is also one of the most menacing of infectious diseases. But it is important to note that there are many forms of the disease, some of which are quite benign or mild.

Meningitis can be caused by either bacteria or viruses or less frequently by fungi, parasites, or other factors. You may hear about aseptic meningitis—this is a general term to describe meningitis that is caused by organisms other than common bacteria.

Viral meningitis is probably the most common form of meningitis. This infection poses little threat to most healthy children and adults. Of the many viruses responsible for meningitis in the United States, enteroviruses are the most common. At Children's Hospital we see viral meningitis mainly in summer and fall.

The symptoms of viral meningitis are usually less severe than those of bacterial meningitis. Even though viral meningitis is usually not serious, its sudden onset can be frightening for a parent or caretaker. One mother describes the onset of her teenage son's bout with viral meningitis:

*I just knew this wasn't an ordinary head-
ache or stomach virus. He kept saying that
he felt like his brain was going to explode
and that the light hurt his eyes. He threw
up several times but it didn't ease his nausea. I had never seen him that sick before.*

Typical of many viral meningitis patients, this teen
was hospitalized for a few days but was symptom
free by the third day. Older children and teens
may be unusually tired for weeks after all other
symptoms have disappeared.

In contrast to viral meningitis, bacterial meningitis is quite serious and can even be life-
threatening. It is one of the more serious illnesses
in infants and young children because of the mor-
tality rate and the incidence of severe long-term
neurologic effects. The incidence of bacterial
meningitis in children peaks between six and
twelve months of age because death or disability
is a possibility with this infection. Since the early
1990s a very effective vaccine has been responsible for the disappearance of *Haemophilus
influenzae* type B (Hib), which had previously
been a major cause of meningitis in children
younger than five years old.

Today pneumococcal and meningococcal
meningitis are the most common serious types
of bacterial meningitis among young people.
More boys get meningitis than girls, but the reason for that is not clear.

Serious complications of bacterial meningitis
result from an increase of pressure on the brain
and inflammation from the infection. If the
nerves leaving the brain are damaged, there may
be developments such as hearing loss or mental
retardation. Upon recovery, your child will have
his hearing tested to make certain there has not
been any hearing loss.

## Causes

Viral meningitis, like the common cold, is caused
by a virus. Typically the enteroviruses, which live
in the intestine, are the cause. These viruses are
spread by the fecal-oral route. The virus enters
into the central nervous system and causes
inflammation of the lining of the brain and spinal cord. Bacteria can also cause meningitis.
Although up to 5 to 10 percent of the general
population carry meningococcal bacteria in the
nose and throat and the upper respiratory tract
as well, very few develop the disease. The disease occurs when the bacteria leave the respiratory tract and travel through the bloodstream to
the meninges.

## How It Spreads

Viral meningitis is spread by contact with infected
feces or nose and throat secretions through coughing and sneezing. Most children carry the virus
without getting the disease, and no one knows
why only a few children become ill.

Bacterial meningitis, for the most part,
occurs in single cases, but it can be epidemic.
That is why it is so important to determine the
cause of the meningitis right away. Meningococcal meningitis is one type of bacterial infection
spread by nose and throat secretions, although
these bacteria cannot usually live for more than
a few minutes outside the body.

While this condition may occur at any age,
the risk of infection increases with the number
of people your child comes in contact with. This
explains why meningococcal meningitis occurs
mainly among school-age children and adolescents. We see it, for example, in child-care centers, dormitories, or in the armed forces—areas
in which there is close personal contact.

A person who has had intimate or direct exposure to a meningococcal meningitis patient within seven days is at risk for contracting the disease. If your child is diagnosed with meningococcal meningitis, your physician may want you to take preventive medication, especially if there are other young children in the household who might be susceptible. Exposure includes being touched or kissed, sharing dishes or silverware, or droplet contamination from nose, throat, or any secretions or excretions from the infected child's body.

If your child requires hospitalization, she will be placed in isolation for the first twenty-four to forty-eight hours.

## Incubation Period

Incubation varies with each virus and is not completely understood. The meningitis caused by enteroviruses has an incubation period of three to six days; however, carriers or sick children carry the virus in their feces before they become sick and also for weeks after they recover. Incubation periods of other viral agents vary and range from four to twenty-one days.

## Symptoms

It is easy to ignore the early signs of meningitis because your child may experience only minor cold or gastrointestinal symptoms for a few days. And because meningitis is relatively rare, it is not readily considered a cause of the problem. If your child has been sick, the medication may mask meningitis symptoms. The type of organism that causes the infection also influences the symptoms. Symptoms may vary if the disease is an isolated infection or a complication of another illness or injury.

The most striking symptoms of meningitis are a severe headache and stiff neck, generally accompanied by a high fever and sometimes a rash. Most cases of viral meningitis run a short, uneventful course. The symptoms usually last from three to fourteen days.

The symptoms that your child displays with acute bacterial meningitis depend largely on his age. With an infant, the signs of meningitis are usually subtle. Your baby may not want to eat. He may be lethargic, irritable, and may not want to be cuddled. He may or may not have mild fever symptoms. Some parents report a high-pitched cry, a vacant stare, and a bulging and tense fontanel (soft spot on the head). It is apparent that your baby is not well, but it may be difficult to figure out what is going on.

With an older child, the onset of meningitis is likely to be abrupt—fever, chills, stiff neck, and severe headache and vomiting associated with or quickly followed by alterations in senses. Sometimes a seizure is the initial symptom. Other symptoms include extreme irritability and agitation, photophobia (sensitivity to light), delirium, hallucinations, aggressive or maniacal behavior, drowsiness, stupor, and coma.

You should contact your doctor immediately if your child has a fever *and* a severe sudden headache accompanied by mental changes, neck/back stiffness, or rashes on the armpits, groin, ankles, and any place where you can apply pressure. Sometimes the rash may appear as tiny red spots, or it may resemble bruises.

## Diagnosis

It is critical to diagnose meningitis quickly because your doctor must know what is causing the disease. Bacterial meningitis requires immediate attention and treatment. That is why your

child will most likely be hospitalized when any
meningitis is suspected. Meningitis is very difficult to diagnose in newborn and premature
infants because the symptoms are not as visible
as in older children.

The diagnosis is confirmed by performing a
spinal tap (lumbar puncture). This is a safe and
relatively simple procedure that involves intro-
ducing a thin needle into the spinal canal—
below the level of the spinal cord—and
sampling less than one teaspoon of the cerebrospinal fluid (CSF), which normally appears

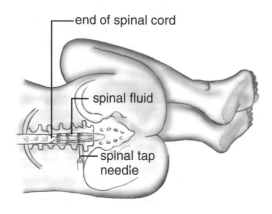

*A spinal tap is taken from the space below the
spinal cord so that the needle will not touch the
spinal cord.*

crystal clear and contains few or no white blood
cells. When meningitis is present, the CSF contains numerous white blood cells, a sign of
infection or inflammation of the meninges lining the spinal cord and brain.

Other lab tests may include blood tests, a
urine analysis, and throat culture to determine
which specific virus or bacterium is responsible.
In typical cases of bacterial meningitis, the
offending bacteria can be cultured usually within
forty-eight hours.

Try to keep your child quiet during the diagnostic testing. Speak softly and reassure her that
the spinal tap will hurt just a little (one teenage
boy described the spinal tap as "just like any
needle"). If you are able to remain calm, you will
help your child stay calm also.

## Treatment

Most children with viral meningitis have a mild
illness. There is no medication for treatment
of viral meningitis. More serious cases require
hospitalization and intravenous fluids; however,
even these cases usually last only a few days
and there are rarely complications. Your child
will be treated primarily for symptoms—
acetaminophen for headache, heat for muscle
aches and pains, and positioning for comfort.
If your child experienced vomiting, he may
receive intravenous fluids to restore his elec-
trolyte balance.

Until diagnostic tests rule out a bacterial
infection, your physician will order intravenous
antibiotics and place your child in isolation—
these are precautionary measures. The antibiotics will be stopped as soon as a viral diagnosis is
made. If any severe neurologic signs and symptoms develop, your physician will reevaluate the
diagnosis.

In contrast to viral meningitis, bacterial meningitis is life-threatening and requires immediate treatment. Your child will be hospitalized immediately and given intravenous antibiotics in large doses for a period of seven to fourteen days. The same tests that are used to diagnose any meningitis will be administered to determine the cause. Depending upon your child's condition, he may receive fluids intravenously. A severely ill child may require intensive care therapy and close observation.

## Prevention

There is no vaccine or preventive medicine for viral meningitis. If your child attends a day-care center, school, or camp, stress the importance of hand washing after using the toilet, blowing her nose, and before eating. Because meningitis is caused by viruses and bacteria, be sure that your child gets prompt treatment for upper respiratory infections, middle ear infections, and other infections.

A vaccine now routinely given to infants controls *H. influenzae* type B meningitis (Hib), which was once the most frequent bacterial cause of childhood meningitis. As a result of this routine vaccination, we have seen a drastic reduction of this type of bacterial meningitis by more than 98 percent.

For children an antibiotic called rifampin is effective in preventing most cases of Hib and meningococcal meningitis from occurring after exposure. This prescription antibiotic helps prevent any child or family member who has been exposed from getting the disease. It should be given within twenty-four hours after exposure. Rifampin is given by mouth once a day for several days and may tint urine, tears, and saliva with an orange color. In some situations other antibiotics may be given to prevent infection.

Pneumovax is an effective vaccine in preventing some infections caused by pneumococcus bacteria. It is recommended only for children who are most susceptible to this infection—children with abnormal immune systems, for instance, or those who have certain diseases such as sickle cell disease or kidney disease. Ask your doctor about this vaccine.

In addition, there is a vaccine against some strains or types of the meningococcal bacterial. This vaccine should be given to children who travel to parts of the world (Africa, for example) where these types of meningococci exist.

# MONONUCLEOSIS

***Mononucleosis must be treated by a doctor.***

Also called mono.

## SYMPTOMS

- High fever
- Sore throat
- Swollen glands
- Fatigue
- Runny nose
- Abdominal discomfort

Commonly called mono, mononucleosis is a mild viral infection that was first recognized in 1921. Mononucleosis actually describes a set of symptoms that includes sore throat, fatigue, swollen lymph glands, fever, and enlarged liver and/or spleen. Mono gets its name because the disease is identified by a marked increase in what are referred to as the mononuclear elements of the blood—certain kinds of white cells that have a single (mono) nucleus.

You may recall hearing mono referred to as the "kissing disease." This name actually reflects the way in which the disease spreads—through the saliva or mucous membranes of an infected person. Most often the source of infectious mononucleosis is from intimate contact with family members or playmates.

Mono is relatively common among young persons between twelve and twenty-five years old; yet most people think of it as a teenage disease. And no wonder—the peak age of incidence for cases occurring outside childhood is approximately eighteen years for men and sixteen for women. The classic symptoms of mono are fever, sore throat, and swollen glands and occur in half of cases among fifteen- to twenty-four-year-olds.

Doctors now know that infectious mono is much more common in younger children than previously recognized. Many cases in young children are simply not diagnosed, primarily because these youngsters do not exhibit the fatigue that older people do and when they do have mono, the symptoms are mild much like a cold.

One parent of a boy in middle school recalls,

*He was sick all the time when he was younger—sore throats, swollen glands, fever, bronchial infections, ear infections . . . you name it, he had it. But he never seemed totally wiped out for more than a couple of days. So we were surprised when a blood test recently revealed that, at some point, he had mono. It was never diagnosed.*

We find that infectious mono occurs throughout the year. Compared to other infectious diseases, mono does not usually occur in outbreaks. College students and military people experience a higher rate of mono than the general population, but that is probably because these groups live in close quarters.

Mono does not usually present complications. Occasionally there may be inflammation of the liver (hepatitis), swollen tonsils, or even a swelling in the lining of the brain, but these problems usually clear up quickly. You may hear of someone with mono who had a ruptured spleen, but that can be avoided by avoiding trauma to the enlarged spleen that is common with mono. This explains why doctors advise the patient to avoid contact sports for a while. Sometimes the tonsils get so enlarged that they block the air passage, but steroid drugs can rapidly decrease the swelling.

## Causes

The virus generally responsible for classic infectious mononucleosis is called Epstein-Barr virus (EBV). However, in about 10 percent of infectious mono cases, the cause is other viruses or infectious agents. Once you get EBV, you have it for the rest of your life, although the virus apparently remains dormant after the first illness. By the time most adults reach eighteen years of age, they have been exposed to EBV and are immune. EBV infects up to 95 percent of the world's adult population.

## How It Spreads

Infectious mono spreads through the respiratory secretions of an infected person. It is passed in the saliva, which is why kissing and close contact with family members are often the culprits. Even though mono spreads more among family members than to outsiders, only about one-third of susceptible family members contract EBV from the infected person. Many people believe that mono is highly contagious, but that it is not so. Because mono does not spread easily from touching items that the infected person has touched, the disease is only mildly contagious. The virus spreads faster among children in crowded or closed conditions.

## Incubation Period

Approximately thirty to fifty days elapse from the time of exposure to EBV-associated infectious mononucleosis until the onset of symptoms.

## Symptoms

Infectious mono symptoms develop rather slowly. For the first few days your child may seem to be very tired, but otherwise she will not complain of anything specific. There may be a fever initially, but many children do not have a temperature until several days later. The fever is generally high (103° to 104°F) and accompanies a sore throat and swollen glands. In some cases (but not many), a child may have a small pink rash on the trunk and extremities. We sometimes see this rash after a child, showing symptoms of mono, has been on a course of amoxicillin, ampicillin, or other penicillins for an earlier infection. We do not know why this happens, but it is a fairly reliable characteristic of infectious mono.

The symptoms generally last for two to three weeks and are milder during the third week. The symptoms of general illness and fatigue may take longer to disappear—sometimes several weeks or months in ordinary cases with no complications. Some studies reveal that recovery depends on the emotional state and attitude of the patient—if your child feels stressed or upset by her illness, she may take longer to heal. This is particularly true with teens, who may feel stressed from missing school and social activities. Try to be patient with your child during this illness.

About 50 percent of patients will have an enlarged spleen, and 10 percent will have an enlarged liver. We generally see these symptoms in the early phase, along with other symptoms. We usually see enlarged tonsils in these children as well.

To some teens, mono is a disease with a "label" that means they are engaging in certain activities when, in fact, they are not. A diagnosis of mono can cause anxiety for teens who do not have a boyfriend or girlfriend. Teens really do believe that mono is the "kissing disease," and a diagnosis can be very embarrassing. Be sure to talk to your child about the causes of mono and encourage her to educate her peers.

## Diagnosis

Although EBV is the most common cause of mono, there are other causes. The next most common cause of monolike symptoms is cytomegalovirus (CMV), a herpes virus. Toxoplasmosis, an animal-borne disease (see *Toxoplasmosis*, page 11), also produces symptoms much like a mono infection. Doctors do not always need to make a precise diagnosis of the cause of mono because often these diseases do not require specific treatment.

Blood tests are the most common tests for EBV. There are a number of different tests for EBV that can give your doctor useful information, such as antibody levels and the number of white blood cells present. A "spot test" known as Monospot permits early diagnosis in teenagers and specifically targets infectious mono. The test is not as accurate in preteens.

## Treatment

In the early stages you will want your child to get plenty of bed rest. This may be a problem with adolescents and young adults, who frequently complain of fatigue for weeks and even months after the onset of symptoms but do not want to miss out on activities.

If there is a strep throat infection, your doctor will prescribe penicillin. To treat the sore throat pain, encourage your child to gargle, drink hot or warm drinks, and suck on throat lozenges. If he develops badly swollen glands or tonsils so enlarged that they obstruct the airways, your doctor will prescribe steroids to reduce the swelling. In an extreme case, your child may have to be hospitalized so the medication can be administered intravenously.

Complications with infectious mono are not common, but when they occur, they require attention. In almost all cases of infectious mono, the spleen or liver is involved. It is best to avoid live vaccines until several months after recovery because your child's immune system may not react normally during the disease.

You will want to give your child lots of fluids to offset the dehydrating effects of fever. Since he may lose a significant amount of weight, try to make meals and snacks that are both appetizing and nutritious. Some people think that it is best to have a recovering child ease back into school by attending either half days or some kind of reduced schedule. Your child can return to school when symptoms subside.

Because of the risk of rupturing the spleen, we recommend that your child avoid heavy lifting and contact sports for two months after the first symptoms of mono, even if he does not have an enlarged spleen.

Acetaminophen is preferable to aspirin for fever and pain because of the rare association of EBV with Reye's syndrome (see page 217).

## Prevention

Currently there is no vaccine against EBV. A child with mono should stay home from daycare or school until the symptoms subside and she feels well enough to go back, but isolation and special precautions are not necessary.

# MUMPS

*A vaccine is available to protect your child against mumps. See* **Vaccines,** *page 301, in the Appendices, for a list of all the vaccines your child needs.*

## SYMPTOMS

- Swollen cheeks and upper neck
- Swollen testicles
- Possible fever, headache, nausea, fatigue

Mumps used to be such a common childhood disease that nearly every child caught it before adulthood.

It is usually an innocuous disease, nothing to worry about. A child's face becomes swollen, and a teenage boy's or man's testicles may swell for a while. However, mumps can sometimes be much more serious. Fortunately, it can now be prevented by vaccination. You should routinely have your child immunized against mumps.

After mumps vaccine came into widespread use in 1977, the number of people catching mumps each year decreased dramatically. By the mid-1980s only a few thousand cases of mumps were reported each year to the U.S. Public Health Service's Centers for Disease Control and Prevention in Atlanta.

However, mumps is still around, and it continues to cause outbreaks from time to time. At Marquette University in Milwaukee one year, 178 people caught mumps. And in Chicago over a four-month period, 116 employees at three financial exchanges came down with mumps, most of them young men and women who worked on the trading floors. Three more people

who lived with exchange employees also got it. Many more such outbreaks are likely to occur if we do not continue to vaccinate our children.

The routine use of mumps vaccine has also caused a shift in the age at which people are most likely to catch the disease. Before the vaccine, a person most often got mumps between the ages of five and nine, while in elementary school. Now a person is more likely to get it at an older age. In the outbreak at the Chicago exchanges, the employees catching mumps ranged in age from seventeen to seventy years.

The significance of this age shift is that a person who catches mumps as a teenager or young adult is much more likely to have severe symptoms and be sick longer.

## Cause

Mumps is caused by a virus called the mumps virus. This is one of the many viruses that infect only human beings.

## How It Spreads

People who are infected with mumps virus shed great numbers of virus particles in their saliva and in the other secretions that come from their mouth and nose. Virus particles are spread inside droplets of moisture into the air during coughing or sneezing.

Your child can become infected with mumps virus when she inhales these virus-containing droplets or when she gets them in her mouth. Virus particles can also be spread by contact such as sharing a drinking glass or an eating utensil with an infected person—or by kissing an infected person.

The trouble is that your child usually catches mumps from someone who does not know he is infected. A person coming down with mumps starts shedding virus a day or two or more before he starts to have symptoms. And about a third of infected people never have any symptoms at all or have symptoms so mild that they are never recognized as mumps—yet these people are shedding virus and your child can catch mumps from them.

Once mumps virus particles get into her body, they spread from her nose and mouth into her bloodstream and then may target specific organs, where they settle down and grow and multiply.

## Incubation Period

It usually takes sixteen to eighteen days from the time a person is infected with mumps virus before he has any symptoms, if he is going to have symptoms. It can, however, take as little as twelve days or as long as twenty-five days.

## Symptoms

If your child does develop symptoms, facial swelling is usually the first thing you notice. The mumps virus most often targets the glands producing the saliva that moistens the mouth and helps us digest our food. We have three pairs of salivary glands. The largest ones are just below and in front of the ears. The other, smaller ones are below our jaw in the neck and beneath the floor of the mouth.

Mumps virus most commonly grows and multiplies in the largest salivary glands, the ones near the ears. As the glands become inflamed, your child's face usually starts to swell on one side. Then, two or three days later, the swelling spreads to the other side, reaching a maximum in another two or three days. Your child's cheeks may puff out so much that she resembles a chipmunk. (See figure right.) Or she may have swelling on just one side, just one cheek puffed out. Less often the virus infects the other, smaller salivary glands, and your child may have swelling in her neck, under the jaw.

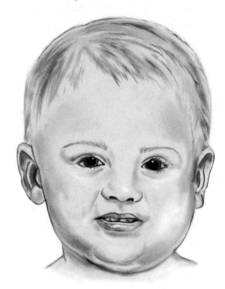

*Facial and upper neck swelling is usually the first sign or indication of mumps.*

Along with the swelling of the face—and sometimes a few days before—your child may also have a low fever and a headache. She may be nauseated and vomiting, lose her appetite, and feel weak and tired.

Your child's swollen salivary glands can be very painful, and they can be even more painful when she opens her mouth, when she tries to chew food or swallow, or when you touch her cheeks. Certain foods—especially acidic ones such as orange juice—may make her glands hurt even more. And the swelling may make it difficult for her to speak clearly. One theory about the origin of the name *mumps* is that it refers to the speech of people with significant swelling: one meaning of the verb *mump* is "to mumble."

As mentioned, however, about one-third of people infected with mumps virus never have any noticeable swelling of their salivary glands. They may just have a low fever or mild headache or no symptoms at all. A person can easily have mumps and never realize it.

## Complications

While usually not serious, mumps can sometimes cause significant complications, particularly among teenagers and adults. Mumps is notorious for the effect it has on males past the age of puberty. In about one out of every three or four teenage boys or adult men, the virus targets the testes, the male reproductive organ where sperm are produced. The infection causes the testicles to swell and become excruciatingly painful and tender and the scrotum to become inflamed and red.

Swelling of the testicles can occur before or after the beginning of facial swelling, or there may be no facial swelling at all. Along with the testicular swelling, the affected person usually has a fever, headache, and nausea. The swelling usually affects just one testicle, but it can affect both.

These symptoms of mumps were described so clearly by the Greek physician Hippocrates in the fifth century B.C. that we know mumps virus has been around at least since those ancient times. "Swelling appeared about the ears, in many on either side, and in the greatest number on both sides," he wrote about people affected in an outbreak. "In some instances earlier, and in others later, inflammations with pain seized sometimes one of the testicles, and sometimes both."

Mumps virus can also infect other glands. In about one-third of females past age fifteen, it can infect the breasts, causing them to swell painfully. The virus can also affect the ovaries, causing swelling and pain in the lower abdomen.

Or the virus can infect the thyroid gland, at the base of the neck, or the pancreas, causing nausea and vomiting and pain in the upper abdomen. If a woman catches mumps during the first three months of pregnancy, it can cause her to have a miscarriage.

In about one out of every ten people who have mumps, the virus invades the central nervous system and causes meningitis, an infection and inflammation of the membranes (meninges) covering the brain and spinal cord. The person usually has a severe headache and an extremely stiff neck, a higher fever, and feels irritable and lethargic. A person can have mumps meningitis without any salivary gland swelling, or have meningitis a week before the swelling or up to three weeks afterward. Adults are more likely to develop mumps meningitis than are young children.

In about one in every 6,000 people, the mumps virus invades the brain and causes encephalitis, an infection of brain tissue itself. Encephalitis is the cause of most deaths due to mumps. Before routine use of mumps vaccine, the disease used to kill about forty people a year in this country. Most of these deaths were among adults.

## Diagnosis

If a physician suspects a person has mumps, a throat swab would be obtained and sent to a laboratory to culture (grow) the virus in order to identify it. Occasionally physicians diagnose mumps by detecting antimumps antibodies in a person's blood.

## Treatment

Unfortunately, there are no medications to treat mumps. In time, mumps will go away on its own as your child's immune system develops enough

## CALL YOUR DOCTOR

- If your child's face becomes swollen.
- If your child develops a swollen, painful testicle.

NOTE: In the latter case, your son may not have mumps but rather a condition called testicular torsion, which requires emergency surgery. This occurs most often in teenagers and is not an infectious disease. Call your doctor immediately or go to your hospital emergency department.

antibodies to overcome all the mumps-virus particles in his body. While this is happening, he needs to rest until any fever and the swelling of his salivary glands or testicles goes down.

You need to make sure that your child takes in plenty of extra fluids to prevent dehydration. He may not feel well enough to drink as much as usual, and he may find it painful to swallow. And if he has any fever, he is losing more fluid than usual from his respiratory tract and his skin. He may also be losing a lot more fluid if he is vomiting. Dehydration can be very dangerous, particularly for small children.

With mumps, you should avoid giving your child citrus or other acidic drinks that may increase the pain in his swollen salivary glands. Using a straw may make it easier for him to drink enough fluid. See *Fluids*, page 290, in the Appendices for more about dehydration and what other fluids to offer and not offer your child.

Since mumps may make it painful to chew and your child may be nauseated, he may lose interest in solid food. Avoid offering him foods that require extra saliva or need a lot of chewing,

such as a steak. Do offer him soft, light, bland foods that he can swallow easily without much chewing.

To relieve the pain of his swollen salivary glands or testes, you can give your child acetaminophen. Acetaminophen both relieves pain and reduces any fever and will help make your child more comfortable. If a teenage boy or young man has especially painful testicular swelling, physicians occasionally prescribe a stronger pain-relieving medication.

Warm or cold compresses applied to your child's face, over his salivary glands, or to the scrotum over his testicles may also help relieve his pain and make him more comfortable. Boys with very swollen testicles may be more comfortable with some sort of support for their testicles, such as snug pants or a small pillow.

A child with mumps should stay home from school as long as he has any fever or any swelling of his salivary glands or testes, not only for his own sake but also to keep him from spreading the virus to anyone else. A person may continue shedding virus for up to nine days after he develops symptoms, and the American Academy of Pediatrics recommends that a child with mumps be kept out of day-care or school for nine days after his salivary glands start to swell.

A person usually recovers from mumps in a week or two. The fever usually lasts three to five days, sometimes longer, and the swelling of the salivary glands goes down in a week or ten days. Swelling of the testicles may last longer, from a few days to several weeks.

Rarely, mumps leaves a person with a lifelong handicap. In the days before the vaccine, when nearly every child had the disease, the virus sometimes spread to the ears, and it caused some permanent loss of hearing in about one out of every 20,000 children. The deafness usually affected only one ear, but sometimes it affected both ears.

Also, if a teenage boy has both testicles involved, the virus can permanently damage both testes and make him sterile, unable to produce sperm and father children. This happens very rarely, only about 2 percent of the time. A boy does not have to worry about becoming sterile if just one of his testicles becomes swollen.

Once your child recovers from mumps, he is immune to the disease for the rest of his life. He cannot get mumps twice. People sometimes are convinced they have had mumps more than once, but it is more likely that they had salivary-gland swelling caused by an infection with another virus or by some other disease.

## *Prevention*

*Both the U.S. Public Health Service and the American Academy of Pediatrics recommend that children routinely be vaccinated against mumps.*

Mumps vaccine produces long-lasting, probably lifelong, immunity to mumps in over 90 percent of people who are vaccinated.

Your child should get a first dose of mumps vaccine when between twelve and fifteen months old. Before the age of about a year, she will not respond to the vaccine and make protective antibodies.

Children usually get mumps vaccine as part of a three-in-one shot called MMR: the first M stands for measles, the second M is for mumps, and the R is for rubella (also called German measles). Currently forty-two states require that children attending day-care be vaccinated against mumps, and forty-three states require that children entering school be immunized.

The U.S. Public Health Service and the Academy of Pediatrics also recommend that your child get a second dose of mumps vaccine—that is, a second MMR shot—between ages four and six, when she enters kindergarten or first grade. However, your child can get a second mumps shot at any age, as long as at least one month has passed since her first shot.

Mumps vaccine consists of live mumps virus that has been weakened. Although the person receiving it develops a very mild mumps infection, she cannot spread the disease to anyone else.

Side effects from the mumps component of the MMR shot are rare. Occasionally a child develops a low fever a week or two after the shot, or her salivary glands swell slightly. The risk of your child having any adverse reaction to mumps vaccine is much less than the risk of her getting serious disease if she does catch mumps.

The U.S. Public Health Service further recommends that all adolescents and adults who are not already immune to mumps also get vaccinated.

You are considered susceptible to mumps—and in need of vaccination—if you were not vaccinated with live-virus vaccine on or after your first birthday. A less-effective, killed-virus vaccine was in use from 1950 through 1978; if that was the only mumps vaccine you received, the Health Service advises that you get vaccinated again.

If you were never vaccinated, you are considered susceptible if you do not have documentation from a physician that you have had the mumps, unless you were born before 1957. Before that date, enough mumps virus was still circulating that almost every child caught mumps, and you probably had the disease whether you knew it or not.

It is particularly important for you and your children to be immune to mumps if you are planning to travel abroad. Mumps virus is more prevalent in much of the rest of the world than it is in the United States.

If you do not know whether you were vaccinated against or had mumps, there is no harm in getting another dose of vaccine. You are not more likely to have side effects if you get another dose.

However, you should not get mumps vaccine if you are pregnant or thinking of becoming pregnant within the next three months. The virus in the vaccine is not known to cause any birth defects, but in theory, the live virus of the vaccine might harm your baby. And you should avoid becoming pregnant for three months after you have had mumps vaccine.

Nor should you get mumps vaccine if you have had a blood transfusion or received immunoglobulin within the past three months, or if you are severely allergic to eggs or to the antibiotic neomycin. Nor should people get mumps vaccine if their immune systems are not normal.

If a teenage boy or adult man who has not previously been vaccinated knows that he has been exposed to mumps, it is too late for the vaccine to help. The vaccine does not work fast enough to keep him from getting the disease. But it is a good idea for him to get vaccinated anyway; it will protect him the next time he encounters mumps virus.

## Resources

You can get more information about mumps and mumps vaccine from the U.S. Public Health Service's Centers for Disease Control and Prevention by calling 1-800-232-SHOT or by connecting to their Web site on the Internet at http://www.cdc.gov.

# PINWORMS

*Pinworms must be treated by a doctor.*

## SYMPTOM

- Itching around the anus at night

Pinworm infections are irritating, but they are not serious and are easily curable. However, it is very common for children to become reinfected again and again. At any one time between 5 and 15 percent of Americans, about 25 million people, mostly preschool and school-age children, are infected with pinworms.

## Cause

The pinworm—*Enterobius vermicularis*—is not a relative of earthworms but is a simpler and much smaller type of worm known as a nematode or roundworm. It is about ¼- to ½-inch long and whitish, like a piece of dental floss. Pinworms live only in the intestinal tracts of human beings.

## How They Spread

A child becomes infected with pinworms when the pinworm eggs get in the mouth and are swallowed. The eggs pass through the stomach to the intestines, where they hatch, mature into adults, and mate. The pregnant female pinworms then migrate, usually at night, out of the intestine to the skin around the anus. There the female pinworm lays her eggs, which cause itching around the anus.

When children scratch the area, they get the eggs on their hands and under their fingernails. The pinworm eggs then spread from child to

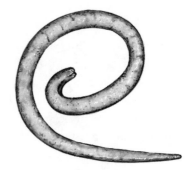

├— Actual size: 3–5 mm —┤
in length

*Pinworm.*

child on their hands or on toys or clothes. Children get the eggs on their fingers, then put their hands to their mouth, and swallow the eggs. Children often reinfect themselves when they bite their nails or suck their thumbs. The eggs can also spread to other members of a family if they share towels, washcloths, or beds.

Pinworm eggs are so light that they float in air; therefore, they can spread when you shake out a towel or sheet. You can inhale them and then swallow them without ever knowing it. You can pick up the infection from the air; you do not necessarily have to put your hands to your mouth.

Contrary to popular belief, people do not pick up pinworms from dogs or cats. The kinds of worms that cats and dogs get are different from pinworms, which, as mentioned, infect only humans.

## Incubation Period

It usually takes four to eight weeks from the time your child swallows pinworm eggs until symptoms appear.

## Symptoms

The classic symptom of pinworms is anal itching when no rash is present in the anal area or on any other part of the body. The itching usually occurs only at night. In very young children, irritability, restlessness, poor sleep, and short attention span may also suggest that pinworms are present.

In girls and women, pinworms may spread up into the vagina and vulva as well and cause a vaginal discharge and itching similar to that associated with a yeast infection.

### CALL YOUR DOCTOR

- If your child complains of itching around his anus only at night and is irritable or has difficulty sleeping.

## Diagnosis

Parents can often diagnose pinworms themselves. If your child has these classic symptoms, your doctor will decide whether it is possible to diagnose the infection over the phone or whether you need to do the tape test.

The preferred method of diagnosis is to apply a piece of clear cellophane tape, sticky side down, across your child's anus; then remove the tape. The tape can be examined for the pinworm eggs. This can be done after he awakens in the morning prior to bathing.

In most cases, though, it is difficult to see the tiny worms. Put the tape in a clean glass jar or small plastic bag and take it to your physician, who can study it under a microscope. At Children's Hospital, we supply parents with a sticky paddle that, after use, is sealed in a tube which can then be mailed in for diagnosis.

Keep in mind, though, that the worms are not active every night. If you do not find anything on the tape the first night but your child still has symptoms, repeat the test for several nights in a row.

## Treatment

Getting rid of pinworms involves both the use of medication and a thorough cleaning of your home, as described below.

Doctors usually prescribe mebendazole or pyrantel pamoate. You give your child one dose of the drug by mouth and then give her a second dose two weeks later. It is important not to forget this second dose; it is needed to kill any newly hatched adult worms and to prevent reinfection.

While your child is being treated, she can continue her normal activities. She does not need to stay home from day-care or school.

However, everyone in your family—whether experiencing symptoms or not—also needs to be treated. Sometimes it is difficult to convince other family members that they can have no symptoms and still be carrying pinworms. But if you only treat your child and she has a recurrence, you can assume that others in your family also have the worms, even if they have no symptoms. Since most infected adults do not have symptoms, this can sometimes create problems. A person without symptoms may say, "I'm not going to take medication. There's nothing wrong with me." However, if you only treat those with symptoms, you will not eradicate the pinworms.

The second part of the treatment consists of a routine house cleaning, concentrating on the bedroom of the infected child. Begin by vacuuming and dusting your child's room. However, extraordinary cleaning is not necessary. Routine washing of bed linens and towels is all that is necessary. You do not need to wash the curtains.

The clothing that your child is wearing at the time you discover the pinworms also needs to be washed. Simply throw everything in your child's hamper into the washing machine. You do not need to wash items she has not worn recently or her out-of-season garments. It is not necessary to use any special disinfectants; just do a routine wash.

If you have wool items that are not machine washable, dry cleaning will kill the pinworms. You can also decontaminate clothing by putting it in a plastic bag for about three weeks.

It is hard to get rid of pinworms, and it is not uncommon for the cleanest houses to have three or four episodes of recurrence.

## Prevention

It is difficult to prevent pinworms from spreading in day-care centers and schools. It is also hard to keep pinworms from running through families. It is not your fault if your child has pinworms, nor can you prevent them from occurring.

The following methods of practical hygiene, however, can help decrease the occurrence of pinworms as well as teach your children healthful practices:

- Teach your children to wash their hands every time they go to the bathroom. Hand washing is even more important than house cleaning.

- Keep your children's fingernails short so that any pinworm eggs cannot lodge under their nails. Also encourage your children to keep their nails clean.

- Insist that everyone in your family wash his or her hands before handling, cooking, and eating food.

- Enlist the help of your day-care provider or babysitter. Have them remind the children to wash their hands after they go to the bathroom and before they eat lunch. Suggest that your day-care center wash the children's toys frequently. See *Recommendations for Day-Care Providers,* page 297, in the Appendices.

# PNEUMONIA

*If your child is having difficulty breathing,
he needs to be evaluated by a doctor.*

## SYMPTOMS

- Coughing more and more
- Breathing harder and faster, difficulty breathing
- Possible fever
- Very runny nose
- Vomiting
- Fatigue

Pneumonia is an infection in the lungs. It can range from being so mild you may not even realize your child has it to so severe that it is potentially life-threatening. These days, however, the overwhelming majority of children with pneumonia recover very nicely, without any long-term effects.

You can think of the lungs as an upside-down tree. The trachea (windpipe) corresponds to the trunk of the tree, and the bronchial tubes to its main branches. As we breathe in, air—with its life-giving oxygen—flows down the windpipe to the bronchial tubes, which divide to direct the air to the lobes of the lungs, three lobes on the right side and two lobes on the left. Then the air tubes redivide again and again, many times, eventually becoming very tiny airways called bronchioles. The bronchioles correspond to the twigs of the tree, and they direct the air to the alveoli (air sacs), which correspond to the leaves or buds. From these air sacs oxygen passes into the bloodstream.

We have millions and millions of these tiny bronchioles and air sacs in our lungs.

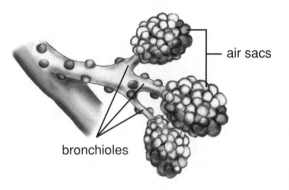

*Enlarged view of bronchioles and air sacs (alveoli).*

When a person has pneumonia, microorganisms grow and multiply in the bronchioles and air sacs, causing the tissues there to become inflamed and swollen. The immune system fights back by sending white cells to the area. Pus forms, composed of mucus and debris from the battle: broken-down white cells, bits of dead germs, fragments of lung tissue. This pus accumulates and physically clogs the bronchioles and fills the air sacs, making it more difficult for the person to breathe and get enough oxygen into the bloodstream.

The amount of pneumonia (the amount of pus that accumulates and interferes with breathing) can range from just a little bit—a small patch of pus that a person might not notice—to a large amount of pus that fills a whole lobe or all the lobes on one side of the lungs or even, in very severe cases of pneumonia, the entire lung.

Pneumonia most commonly strikes at the extremes of our lives, when we are very young and when we are very old. Your child is most likely to get pneumonia when he is under the age of five: every year 40 out of every 1,000 children in this age group have pneumonia. By the time your child reaches his teen years, however, his chances of contracting pneumonia drop dramatically: only 7 out of every 1,000 adolescents between the ages of twelve and fifteen get it each year.

Before the introduction of antibiotics in the mid-twentieth century, pneumonia was the most common cause of death among children. Today it is very rare that a child in this country dies from pneumonia. In developing countries, however, pneumonia is still a major cause of death among children. It kills about 4 million children every year, according to the World Health Organization. This is more than one-fourth of all deaths among children under five, and half the children dying from pneumonia are babies under the age of one year. And among elderly people in this country, pneumonia is still a significant cause of death.

Your child can get pneumonia at any time of the year, but he is most likely to get it during the colder months, winter through early spring. Pneumonia is common enough that in the emergency department at The Children's Hospital of Philadelphia, we usually see several children a day who have it.

## Causes

Pneumonia can be caused by many, many different germs. In children the most frequent causes are the common respiratory viruses.

The virus that most commonly causes pneumonia, particularly in babies and very young children, has a long name: respiratory syncytial virus (RSV). RSV is also the most common cause of bronchiolitis (inflammation of the bronchioles), and it can also cause croup, bronchitis, and middle-ear infections in children. In adults,

however, RSV usually just causes a cold. See *Respiratory Syncytial Virus (RSV) Infections,* page 26, for more about this widespread virus.

Second only to RSV as a cause of viral pneumonia in children are the parainfluenza viruses, which are also common causes of croup and also cause colds, bronchitis, bronchiolitis, and sore throats. Other respiratory viruses that can produce pneumonia include the influenza viruses, the enteroviruses, and the adenoviruses.

Among bacteria, *Streptococcus pneumoniae* is the most common cause of pneumonia in both children and adults. This bacterium is also called pneumococcus and sometimes strep pneumo for short. About 500,000 people in the United States get *S. pneumoniae* pneumonia each year, according to the U.S. Public Health Service's Centers for Disease Control and Prevention. Strep pneumo can also cause sinusitis, meningitis, and middle-ear infections in children. Your child is most likely to get pneumonia from *S. pneumoniae* during the winter or spring.

Other bacteria that sometimes—but much less frequently—cause pneumonia in children include *S. pyogenes* (also called group A streptococcus), which is the organism that produces strep throat, and *Staphylococcus aureus*, which also causes skin infections, food poisoning, and a variety of other diseases.

Another bacterium with another long name, *Haemophilus influenzae* type b, used to cause some pneumonia as well as meningitis in young children. Today, however, thanks to a hemophilus vaccine introduced in 1985, hemophilus type b diseases are uncommon. You should make sure, however, that your baby is immunized with this vaccine. For more about the vaccine, see *Hemophilus Infections,* page 130.

In school-age children, some 10 to 20 percent of pneumonias are caused by a common—and oddball—microbe called *Mycoplasma pneumoniae.* Mycoplasma is neither a virus nor a true bacterium: it can live on its own, while viruses cannot, and it has no cell wall, while bacteria do. *M. pneumoniae* can also cause croup, bronchitis, and middle-ear infections. Pneumonia due to mycoplasma is very rare in children under the age of two or three. Your child can get pneumonia from mycoplasma at any time of the year.

Among the many other organisms causing pneumonia in infants is the bacterium *Chlamydia trachomatis.* Chlamydia is a sexually transmitted germ, and a pregnant woman who is infected can pass the bacteria on to her baby during delivery. Chlamydia is a common cause of pneumonia among babies in their first few months of life.

Many other viruses occasionally cause pneumonia, including the Epstein-Barr, herpes simplex, chickenpox, rubella, and measles viruses. During the most recent resurgence of measles, 8 percent of people of all ages who caught measles—and 11 percent of children under five—also developed pneumonia.

Pneumonia due to the bacterium *Legionella pneumophila*—Legionnaires' disease—gets a lot of publicity because it is so often deadly, but it is extremely rare among children.

In some geographic regions, certain organisms can cause a local type of pneumonia. In parts of California and other southwestern states, a fungus called *Coccidioides immitis* occurs in the soil, and a person can get a pneumonia called coccidioidomycosis or valley fever from inhaling its spores. In Ventura County near Los Angeles in early 1994, there was a sharp jump in the number of people who caught valley fever after a major earthquake stirred up the soil.

Children and adults whose immune systems are not normal—those who have cancer or have had organ transplants and those born with immunodeficiency diseases or who have acquired immunodeficiency syndrome (AIDS)—can develop severe pneumonias from microorganisms that cause little or no trouble in other people. Pneumonia due to an organism called *Pneumocystis carinii* is common among adults and children with AIDS.

## How It Spreads

The most common causes of pneumonia in children—respiratory syncytial virus (RSV), *S. pneumoniae,* and *M. pneumoniae*—are organisms that your child picks up from other children or adults who have these germs growing in their noses and throats. Such infected people shed these organisms in their nose and throat secretions.

When an infected person coughs or sneezes or even just talks, she can spray these secretions—and the virus or bacteria—on anyone nearby. If she gets the germs on her hands, she can spread them to anyone who touches her hands. When this person touches her own nose or mouth or eyes, she can infect herself. An infected person can also spread these germs to another person when they share a drinking glass or when they kiss.

RSV, in particular, spreads in these ways very rapidly from one person to the next. *M. pneumoniae*, on the other hand, spreads from person to person very slowly.

The sneaky thing about some of these organisms is that your child can catch pneumonia from someone who does not have pneumonia. A baby can catch RSV from an adult who only has a cold, and that RSV infection in the baby can turn into pneumonia.

*S. pneumoniae* is even sneakier. It often lives in our noses and throats without causing any symptoms. Some 25 to 50 percent of normal, healthy children thus carry strep pneumo without being sick, and even among adults who have no contact with children, about 5 percent are carriers of strep pneumo. Your child can get *S. pneumoniae* pneumonia from another child or adult who is not sick at all.

Both RSV and parainfluenza virus can remain alive on surfaces for long periods of time, six to eight hours for RSV and up to ten hours for parainfluenza virus. If a person with an RSV cold sets a used tissue down on a bedside table, a toddler can come along hours later, touch the table, get virus on his hands, and catch an RSV infection.

Once RSV particles get inside a child's body, they settle down in his nose and throat, and as they multiply, they spread from one cell to the next. If they travel down as far as his lungs, he may develop pneumonia. The bacterium *S. pneumoniae*, on the other hand, may spread from a child's throat to his lungs via his bloodstream. Or he may inhale a droplet of contaminated secretions directly into his lungs.

## Incubation Period

If your baby or toddler becomes infected with respiratory syncytial virus (RSV), pneumonia may develop within two to six days, but it can take from as few as two days to as many as eight.

With *S. pneumoniae*, the incubation period is quite variable. With *M. pneumoniae*, it is usually several weeks.

## Symptoms

As the virus or bacterium multiplies in a child's lungs and causes pus to clog his bronchioles and air sacs, he coughs more and more. And to get enough oxygen, he instinctively starts breathing harder and faster than usual. These symptoms, as mentioned earlier, can range from being so mild you may not even notice them to so severe that they can be frightening. A child's symptoms can also vary with the organism that is causing his pneumonia.

If your child has pneumonia caused by *S. pneumoniae* or other bacteria, it usually starts more suddenly and is more severe than pneumonia due to a virus. Over a few hours a child can change from being perfectly well to being obviously very sick. He almost always has a fever, which can reach 102°F or more. He usually loses interest in eating and becomes much less active. Sometimes *S. pneumoniae* pneumonia hits so fast that doctors call it galloping pneumonia.

In more severe cases the strep pneumo bacteria sometimes spread outside a child's lung and infect and inflame the membrane that covers the outside surface of the lungs and lines the inside surface of the chest wall. This membrane is called the pleura, and inflammation of the pleura is called pleurisy. When a child has pleurisy, he feels pain in his chest whenever he coughs or takes a deep breath.

Sometimes so much pus forms in a child's lungs that it escapes from his lungs and accumulates in his chest cavity. Physicians call such an accumulation of pus an empyema. Again, the child feels pain in the part of his chest where he has the empyema whenever he coughs or breathes deeply, and you may notice that he holds his side, his elbow pressed into his ribs, to help keep his pain under control.

Children who have sickle cell anemia tend to get *S. pneumoniae* pneumonia more severely than other children, as do children who have no spleens, those who have certain types of kidney disease, and those whose immune systems are not normal.

If your child has pneumonia due to respiratory syncytial virus (RSV) or another respiratory

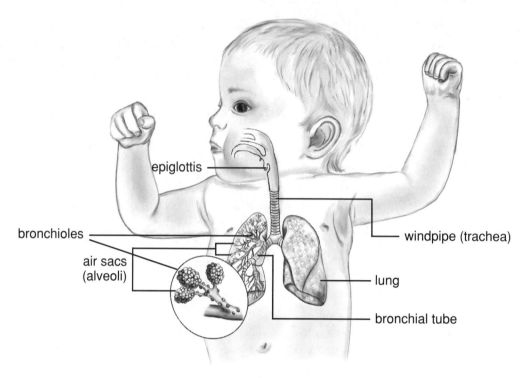

*The respiratory tract.*

virus, the pneumonia usually develops more gradually than bacterial pneumonia does. With RSV pneumonia, your baby or toddler usually has a very, very runny nose, with large amounts of clear mucus running out, for two or three days. Then, as the virus spreads from her nose and throat down into her lungs, she gradually gets worse. She starts coughing, several coughs in a row that may awaken her at night. After coughing, she may vomit; the coughing sets off a reflex that triggers vomiting. In contrast to bacterial pneumonia, her fever may or may not be high. By the third or fourth day, she is breathing faster and is also likely to wheeze—make a whistling sound—as she breathes.

RSV pneumonia is very similar to bronchiolitis due to RSV, but RSV pneumonia is usually more severe than bronchiolitis. See *Bronchiolitis*, page 21.

However, RSV pneumonia is generally more likely to be mild than is pneumonia due to *S. pneumoniae* or other bacteria. Both viral pneumonia and bacterial pneumonia can range from very mild to very severe, but a smaller percentage of children with RSV pneumonia have it severely than is the case with *S. pneumoniae* pneumonia.

As with *S. pneumoniae* pneumonia, children with certain other diseases tend to get RSV pneumonia more severely: children who have congenital heart disease, those whose immune systems are not normal, and particularly babies who were born prematurely, spent time on a respirator, and have a lingering lung disease called bronchopulmonary dysplasia.

If your child has pneumonia due to *M. pneumoniae*, it typically develops even more gradually than viral pneumonia and is usually even milder. Physicians call it walking pneumonia because the infected person usually does not feel or look all that sick. Your child usually can continue his normal activities, going to school, playing with other children, socializing with friends. He may not have much fever; it may reach 101°F or so from time to time. But he coughs and coughs for a week or ten days or more, and he may breathe somewhat faster than usual. He does not eat as well, and when he tries to run about or engage in other physical activity, he finds he does not have as much energy as usual.

With any pneumonia, as pus clogs a child's bronchioles and air sacs, he not only breathes faster but may have so much difficulty breathing that he develops respiratory distress. When he breathes out, at the very end of each breath he may make a grunting sound as he instinctively tries to keep his clogged air sacs open. As he tries to get more air, his nostrils may flare out at the sides. He may use extra muscles, muscles he does not usually use for respiration, to help him breathe and thus develop what are called retractions. Each time he takes a breath, you may see the muscles in the spaces between his ribs and also those in the spaces at the base of his neck, above the collarbone, pulling in (retracting). He may also use his abdominal muscles to help him breathe, causing his breastbone to sink down.

With less air getting to his air sacs, less oxygen may be passing into his bloodstream and reaching his brain and other tissues. He may start turning grayish or bluish around the mouth and at the tips of his fingers.

His behavior may also change. Instead of smiling and playing, he may become limp and lethargic and less responsive. He just concentrates on breathing.

If a child has a very severe pneumonia, he may go into respiratory failure: he may pause from time to time in his breathing or even stop breathing completely.

## Diagnosis

When your pediatrician listens to a child's chest with his stethoscope, what he hears may cause him to suspect that she has pneumonia and, if so, also give him a clue—but only a clue—about what is causing it, whether it is caused by a virus or bacterium.

If he hears that a child is wheezing all over her lungs as she breathes, her pneumonia is more likely to be caused by a virus. And if your child is a baby or toddler and it is November, December, or January, the doctor is likely to suspect her pneumonia is caused by respiratory syncytial virus (RSV).

If he hears a sound in only one part of the lungs—a high-pitched squeak or cracking sound, say, at the back right—a child's pneumonia is more likely to be caused by bacteria, particularly if she also has a high fever and is fairly sick.

To find out for sure whether a child has pneumonia, the doctor has an X-ray taken of her chest. If she does have pneumonia, the infection in her bronchioles and air sacs shows up as white patches on the X-ray.

The X-ray may also provide a clue about the cause of a child's pneumonia. In viral pneumonia, the X-ray is likely to look wispy and spread over more than one area of a child's lungs. In bacterial pneumonia, the pus is more likely to be concentrated in one area. If pus fills a whole lobe or more of a child's lungs, physicians say the child has lobar pneumonia.

## CALL YOUR DOCTOR

- If your child is breathing faster than usual or you are concerned about the way she is breathing.

- If your child has a cough that is getting worse.

- If your child has a fever, that is, a temperature of 101°F or more.

- If your child has signs of respiratory distress: her nostrils are flaring out and she is pulling in (retracting) the muscles between her ribs and at the base of her neck as she breathes.

**Pneumonia usually does not develop so rapidly that you need to call 911, but do CALL 911 or take your child to your hospital emergency room:**

- If your child is making a grunting sound at the end of each breath as she breathes out.

- If your child is struggling to breathe and gasping as she breathes.

- If your child has a grayish or bluish tinge around her mouth or at the tips of her fingers.

- If your child is lethargic or unresponsive.

- If your infant or child pauses in her breathing for more than ten to fifteen seconds.

If your child has walking pneumonia due to *M. pneumoniae*, her X-ray may look worse than she does. The shadows may be extensive on both sides of her lungs; yet she neither looks nor feels nor acts all that sick.

A child's X-ray may show that the infection is not so much in her bronchioles and air sacs as in the supporting tissue between them. Physicians call this type of lung infection pneumonitis. Pneumonitis is usually caused by a virus, and it is usually a milder disease than pneumonia.

When a teenager has pneumonia, to try to identify what organism is causing the disease, at Children's Hospital we often ask him to try to cough up a sample of pus from his lungs. Such a sample is called sputum. Then the lab studies the sputum under a microscope and also attempts to culture (grow) *S. pneumoniae* or other bacteria from the sample.

In younger children, however, we often are never able to identify what organism is causing their pneumonia because children under the age of nine or ten are not able to cough up such a sputum sample.

We can sometimes get another clue about the cause of a child's pneumonia from blood tests. The lab may be able to culture bacteria from his blood, but most of the time, children with pneumonia do not have bacteria in their blood. If a child's white-cell count is very high, his pneumonia is more likely caused by bacteria than a virus.

If a child is so sick that we must admit him to the hospital and we suspect his pneumonia is caused by RSV, we suction a sample of mucus from his nose, and our lab does a rapid test for RSV. RSV spreads so easily that the hospital staff needs to know if a child has this virus. If he does, we must take special infection-control precautions to keep the virus from traveling to other sick children in the hospital.

## Treatment

If your child has pneumonia caused by respiratory syncytial virus (RSV) or any other virus, she does not need to take any antibiotic. Antibiotics do not work against viruses; they do not kill viruses.

If your pediatrician believes or is able to prove that your child has pneumonia caused by a bacterium, however, she *does* need to take an antibiotic. At Children's Hospital, if a child is not too sick, if she is eating and drinking well and not vomiting, the pediatricians prescribe a course of antibiotics she can take at home, by mouth, for a period of seven to ten days. There are many possible antibiotics we can prescribe that are effective against a broad range of bacteria, that can kill not only *S. pneumoniae* but also other bacteria that may be involved.

If a child has walking pneumonia due to *M. pneumoniae*, the pediatricians usually prescribe the antibiotic like erythromycin for seven to ten days.

Most children who have pneumonia have the disease mildly enough that they can be treated at home.

## Medications

You should continue to have your child take any oral antibiotic your pediatrician has prescribed. Your child should take at least a seven- to ten-day course of antibiotic to kill all the bacteria in his body. Make sure that he takes all the pills, even if he begins to look and feel better before he finishes them.

If your child has a fever and is uncomfortable, you can give him acetaminophen.

If a child is coughing so much at night that it keeps him awake, we usually suggest giving him a cough suppressant containing dextromethorphan, but only at bedtime and only for a few days. However, you should never give any cough medicine to babies under a year.

## Fluids

Be sure to give your child plenty of extra fluids to keep him from becoming dangerously dehydrated. When a child has pneumonia, he loses more fluid than usual because he is breathing faster, producing more secretions, and may have a fever. He also may not feel well enough to drink as much as usual on his own. Babies particularly, because they are so small, can become dehydrated very quickly. See *Fluids*, page 290, in the Appendices for information about what fluids to give children of different ages.

## Humidity

Use a humidifier in your child's bedroom to increase the moisture content of the air he is breathing. The extra humidity will not reach down into his lungs as far as his inflamed air sacs, but it will help with any upper-respiratory symptoms he has. See *Humidity*, page 293, in the Appendices for more information about humidity and humidifiers.

## Rest

It is important that a child with pneumonia get plenty of rest while his body and immune system are fighting off the viral or bacterial infection. Wait until your child's fever is down, he is coughing less, and his appetite and energy level are back up nearly to his usual level before sending him back to his day-care center or school.

\* \* \*

If your child has bacterial pneumonia and is taking an antibiotic, he usually will improve dramatically within the first twenty-four or forty-eight hours. Bacterial pneumonia usually starts fast and, with antibiotic treatment, usually also goes away fast.

Viral pneumonia, which develops more gradually, also goes away more gradually. If your child has viral pneumonia, he should get better—cough less and wheeze less—over a period of several days as the virus runs its course.

Walking pneumonia due to *M. pneumoniae*, which develops more slowly than bacterial pneumonia, also responds more slowly to the antibiotic. If your child has walking pneumonia, once he starts the erythromycin, he should gradually improve over the next four or five days.

Whatever the cause of your child's pneumonia, however, within forty-eight to seventy-two hours you should start to see some improvement in his symptoms. He should be on the mend and feeling somewhat better. He should be breathing more easily and coughing less, his fever should be coming down, and his energy level should be returning to normal.

If your child's symptoms are *not* showing some improvement within forty-eight to seventy-two hours, you should definitely call your doctor again.

With children who have bacterial pneumonia, at Children's Hospital we insist on seeing them again, for a follow-up examination, twenty-four or forty-eight hours after they start treatment, to make sure they are indeed getting better. If a child is not improving, she may need to take a different antibiotic or be admitted to the hospital.

## Hospitalization

About 10 percent of the children we see with pneumonia at Children's Hospital are sick enough that we need to admit them to the hospital. The children we are most likely to admit are those who also have other, chronic diseases, such as sickle cell anemia, congenital heart disease, or chronic lung disease, or whose immune systems are not normal. We also usually admit babies under six months old.

Respiratory syncytial virus (RSV) alone is responsible for 90,000 infants and young children being hospitalized for pneumonia and bronchiolitis each year in the United States; 16 out of every 1,000 infants who have RSV pneumonia or bronchiolitis need to be hospitalized.

In the hospital a child can receive antibiotics intravenously and also intravenous fluids if she is dehydrated. Our staff can periodically measure the oxygen level in her blood and give her extra oxygen if she needs it. If a child with bacterial pneumonia has an empyema—a pocket of pus outside her lungs, in her chest cavity—that shows on an X-ray, the physicians can insert a tube into her chest to drain out the pus.

If a child has severe RSV pneumonia, we occasionally prescribe an antiviral drug called ribavirin. Ribavirin is given as a mist and must be administered in the hospital. It is not always effective and therefore is used only in the sickest of children, where even a little benefit is important.

Of the children admitted to Children's Hospital for pneumonia, about one out of every 100 is so severely ill that she must be treated in an intensive care unit, where we can monitor her respiration and heart rate closely. A very, very few children with pneumonia are so critically ill that they need to be on a respirator to help them breathe.

Most children with pneumonia stay in the hospital two to four days, occasionally longer.

Before the introduction of antibiotics, *S. pneumoniae* pneumonia used to kill about 25 percent of the people who had it. Today it is very, very rare for it to kill an otherwise healthy child. Most deaths from *S. pneumoniae* pneumonia occur among elderly people.

Pneumonias due to other bacteria, however, while less common, are more likely to be deadly. It was pneumonia due to *Streptococcus pyogenes* (group A streptococcus) that killed Jim Henson, the creator of the Muppets, at the age of fifty-three.

RSV pneumonia and bronchiolitis, according to the U.S. Public Health Service's Centers for Disease Control and Prevention, together kill an estimated 4,500 babies and young children in the United States each year. These are usually babies who also have some other, chronic disease, such as lung disease or congenital heart disease. It is very rare that RSV pneumonia kills an otherwise healthy baby.

## Prevention

Remember that the microbes most commonly causing pneumonia in children—respiratory syncytial virus (RSV), *S. pneumoniae,* and *M. pneumoniae*—are organisms that your child picks up by coming in contact with nose and throat secretions from an infected person, who may not be sick at all.

Therefore, teach everyone in your household to cover their nose and mouth whenever they cough or sneeze so they do not spray these germs onto others.

Be sure that everyone discards used tissues in a way that they will not come in contact with anyone else. Used tissues should not be left on tabletops or other surfaces.

Teach your children not to drink from the same glass as another person, particularly when that person has a respiratory infection. And when someone is sick, they should not kiss her until she is well again.

Most important of all, teach your children to wash their hands frequently. You never know what your children might pick up on their hands as they go about their daily activities and touch toys, doorknobs, telephones, and other surfaces.

Since your baby or toddler can get RSV pneumonia from an older child or adult who merely has a cold, try to keep him away, as much as possible, from his older brothers or sisters—or anyone else—whenever they have a respiratory infection.

You should definitely get your baby immunized against *Haemophilus influenzae* type b bacteria, to keep him from getting not only hemophilus pneumonia but also meningitis and the other serious diseases this germ can cause.

*Both the U.S. Public Health Service and the American Academy of Pediatrics recommend that all children routinely be vaccinated against hemophilus type b.*

Your baby should get a series of three or four shots (depending on the particular vaccine preparation your doctor uses), starting when he is two months old. See "Prevention," page 133, in *Hemophilus Infections* for more about this vaccine.

There is also a vaccine against *S. pneumoniae,* which prevents not only pneumonia but also meningitis and other infections caused by this bacterium. However, this vaccine is *not* recommended for normal, healthy children. It is not necessary for them.

This vaccine *is* recommended—by both the U.S. Public Health Service and the American Academy of Pediatrics—for children two years old or older who have conditions that put them at greater risk of getting *S. pneumoniae* pneumonia severely: children who have sickle cell anemia, who have no spleens, who have certain kidney diseases, or whose immune systems are not normal, including children infected with human immunodeficiency virus (HIV).

The U.S. Public Health Service also recommends that all adults age sixty-five and older be immunized with *S. pneumoniae* vaccine.

# POLIOMYELITIS

*A vaccine is available to protect your child against poliomyelitis. See Vaccines, page 301, in the Appendices, for a list of all the vaccines your child needs.*

*Paralytic polio must be treated by a doctor in a hospital.*

Also called polio.

## SYMPTOMS

- Stiff neck
- Fever
- Severe headache
- Stiff muscles
- Permanent paralysis

Poliomyelitis is a potentially serious disease of a person's nerves and muscles. Polio can kill or leave a person paralyzed for life. Fortunately, poliomyelitis can be prevented by vaccination. You should routinely get your baby immunized against polio, beginning at about two months of age.

In the late 1940s and early 1950s, tens of thousands of people in the United States caught polio every year. The peak was reached in 1952, when 57,879 cases were reported to the U.S. Public Health Service's Centers for Disease Control and Prevention (CDC) in Atlanta. Most of these polio victims were children, which is why polio also used to be called infantile paralysis.

Parents were so terrified of polio—as people now in their fifties and sixties and older remember well—that during polio season, in late summer and early fall, many kept their children home from public places. Authorities in some communities closed public swimming pools and movie theaters and did not open the schools until well into the fall, after polio season had passed.

*Thanks to vaccination introduced in 1955, poliomyelitis today has been eliminated from the United States and the rest of the Western Hemisphere.*

Poliomyelitis has not disappeared, however, from developing nations. Many thousands of people, particularly in Africa and Asia, still get polio every year, and there are occasional outbreaks in industrialized countries. In 1992 and 1993, seventy-one unvaccinated people in the Netherlands contracted polio. If we do not continue vaccinating our children, polio could return to the United States at any time.

## Causes

There are three viruses that cause poliomyelitis, called polioviruses types 1, 2, and 3. These viruses make their home only in human beings.

In the late 1940s, poliovirus was first grown in the laboratory by John Enders, Thomas Weller, and Frederick Robbins of Harvard University. This was considered such a crucial step toward the development of polio vaccine that the three scientists won the 1954 Nobel Prize in Physiology and Medicine for their accomplishment.

Thanks to vaccination, all three of these polioviruses themselves have now been eradicated from North America. However, one of them—poliovirus type 3—did recently return. Unvaccinated Canadians who visited the Netherlands at the time of the 1993 outbreak also became infected and unwittingly carried poliovirus particles in their bodies back to their homes in southern Alberta. Investigators isolated poliovirus 3 particles from twenty-one people, most of them children. Fortunately, none of these people developed active polio, nor did they spread it to anyone else.

## How It Spreads

People who are infected with a poliovirus have virus particles growing and multiplying in their throat and intestinal tract. They shed these virus particles in large numbers in their throat secretions and in their stools.

A person usually catches poliomyelitis from someone who has absolutely no signs of the disease. Ninety to 95 percent of infected people never have any symptoms at all and are not aware that they are shedding the virus.

A person can become infected if a poliovirus gets into the mouth, and the virus usually gets into the mouth from a person's hands. Young children who are infected and not yet toilet trained can easily get poliovirus particles on their fingers and spread the virus to any other children they touch. When these other children put their fingers in their mouth, as children do, they can become infected. This is one of the many reasons to encourage your children to wash their hands frequently, particularly after going to the toilet and before eating.

If a person gets poliovirus particles in his mouth, they start growing and multiplying in his throat. He also swallows virus particles, which pass through his stomach and settle down in his intestines, where they also grow and multiply.

## Incubation Period

If a person is infected with a poliovirus, it usually takes one to three weeks for any paralysis to develop, if it does develop, although it can take as little as four days.

## Symptoms

Ninety to 95 percent of people infected with a poliovirus, as mentioned, never develop any symptoms at all and never know they are infected.

Another 4 to 8 percent have minor symptoms similar to those caused by so many other viruses: a low fever, a sore throat, a headache, loss of appetite, some stomach upset, and nausea. These symptoms usually last one to three days and are usually so mild that a person has no reason to see a doctor.

A few days after these minor symptoms, in 1 to 5 percent of infected people, poliovirus particles get into the bloodstream and, from there, invade the central nervous system and cause meningitis, an infection of the membranes (meninges) covering the brain and spinal cord. These people have a higher fever, severe headache, a very stiff neck, and also extreme stiffness in their back and legs, but no paralysis. This form of the disease is sometimes called nonparalytic poliomyelitis.

Only 1 or 2 percent or less of infected people, a few days after the minor symptoms, develop paralytic poliomyelitis. The virus enters the nerve cells in the person's spinal cord that activate and control his muscles, and as the virus multiplies, it damages and destroys these nerve cells. The person's muscles become so weak that he is unable to move his limbs. Sometimes the paralysis affects just one limb, one arm or one leg, but it can paralyze all four at once.

The paralysis sometimes develops gradually, over several days, or sometimes a person becomes completely paralyzed in an arm or leg within a few hours. He also has intense pain and spasms in the affected muscles. The virus may also destroy nerves in his head, and he may become unable to cough or to swallow or even to speak.

The most serious form of poliomyelitis occurs when the virus damages the nerves controlling the respiratory muscles in the chest or the center in the brain that controls breathing, and the person becomes unable to breathe on his own.

## CALL YOUR DOCTOR

**Your child is very unlikely to contract poliomyelitis in the United States, but do call your doctor—**

- If your child develops a severe headache, a very stiff neck, or if her muscles become weak or painful or paralyzed.

- If your baby is being vaccinated against polio and you are not sure whether you are fully immunized against the disease. You may want to get vaccinated too.

- If you are planning a family trip abroad to any countries where polio is prevalent. You should make sure that everyone in your family is immunized.

## Diagnosis

There are conditions other than poliomyelitis, including infections with some other, common viruses, that can also cause a person's muscles to become weak or paralyzed.

To distinguish poliomyelitis from other causes of paralysis, at The Children's Hospital of Philadelphia, if we were to see a child or teenager with a paralytic disease, we would obtain samples of his nose and throat secretions and of his feces. We would also do a lumbar puncture (spinal tap) to obtain a sample of the child's spinal fluid. (For information about this procedure, see "Diagnosis," page 185, in *Meningitis*.) We would then

have our laboratory try to culture (grow) and isolate the virus from these samples in order to identify it.

## Treatment

There are no drugs that can help a person overcome any of the polioviruses. There are no antibiotics that can kill polioviruses—or any other virus—nor are there any antiviral drugs available.

A person who does get paralytic poliomyelitis usually must be hospitalized for long periods of time. To prevent her body from becoming permanently deformed, she usually must lie on a firm bed, with her limbs kept in alignment with splints. She usually needs sedatives and pain-relieving drugs to help withstand the muscle pain. Therapy often includes hot packs and warm baths to help ease the pain and stiffness of her muscles. If she cannot swallow, she may need to be fed with a tube.

Polio victims who cannot breathe on their own must be on artificial respirators, sometimes for months and even years. During the polio epidemics of the 1940s and 1950s, many victims had to live inside large tanklike respirators called iron lungs, which enclosed their entire body. (Today's respirators are smaller and much less cumbersome.)

Death from poliomyelitis is usually caused by failure of a person's respiratory system. The person becomes unable to breathe even with the aid of a mechanical respirator. Today in countries where polio still exists, it kills about four of every 100 people who have the kind of polio that affects breathing.

People who survive poliomyelitis often need to undergo lengthy physical therapy and rehabilitation, once their pain has gone, and sometimes surgery, to regain as much strength and motion as possible in their affected muscles. Some people with paralytic polio do recover completely, but many are left permanently and severely crippled.

If you have watched renowned violinist Itzhak Perlman, on television or in person, struggle across a stage on his crutches, you have seen what polio can do to a person; Perlman contracted polio when he was four years old. Probably polio's most famous victim was Franklin Delano Roosevelt, president of the United States from 1932 to 1945. He caught polio at the age of thirty-nine and lost much of the use of his legs. Countless other polio survivors were doomed to live out their lives in wheelchairs or on respirators.

Today a number of people who had polio back in the 1940s and 1950s, when they were children, are finding that they are now experiencing new symptoms. Their muscles are becoming weak and easily fatigued, and some are having difficulty breathing. Some who were able to walk without any aid now need braces and crutches or even wheelchairs. Postpolio syndrome, this is called. It is probably not caused by a reaction of the virus, most experts believe, but by deterioration of damaged nerve cells as these people, now in their fifties and sixties and older, are aging.

## Prevention

*Both the U.S. Public Health Service and the American Academy of Pediatrics recommend that children routinely be vaccinated against poliomyelitis.*

Two types of polio vaccine are now in use, and there are important differences between them (discussed below) that you should know about. Both types of polio vaccine will protect your child against all three polioviruses.

Whichever type of polio vaccine your pediatrician suggests, your child needs four doses.

He should get the first dose when he is about two months old, the second when he is four months old, and the third when he is between six and eighteen months of age, depending on the vaccine type. Almost all states require that children attending day care be immunized against poliomyelitis.

Your child then needs a fourth, booster dose of polio vaccine before he goes to school, when he is between the ages of four and six years. *All fifty states require that schoolchildren be immunized against poliomyelitis.*

Of the two types of vaccine, one is the type originally developed by Dr. Jonas Salk and first licensed in 1955. Your child gets this vaccine as an injection. When the Salk vaccine was first introduced, it produced an immediate and dramatic decrease in the number of people paralyzed by polio. The number of cases reported to the U.S. Public Health Service's Centers for Disease Control and Prevention (CDC) dropped from tens of thousands in the 1940s and 1950s to only 2,525 in 1960.

The Salk-type vaccine is very safe. The polioviruses in it have been killed; they have been inactivated chemically (so the vaccine is sometimes called IPV, for "inactivated poliovirus vaccine"). Your child cannot get poliomyelitis from this vaccine. The only side effect it is known to produce is some slight soreness and redness at the site of the injection. However, this vaccine contains trace amounts of streptomycin and neomycin; if your child is severely allergic to either of these antibiotics, he should not be given this vaccine.

The other polio vaccine is the type developed by Dr. Albert Sabin and introduced six years after the Salk vaccine, in 1961. This vaccine consists of live polioviruses that have been weakened enough that they do not cause poliomyelitis. Your child takes this vaccine not as a shot but by mouth (so the vaccine is sometimes called OPV, for "oral poliovirus vaccine"). When first introduced, the Sabin vaccine produced a further, dramatic drop in the number of people contracting polio. By the late 1960s only a few dozen cases were being reported to the CDC each year.

The Sabin polio vaccine is very effective. The live viruses multiply in your child's throat and intestines, and this causes his immune system to develop antipoliovirus antibodies, right there on the spot, where polioviruses like to grow.

Also, a child vaccinated with this oral live-virus vaccine sheds the weakened polio vaccine viruses in his throat secretions and stools for several weeks after his vaccination, sometimes for months. He can thus spread the vaccine viruses to others around him. You can get the virus particles in your mouth when you kiss him or on your hands when you change his diapers, and from your hands you can get the virus into your mouth. This means that you and other members of the household also become infected by the vaccine viruses. This bolsters everyone's own immunity to polio.

Until 1997 the U.S. Public Health Service and the American Academy of Pediatrics recommended that children receive the oral live-virus vaccine for all four of their doses of polio vaccine.

Unfortunately, the live viruses in the oral vaccine very, very rarely can change into a disease-producing form and actually cause someone not previously vaccinated to get paralytic polio. During the 1980s and early 1990s, eight or nine Americans a year caught polio this way. (No one has caught polio in this country from wild polio virus, as it is called to distinguish it from vaccine virus, since 1979.) While this is obviously tragic for these people, you have to remember that before the vaccines, tens of thousands of people used to become paralyzed every year.

In 1997, to reduce the number of people getting polio from the oral live-virus vaccine, the Public Health Service and the Academy of Pediatrics made a major change in their recommendations. There are now three different vaccine schedules that physicians can select from, depending on, among other factors, the age of the person being vaccinated and her vaccine history, that is, which vaccines she has previously received.

One schedule—a new one—calls for two doses of the killed-virus vaccine at two and four months of age, followed by two doses of the live-virus vaccine at twelve to eighteen months and four to six years, that is, two injections followed by two oral doses. With this combination schedule, a child will develop some protective antipoliovirus antibodies before she takes her first dose of live-virus vaccine.

A second approved schedule is, as before, four doses of live-virus vaccine. These doses are all given by mouth, at two and four months of age, between six and eighteen months, and between four and six years.

The third schedule is four doses of the killed-virus vaccine, that is, four injections. This regimen is absolutely safe; there is no chance of getting polio with this schedule. This schedule is recommended for children and adults whose immune systems are not normal. These include people who have cancer, who are infected with the AIDS virus, or who are on long-term therapy with corticosteroids. Children and adults who live with people whose immune systems are not normal should also get the killed-virus vaccine. And if your baby has just received the oral live-virus vaccine, you should keep him away from anyone whose immune system is not normal.

The U.S. Public Health Service also recommends that certain adults be immunized against poliomyelitis, among them, parents who have not been vaccinated against polio and whose children will be receiving the oral live-virus vaccine. The U.S. Public Health Service also recommends that adults traveling to developing countries where polio is prevalent make sure that they are vaccinated. Even adults who have recovered from polio need to be vaccinated. Survivors develop immunity only to the one type of poliovirus that infected them. Theoretically, they could catch polio again from either of the other two polioviruses.

Currently the U.S. Public Health Service recommends that people visiting Africa, India, Southeast Asia, and most of the nations of the former Soviet Union, among many other places, be immunized against polio. And you should know that while the polio season in the United States used to be late summer and early fall, in the tropics you can catch polio at other times of the year.

## Resources

To find out whether polio is a threat in any country you plan to visit, you can call the U.S. Public Health Service's Centers for Disease Control and Prevention's (CDC) International Travelers' Hotline at 1-888-232-3228.

For more information about polio and the polio vaccines, you can call CDC's automated voice system at 1-800-232-SHOT. You can also obtain travel and vaccine information by connecting to CDC's home page on the Internet at http://www.cdc.gov.

# REYE'S SYNDROME

*Reye's syndrome must be treated by a doctor.*

## SYMPTOMS

- Sudden and dramatic onset
- Vomiting
- Lethargic and disoriented
- Hyperventilation (breathing rapidly)
- Dilated pupils
- Agitated or irrational behavior alternating with deep sleep
- Hallucination
- Coma

Reye's (pronounced "rise") syndrome is a childhood disorder characterized by vomiting, disorientation, and a progressive loss of consciousness. Although most parents are familiar with Reye's syndrome because of its alleged link with the use of aspirin during viral infections, few know very much about the actual disorder. That is not surprising because the syndrome itself is still not well understood.

Reye's syndrome was first named when a doctor in North Carolina in the early 1960s reported an epidemic of more than a dozen fatal cases of an encephalitislike illness during an influenza B outbreak. Although this was not the first time the syndrome had been reported, it was finally identified, characterized, and given a name.

Several drugs, including aspirin and anti-vomiting medications, have been linked to this disorder. In 1984 the surgeon general of the United States recommended that aspirin therapy be avoided in young children who have chickenpox or any other flulike illness. Although the association between Reye's syndrome and aspirin continues to be questioned and there is no conclusive proof of a link, we have seen a tremendous decline in the number of cases since this warning was made public.

Reye's syndrome generally affects children between four and sixteen years of age. Despite the warnings, it is rather rare—just one case per million persons. The disorder is usually benign, and most children recover from Reye's syndrome without any major problems. However, some children with a severe illness may have complications such as seizures, psychomotor (the motor, or movement, effects of the brain or mind) retardation, or speech abnormalities. A severe or untreated case of Reye's syndrome, in which there is massive brain swelling and rapid changes in the child's neurologic and body functions, may result in death.

## Causes

Reye's syndrome is not caused directly by an infection. Instead, the syndrome is the result of an infection-related injury to an important component of the cells of the liver and brain. Although we are not certain of the origin of the illness, nearly all cases of Reye's syndrome are associated with a viral infection—either the flu or an upper respiratory infection, for example. In 10 percent of Reye's syndrome cases, chickenpox is generally the most recognizable of the diseases that precedes it.

## How It Spreads

Reye's syndrome itself is not contagious. But the illness that precedes it, such as chickenpox, can spread from person to person.

## Incubation Period

Symptoms may begin three to eight days after the first sign of a chickenpox rash. However, you may see symptoms of Reye's syndrome at any time within the two-month period following a viral illness.

## Symptoms

Symptoms will appear dramatically and rapidly. Initially, your child will begin to vomit. Within the next day or two, he will become lethargic and disoriented. You may see him start to hyperventilate (breathe rapidly), and his pupils will be dilated. He will become very agitated or irrational. This behavior will alternate with periods of deep sleep. In some cases your child may hallucinate. In more serious cases he may become comatose.

Initially, Reye's syndrome can be quite frightening. For the first forty-eight to seventy-two hours after the onset of symptoms, your child's condition will deteriorate. Then he will plateau for another twenty-four to forty-eight hours. However, unless there are severe complications, he will rapidly recover within the next five to ten days.

### CALL YOUR DOCTOR

- If your child has recently had a cold or flu and, after recovering, begins to show symptoms of vomiting and nausea or altered consciousness.

## Diagnosis

There is no single lab test to confirm Reye's syndrome, but lab tests can reveal several abnormalities typical of this condition. Your doctor will want to check your child's liver function because the liver in children with Reye's syndrome undergoes certain changes.

If your doctor suspects brain swelling—the most serious complication of Reye's syndrome—she may order a CAT scan, blood work, and possibly a spinal tap. Brain-wave tests (electroencephalograms) also reveal abnormalities that characterize the severity of the disorder.

## Treatment

If your child has Reye's syndrome, she will be treated in the hospital. A child who is severely ill needs to be in an intensive care unit, where she can be treated by specialists experienced with this disease.

Treatment is aimed largely at managing the symptoms rather than curing the illness. Your doctor will want to treat the brain swelling, correct blood and fluid abnormalities, and prevent complications. Because it is important to maintain the proper fluids and nutritional balance, your child will probably receive intravenous fluids.

The most important factor in treating this disorder is early diagnosis and aggressive therapy. Most children respond to treatment within forty-eight to seventy-two hours.

## Prevention

Children with chickenpox should not receive salicylates (aspirin or certain antacids) because they increase the risk of subsequent Reye's syndrome. Be sure you check labels—you may not always realize that salicylates are contained in an over-the-counter preparation. To control your child's fever, use acetaminophen. In general, it is a good practice to avoid using aspirin for any illness in children younger than age twelve.

# RINGWORM

Also called tinea.

## SYMPTOMS

- Ringlike rash or sores almost anywhere on the body, often scaly and itchy
- Circular bald patches in the hair

Ringworm—which is not caused by worms and does not always resemble rings—is a common fungus infection of the scalp and of the skin elsewhere on the body. While ringworm can be annoying, it is rarely serious. It almost always can be cured quickly and easily.

The disease has a long history. Ringworm was first described around A.D. 30. In the early nineteenth century, it became the first human disease that physicians discovered is caused by an infection—that is, by a living microorganism.

While people of any age can catch ringworm, ringworm of the scalp is much more common in children. It is the most common form of ringworm in children and most frequently affects those between the ages of five and ten. For some reason, boys are about three times more likely than girls to develop scalp ringworm.

## Causes

About a dozen different fungi belonging to a group called the dermatophytes cause ringworm. *Dermato-* means "skin," and *-phyte* means "plant" (although fungi are no longer classified as plants). Three groups of dermatophytes—*Trichophyton, Epidermophyton,* and *Microsporum*—are responsible for ringworm, and just one—*Trichophyton tonsurans*—causes 90 percent of scalp ringworm in this country.

These dermatophytic fungi live on the outermost layer of skin, a layer that consists of dead cells that are continually flaking off. Some dermatophytes live almost exclusively on the skin of human beings. Others primarily infect other animals, including house pets and farm animals, but they can also infect us. One, called *Microsporum canis,* infects dogs, cats, and also people.

## How It Spreads

People, pets, and other animals that are infected with any of the dermatophytes shed bits and pieces of fungus on flakes of their dead skin. You can pick up the fungus by touching the skin of an infected person. Fragments of fungi can also persist for days on inanimate objects such as towels, clothing, sheets, furniture, and other surfaces. A child can catch ringworm by sleeping in the same bed as an infected child.

The fungi causing scalp ringworm can also spread from one child to another on combs, brushes, barrettes, hair ribbons, telephones, and hats, and other headgear. A very young child may catch the fungus by patting the head of an infected playmate and then putting her hands in her own hair. Tight braiding and other hairstyles that expose sections of a child's scalp give the fungus room to grow. And applying gels, pomades, and other sticky dressings to a child's hair can make it easier for the fungus to gain a foothold.

Young animals, like young children, are especially susceptible to ringworm, and the fungus passes easily from kittens to those who cuddle them. One study found that in 32 percent of households with infected cats, one or more members of the family developed ringworm traceable to the cat. People have also caught ringworm from horses and cattle, which can leave bits of fungus behind when they rub against fences and gates.

Even a minor skin injury can predispose a person to developing ringworm. The infection is also more prevalent in warm, humid climates.

## Incubation Period

Your child may show signs of ringworm a few days or weeks after being exposed to one of the fungi, or she can carry a fungus for months or years before developing any symptoms.

## Symptoms

Typically ringworm *does* look like a ring. The infection starts as a small, roundish, reddish sore almost anywhere on your child's body. As the fungus continues to grow, it spreads outward in all directions, causing the spot to become larger and larger. The center of the sore tends to heal and the fungus to disappear from it, resulting in a reddish ring with fairly sharply defined edges surrounding a clear area. The lesion is often scaly and itches and makes your child uncomfortable. However, ringworm does not otherwise make him feel sick.

When a ringworm fungus grows on your child's scalp, it grows not only on the surface of his scalp but also in his hair follicles (or roots), and it actually invades the inside of his hair shafts. This causes hairs to break off, usually near the roots, and your child develops bald patches that are usually circular. (See above right.) The itching and scaling on his scalp can be mistaken for dandruff.

Sometimes a child's bald places are studded with broken-off hairs that look like black dots. This is called black-dot ringworm and is the type of scalp ringworm we most commonly see on children at Children's Hospital. Sometimes a child develops patches where infected hairs turn

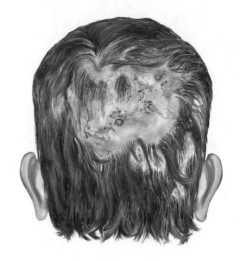

*Ringworm on the scalp.*

gray and dull; this is called gray-patch ringworm. Sometimes the sores on his scalp become severely inflamed and form raised, red, oozing, pus-filled lesions called kerions. Kerions are usually a sign that a child is especially sensitive to the infecting fungus. If a child's scalp ringworm is not treated appropriately, it can persist and may cause scarring and permanent loss of hair.

Your pediatrician is likely to use the term *tinea* for this infection. *Tinea* is from the Latin word for "worm" and has been used since the Middle Ages to mean "ringworm." *Tinea* is also Latin for "moth," and ringworm sores in hair do sometimes look like the holes that clothes moths make in woolen material.

When a ringworm fungus grows elsewhere on a person's body instead of the scalp, it does not always look like a ring. Its appearance can be quite variable. Sometimes the lesion does not clear in the center but remains a solid, reddish area. Sometimes it forms concentric rings, or a person may have multiple rings on many parts of his body. The sores may become crusty or develop into kerions, as on the scalp. Like scalp ringworm, if body ringworm is not treated, it can last for years.

When a ringworm fungus grows on the feet and between the toes, it is called athlete's foot. See *Athlete's Foot*, page 14. When a fungus grows on the skin in the groin, it is often called jock itch. See *Jock Itch,* page 159.

---

**CALL YOUR DOCTOR**

- If your child's hair begins to fall out.

- If your child develops sores on his scalp or it becomes inflamed or oozes pus.

- If your child's scalp continues to flake even after several shampoos with an over-the-counter dandruff shampoo.

- If your child develops one or more patches of sores elsewhere on her body that persist, or her skin becomes itchy and inflamed.

---

## Diagnosis

Ringworm of the scalp should be considered whenever a child loses hair.

To determine whether your child's sores are caused by ringworm and, if so, by which fungus, your pediatrician needs to obtain a sample of the fungus. She first cleanses your child's scalp or skin with alcohol. Then she uses a scalpel, clean toothbrush, or wet cotton swab to collect infected hairs and flakes of skin. This procedure does not take long and does not hurt. The laboratory examines the hairs and flakes under a microscope and may also try to culture (grow) the fungus in order to identify it.

## Treatment

If your child has ringworm of the scalp, she needs to take an antifungal medication by mouth to cure her infection. Remember: the fungus is growing *inside* her hair roots. Medication applied directly on her hair and scalp will not penetrate the hair shafts and kill the fungus.

Doctors most often prescribe a medication called griseofulvin to treat scalp ringworm. Griseofulvin works best if you give it to your child *after* a meal that includes a fatty food such as ice cream, peanut butter, or whole milk. Fatty foods aid in the medicine's absorption from your child's digestive tract.

Your pediatrician will probably also suggest that you wash your child's hair with a shampoo containing selenium sulfide. This reduces the amount of itching and flaking and lessens the likelihood that your child will infect someone else.

While your child is taking the antifungal medication, she may go to her day-care center or school and enjoy her regular activities. There is no need to cut her hair. But if you take your child to a barber or hairdresser, be sure to tell him that your child has a contagious infection.

These antifungal medications work slowly, and your child will probably need to take the medicine and use the special shampoo for six weeks, perhaps longer. She continues to be contagious as long as you can see any sores or patches on her scalp.

If your child has ringworm elsewhere on the body, other than the scalp, however, it usually *can* be cured with an antifungal medication that you apply directly on the sores. When a fungus just causes body ringworm, it remains on the surface of the skin and does not penetrate into the hair follicles or down into deeper layers of the skin. There are a number of over-the-counter fungus-killing medications that your doctor can choose to recommend, among them miconazole and clotrimazole.

It is very important to use only the medication your pediatrician recommends. Using the wrong one can make matters worse: your child's infection may last longer.

If your child has extensive ringworm on several parts of her body, or if her symptoms fail to improve within a few days after treatment begins, your pediatrician may prescribe an oral antifungal medication.

Bathe your child every day and gently remove loose scabs and crusts from her skin. Wash your hands in hot soapy water before and after you touch her skin and before and after applying ointment. Try to keep her from picking at her sores; this could spread the fungus or lead to a secondary bacterial infection. If she has extensive body ringworm, she might be more comfortable in loose-fitting clothes. Again, she will be able to infect others as long as she has sores on her skin.

With either scalp or body ringworm, call your physician again if your child's sores do not begin to clear up within a week after you begin using the treatment. If your child develops a rash, upset stomach, or headache, she may be having a reaction to the medication; call your doctor.

## Prevention

You can help keep your child from getting ringworm by keeping his hair and skin clean and dry. Your child should have and use his own hairbrush and comb. Teach him not to share or borrow grooming items, headphones, or caps. Teach him also to be careful not to pick up someone else's towel during a game or in the locker room.

Remember that your child can catch ringworm from pets and other animals. If your cat or dog shows any signs of possible ringworm—scaly, itchy, hairless areas on its fur or skin—see your veterinarian promptly.

# ROSEOLA

## SYMPTOMS

- High fever
- Pink rash after fever subsides
- Runny nose
- Irritability
- Droopy or puffy eyelids

Roseola is sometimes called baby measles because of its characteristic red rash that resembles that of measles. The illness occurs most commonly in children between the ages of six months and two years of age. We rarely see it before three months or after four years of age.

What distinguishes roseola from other diseases is the timing of the appearance of the rash, which follows a high fever that lasts for three to five days. The pink, spotty rash appears after the fever subsides, and it can last anywhere from hours to days. As the mother of a three-year-old described it,

> When his temperature went back to normal, I thought Justin was over whatever it was he had. Then, all of a sudden, this rash appeared all over his middle. We were sure it was measles. I called our pediatrician, who said it sounded like roseola. She told us to let her know if the rash continued to spread. To our surprise, it was completely gone by the evening.

Their pediatrician knew that in measles, children always have a fever when the rash develops. While roseola is a nuisance, it is basically harmless.

In fact, your child will probably feel fine and will be as playful as usual except during the initial feverish days. The disease is self-limiting, which means that it goes away by itself and does not require medical intervention. Complications are rare.

While most children get roseola one time, we sometimes see a reactivation of this virus in immunocompromised patients. Complications for these particular patients may include encephalitis, pneumonia, and bone marrow suppression.

## Causes

This illness is caused by a common virus called human herpes virus 6 (HHV-6), a member of the herpes virus family. It is now believed that roseola may also be caused by HHV-7 as well.

## How It Spreads

Although humans are the only known hosts, roseola is not very contagious. It is probably easiest to catch during the fever phase. Most likely your child will get roseola from the respiratory secretions of someone else in the family or a caretaker who has no obvious symptoms.

## Incubation Period

The first symptoms usually occur about nine days from the time of exposure, but the incubation period may actually be anywhere from five days to two weeks.

## Symptoms

Initially, roseola seems like a bad cold. Your child will have a high fever that lasts three to five days and a runny nose. She may seem irritable or fussy and refuse to eat. In some children, the eyelids appear droopy or slightly puffy. When the fever subsides, a slightly raised pink, spotty rash appears mainly on the face and upper body and then begins to fade. The rash typically lasts for about twenty-four to forty-eight hours, but it may disappear after just a few hours.

---

### CALL YOUR DOCTOR

- If the rash does not disappear or appears to be getting worse.

---

## Diagnosis

The key to diagnosis is the fact that the rash appears once the fever is gone. Most parents are able to diagnose roseola without a visit to the doctor. When a rash appears after a fever has subsided, it becomes clear that your child has roseola.

## Treatment

There is no treatment for roseola, which is a viral infection. You should treat your child's symptoms and try to keep him comfortable. Use the recommended dosage of acetaminophen for fever. You may want to dress your child in lightweight clothing and give him a tepid (barely cool) sponge bath if his temperature goes over 103°F. Encourage him to drink lots of fluids. As soon as the rash is gone, your child may resume normal activities.

## Prevention

There is no way to prevent roseola.

# RUBELLA

*A vaccine in available to protect your child against rubella. See* **Vaccines,** *page 301, in the Appendices for a list of all the vaccines your child needs.*

Also called German measles and three-day measles.

## SYMPTOMS

- Rash

- Swollen lymph glands

- Possible low fever, headache, slight sore throat, runny nose, cough, red eyes

- If a woman is pregnant and not immune to rubella, possible miscarriage, stillbirth, severe birth defects

Rubella is a mild and generally harmless rash disease if you get it when you are a child.

If you catch rubella while you are pregnant, however, it can have devastating consequences. It can cause a woman to have a miscarriage or her baby to be stillborn, or her child may be born with severe birth defects: he may be deaf or blind or have a deformed heart or damaged brain. Fortunately, rubella can be prevented by vaccination. You should routinely have your child immunized against rubella.

Before the introduction of rubella vaccine, 47,000 to 58,000 cases of rubella were reported each year to the U.S. Public Health Service's Centers for Disease Control and Prevention (CDC). No doubt many more people had the disease, but for some reason it was not reported.

During the last big rubella epidemic, in 1964 and 1965, the disease killed more than 8,000 babies in this country, either before they were born or soon thereafter, and about 20,000 babies were born with serious lifelong handicaps.

Since rubella vaccine was introduced in 1969, the number of reported cases in the United States has decreased dramatically to only a few hundred a year in most years. In addition, the number of babies born with defects due to congenital rubella has dropped to only a handful a year, usually fewer than a dozen.

However, rubella still causes trouble among people who have not been vaccinated. In the early 1990s outbreaks occurred among Amish people in at least six states. In Lancaster County, Pennsylvania, in one three-month period, nine Amish women who caught rubella while they were pregnant subsequently had miscarriages or delivered stillborn babies, and eleven more women gave birth to babies with severe defects. If we do not continue vaccinating our children, more such outbreaks can occur, and more babies will be born with handicaps.

Before the use of rubella vaccine, a person most commonly caught the disease while in elementary school, between the ages of five and nine years. Today teenagers and young adults who have not been vaccinated are the ones most apt to get rubella, the very age group most likely to become pregnant.

About 10 percent of American women in their child-bearing years remain susceptible to rubella, says the CDC, because they have neither had the disease naturally nor been vaccinated. These women risk losing a baby or giving birth to a child with severe defects. If you are one of these women, you should arrange to be vaccinated before you become pregnant.

## Cause

Rubella is caused by a virus simply called rubella virus. Rubella virus makes its home and multiplies only in the bodies of humans.

## How It Spreads

People who are infected with rubella shed virus particles in great quantities in the secretions that come from their nose and throat. They can spray droplets of moisture containing these virus particles into the air whenever they cough or sneeze or even when they simply talk.

Your child can become infected with rubella virus when she breathes in these virus-containing droplets or when she gets them in her mouth. She also can catch rubella by having direct contact with an infected person's saliva, that is, by kissing or by sharing a drinking glass or a spoon.

What helps spread rubella virus is that as many as half of infected people never develop any symptoms, and even those who do have symptoms shed virus particles for up to a week *before* they get sick. Your child can catch rubella from someone who has no idea he is shedding rubella virus particles.

When a woman catches rubella while she is pregnant, the virus particles can spread from her bloodstream into the placenta and, from there, into the tissues of her developing baby. The virus produces an infection in the baby that persists throughout the pregnancy. The risk of this rubella infection damaging the baby is greatest during the first three months of pregnancy. Up to 85 percent of babies infected with rubella in these early months are born with congenital defects.

Since a pregnant woman can catch rubella from someone who has no symptoms and does not know he is infected, and since she in turn may have no symptoms, her baby can be in danger and no one realizes it until the baby is born.

A baby infected with rubella virus in the womb not only is born infected but also continues to be infected for many months, sometimes until he is a year or more old. He sheds virus particles in his nose and throat secretions and also in his urine and can spread the virus to anyone around him who is not already immune.

## Incubation Period

If your child is exposed to rubella, it usually takes fourteen to twenty-one days to develop symptoms, if she does have symptoms.

## Symptoms

When a child catches rubella after his birth, usually the first sign—if he has any symptoms—is that he breaks out in the rash.

The rash is usually pinkish and starts on his face. Over the next twenty-four hours, it spreads downward over his neck to his trunk and arms and legs until it covers his entire body. The spots usually remain separate, not running together, and they often itch. However, a person can have rubella and not have any rash at all.

Along with the rash, a child usually has swollen lymph nodes ("swollen glands") behind his ears and at the back of his head and neck. He may have a low fever (101° to 102°F), a headache, a slight sore throat, a runny nose, and a cough. His eyes may hurt and become red.

A teenager, on the other hand, usually has these symptoms for a few days *before* he breaks out in the rash. With the rash, teenagers and adults—especially women—often have some arthritis, that is, pain or swelling or stiffness in their joints, particularly those in their wrists, fingers, and knees. Occasionally the pain can be severe.

Very rarely, rubella after birth can lead to other complications. One out of 3,000 children develops a blood-clotting disorder called thrombocytopenia. One out of 6,000 people, more often adults and more often females, develops encephalitis, an infection and inflammation of the brain.

If this were all that rubella did, we would not be so concerned about vaccinating children against it. In contrast to rubella after birth, congenital rubella can be catastrophic. Remember: if a woman has rubella early in pregnancy, the chances are 85 percent that her baby will be born with defects. As the virus grows and multiplies in her fetus, it can interfere with the normal development of many different organs and also permanently damage them. Babies born infected with rubella virus often have more than one problem.

The most common handicap is some degree of deafness, caused when the virus damages a baby's developing ears. More than 80 percent of babies born with rubella have some impairment of their hearing.

The virus can also damage a baby's eyes. Some babies born with rubella have eyes that are abnormally small, a condition called microophthalmia. About one-third have cataracts, cloudiness of the lenses of their eyes. Others have glaucoma, an increase in the pressure of the fluid within the eyes. Glaucoma can cause a child to become blind.

Nearly half of babies born with rubella have structural malformations of their heart that may be life-threatening. Many have abnormal holes between the chambers of their heart or a narrowing of the opening to the artery leading to their lungs.

Many babies born with rubella are mentally retarded, some severely so. And these babies are usually also small for their gestational age and, after birth, continue to grow more slowly than normal babies.

---

### CALL YOUR DOCTOR

- If your child has a rash and also has a fever (101° or above) or complains of feeling sick.

- If you are not immune to rubella or do not know whether you are immune, particularly if you are a woman of child-bearing age. You may need to be vaccinated against the virus.

---

## Diagnosis

When a child catches rubella after birth, her rash and other symptoms are similar to those caused by many other common viruses, such as the enteroviruses and the adenoviruses. These days, with the widespread use of rubella vaccine, such symptoms are much more likely to be caused by one of these other viruses. Allergies can also cause rashes that resemble the rubella rash. The only way to be sure that a person has rubella is by laboratory testing.

At Children's Hospital we usually test for rubella only when a baby is born with symptoms that could have been caused by a congenital rubella infection. We both test her blood for antirubella antibodies and also try to culture (grow) the virus from her nose and throat secretions and from her urine.

## Treatment

If your child catches rubella after his birth, he does not need any specific treatment. He does not need to take any antibiotics. Antibiotics do not kill rubella virus or any other virus. Nor are there any antiviral drugs available that can kill rubella virus.

Your child's own immune system will, in time, make enough antibodies to overcome and destroy all the rubella virus particles in his body. While this is happening, your child may or may not need to rest in bed, depending on whether he has any fever and how sick or tired he feels.

If your child has a fever and is uncomfortable, you can give him acetaminophen. Acetaminophen both reduces fever and relieves pain.

A child's fever, if any, usually goes away in a day or two, and his rash usually begins to fade on the second day. The rash clears the same way it came, from head to toe, disappearing first from his face and then from the rest of his body. The rash is usually gone by the end of the third day, although it sometimes lasts longer. This is why rubella is also called three-day measles, in contrast to regular measles, in which the rash usually lasts six to seven days.

However, a child continues to shed virus particles—and can continue to spread rubella—for several days after his rash disappears. To keep him from infecting anyone else, the American Academy of Pediatrics recommends that you keep your child home from day care or school for seven days after the rash first appears.

And throughout these seven days, be sure to keep him away from any woman who may be pregnant and might not be immune to rubella.

A child's lymph nodes may remain swollen for several weeks. Infected adults who have arthritic pains in their joints may continue to have these pains for several months, but usually the pain disappears eventually.

# Born with Rubella

Babies who are born with congenital rubella, on the other hand, may need extensive treatments. Even then, many do not survive their first year of life.

A baby with a congenital heart malformation may need immediate surgery to repair her defect and save her life. A baby born with glaucoma needs medical treatment to prevent blindness. A baby who has cataracts needs eye surgery to remove her clouded lenses. Children who are deaf or partially deaf require evaluation of their hearing, hearing aids, and special education.

Even babies infected with rubella who seem normal need to be examined periodically during their first few years of life to make sure that no subtle problems are overlooked.

Because babies born with rubella continue to shed virus particles from their nose and throat and in their urine for many months, sometimes for a year or more, they, too, should be kept away from any woman who is pregnant and may not be immune to the disease.

Many babies born with rubella are so handicapped that they are never able to lead normal lives. When the men and women born with congenital rubella during the 1964–65 epidemic reached their twenties, only one-third were able to live on their own. Another third lived at home but required substantial help from their families. And the remaining third were so severely disabled they needed to live in institutions.

# *Prevention*

*Both the U.S. Public Health Service and the American Academy of Pediatrics recommend that children routinely be vaccinated against rubella.*

The reason for vaccinating children is to reduce the total amount of rubella virus in circulation and to keep children from catching rubella and spreading the virus to pregnant women. The reason for vaccinating males as well as females is the same: to keep them from giving rubella to pregnant women. And when vaccinated girls grow up and have children of their own, they will be immune to rubella and thus run no risk of bearing a rubella-damaged baby themselves.

Your child should get his first dose of rubella vaccine when he is between the ages of twelve and fifteen months. Almost all states require that children attending day-care centers be immunized against rubella.

Children usually receive rubella vaccine as part of a three-in-one shot called MMR. The first M stands for measles; the second M is for mumps; and the R, of course, is for rubella.

Your child then needs a second MMR shot when he is four to six years old, just before he enters kindergarten. *All fifty states require that schoolchildren be immunized against rubella.*

The U.S. Public Health Service also recommends that everyone, teenagers and adults, males as well as females—but particularly women of child-bearing age—be vaccinated against rubella unless they are already immune. Vaccination of susceptible women of child-bearing age, advises the Health Service, should be part of routine medical care. However, you should not get rubella vaccine if you are already pregnant.

Rubella vaccine consists of live rubella virus that has been weakened. This is the reason you should not be vaccinated against rubella while you are pregnant. There is no evidence that the vaccine virus has ever caused birth defects, but since it is theoretically possible, both the Health Service and the Academy of Pediatrics recommend that pregnant women play it safe and not take the vaccine. You should also avoid becoming pregnant for three months after you get rubella vaccine.

Other people who should not be vaccinated with live-virus rubella vaccine are those whose immune systems are not normal, including those born with immunodeficiency diseases, those who have certain cancers, and those who are undergoing long-term treatment with corticosteroids. Nor should you receive rubella vaccine if you are severely allergic to the antibiotic neomycin.

You are considered immune to rubella if you were ever vaccinated. However, because rubella vaccine was introduced only in 1969, many women now in their child-bearing years were not vaccinated as children and are not immune. About 10 percent of women in this age group, remember, are still susceptible to rubella.

You are also considered immune to rubella if you have had the disease. However, because so many other viruses cause similar symptoms, you cannot be sure you have had rubella unless your doctor confirmed the diagnosis with a blood test.

If you do not have documentation that you have been vaccinated or that you have had rubella, both the U.S. Public Health Service and American Academy of Pediatrics advise that you should be vaccinated. There is no harm in getting a rubella shot if you are already immune.

It is particularly important to be immune to rubella if you are planning to travel abroad. "All women travelers," says the Public Health Service, "particularly those of childbearing age, should be immune before leaving the United States."

While children need two MMR shots, adults need only one dose of rubella vaccine. Rubella vaccine produces long-term, probably lifelong immunity to the disease in more than 90 percent of people who are vaccinated.

About 10 percent of children have some side effects from the rubella component of the MMR shot: a rash, a fever, or swollen lymph nodes.

These side effects usually develop within a week or two after the shot and last a day or two. About one child out of 100 has some pain or stiffness in his joints, which may last a few days to a few weeks.

Adults—again, particularly women—are more likely to experience side effects from a rubella shot. About 25 percent of adult women have some pain in their joints. This usually begins one to three weeks after the shot and lasts for a few days.

After your child has an MMR shot, he will shed small amounts of the vaccine virus from his throat for seven to twenty-eight days, but there is no evidence that any recently vaccinated child has ever spread the vaccine virus to anyone else. There is no danger in your child getting his MMR shot if you are pregnant and not sure about your own immune status.

If you are vaccinated against rubella while you are breastfeeding, however, you may—rarely—spread the vaccine virus to your baby in your breast milk. Your baby may develop a mild case of rubella but should not become seriously ill. Indeed, breastfeeding mothers who are not immune, says the Health Service, *should* be vaccinated against rubella.

If a woman does catch rubella while she is pregnant, there is little that can be done. Remember: if she has the disease during the first three months of pregnancy, the odds are high—85 percent—that her baby will have birth defects. Some women have chosen to terminate their pregnancies by abortion. During the 1964–65 rubella epidemic, 5,000 therapeutic abortions were performed to prevent the birth of babies damaged by rubella.

## Resources

For more information about rubella and rubella vaccine, you can call the U.S. Public Health Service's Centers for Disease Control and Prevention (CDC) at 1-800-232-SHOT or you can connect to CDC's home page on the Internet at http://www.cdc.gov.

# SALMONELLA INFECTIONS

Also called salmonellosis. The ending *-osis* means "disease."

## SYMPTOMS

- Diarrhea, possibly bloody or with mucus

- Possible abdominal cramps, vomiting, fever

- Uncommonly, infection of bloodstream, inflammation of bone or joint, meningitis

Salmonella bacteria are among the most common causes of diarrhea and food poisoning. Salmonella is the reason people should avoid eating raw or undercooked eggs and one of the reasons you should avoid raw or undercooked meat or poultry.

Some 2 to 4 million people in the United States develop salmonella infections every year, according to the U.S. Public Health Service's Centers for Disease Control and Prevention (CDC), and in recent years the number of people catching salmonella disease has been increasing. Salmonella is a frequent cause of food poisoning outbreaks; dozens of such outbreaks—in restaurants, at picnics, at conventions, in nursing homes—are reported each year to the CDC.

Diarrhea due to salmonella is most common in young children under five years old, particularly in babies under a year. At The Children's Hospital of Philadelphia, we see about 150 to 200 children a year who have salmonella infections.

## Causes

Salmonella infections are caused by several species of bacteria named after an American scientist, Daniel E. Salmon, one of the early investigators of the organisms.

One species of salmonella, *Salmonella typhi*, is the cause of typhoid fever. This disease is now rare in the United States. Only a few hundred people have it each year, most of them adults and most of them people who caught the disease while traveling abroad.

There are a number of other species and more than 2,000 strains of salmonella that do not cause typhoid but instead cause diarrhea and occasionally other diseases. These other, nontyphoid salmonella infections are the ones your child is likely to encounter and the ones we are discussing here.

These salmonella bacteria live and multiply in the intestinal tracts of a wide variety of farm animals, including cattle, pigs, sheep, chickens, and turkeys. The animals may or may not be sick themselves.

## How They Spread

Animals that are infected with salmonella shed the bacteria in their feces. Your child can become infected with salmonella when he gets the bacteria in his mouth and swallows them.

People most commonly ingest salmonella bacteria in food. When infected animals are slaughtered, bacteria can get from their feces onto their flesh. Almost any food of animal origin—particularly meat, poultry, and eggs—can thus be contaminated with salmonella, and your child can become infected with the bacteria if he eats the food raw or undercooked.

People have gotten salmonella poisoning from undercooked roast beef (many people like it rare), chicken, and turkey, as well as from ham, pork, fish, shellfish, and many other foods. About 1 percent of raw beef and 5 to 7 percent of ground beef contain salmonella, according to the U.S. Department of Agriculture, and about 20 percent of raw chicken has the bacteria on it.

Your child can also become infected with salmonella from drinking raw, unpasteurized milk. In one outbreak in Chicago, a slip-up in a milk-processing plant allowed raw milk contaminated with salmonella to mix with supposedly pasteurized milk. Some 150,000 people became sick, and 2,777 people were hospitalized.

Salmonella can get onto the outside of an eggshell, from chicken feces, and they also can be inside an egg. They can infect the ovaries of seemingly healthy hens, which then can deposit the germs inside the shell before it hardens. In the northeastern part of the country especially, one out of every 10,000 eggs, according to the U.S. Public Health Service, may have salmonella inside the shell. In other parts of the country, contaminated eggs seem to be less common.

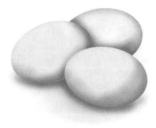

*Raw eggs can be contaminated with salmonella bacteria.*

Raw eggs were responsible for one of the largest outbreaks of salmonella food poisoning to date. More than 200,000 people in forty-one states became ill recently after eating a national brand of ice cream. It turned out that trucks carrying the ice cream had previously been used to carry raw eggs. People have also gotten salmonella poisoning from raw or undercooked eggs in scrambled eggs, omelets, egg salad and sandwiches, Caesar salad dressing, hollandaise sauce, cookie batter, turkey stuffing, and homemade eggnog and mayonnaise. Commercial eggnog and mayonnaise are safe to eat because they are made with pasteurized eggs.

Fruits and vegetables are not common sources of salmonella, but animal feces may contaminate them if they are on the ground. Contaminated cantaloupes from Texas once sickened 400 people in twenty-three states.

Salmonella can also get into food from the hands of infected people. You can carry the bacteria in your intestinal tract without knowing it, without having any symptoms of diarrhea. If you do not wash your hands thoroughly after using the toilet and before preparing food, you may have the bacteria on your hands and can spread them to others. Flies can also deposit salmonella on food if they first land on animal or human feces containing the bacteria or if they are carrying them in their own gut and shedding them in their feces.

You can also spread salmonella in your own kitchen if you use the same knife or cutting board you used for meat or poultry to prepare other foods—slicing tomatoes for salad, say—without washing the knife and board first. You can also contaminate cooked meat if you serve it on the same platter that held the raw meat.

A person can catch salmonella from drinking water that has been polluted with animal or human feces. Occasionally salmonella gets into community water supplies. Wild-bird droppings once contaminated a water-storage tower in Missouri; 625 people became sick, and 15 people had to be hospitalized.

Salmonella bacteria are among the many germs that can cause people to develop traveler's diarrhea when they eat contaminated food or drink polluted water while they are traveling abroad in developing countries.

Your child can catch salmonella directly from pet birds and reptiles (lizards, snakes, and turtles). Some 90 percent of reptiles, according to the U.S. Public Health Service, may carry salmonella in their intestines, without having any symptoms, and shed the bacteria in their feces. Infants have caught salmonella infections from reptiles without having any direct contact with them. Pet turtles used to spread so much salmonella that the Food and Drug Administration now bans their interstate shipment. Children have also caught salmonella from baby chicks and ducklings they received as Easter presents.

Once your child swallows salmonella bacteria, they pass through his stomach into the intestinal tract, where they grow and multiply.

## Incubation Period

It usually takes from six hours to two days for a person to become sick—if he is going to become sick—after ingesting salmonella bacteria, but it can take up to ten days.

## Symptoms

As salmonella bacteria grow and multiply in your child's intestinal tract, she may never have any symptoms at all, or she may have only mild diarrhea, a few loose stools. On the other hand, your child may have frequent bowel movements throughout the day, and her stools may be streaked with blood or with mucus. She may experience cramps in her abdomen, she may be vomiting, and she may or may not have a fever.

The danger of any diarrhea, whether due to salmonella or another organism, is that it can cause your child's body to become dehydrated. She is losing extra fluid through her frequent stools and any vomiting and, if she has a fever, through increased evaporation from her skin. Babies particularly, because they are so small, can very quickly develop serious—even life-threatening—dehydration. See *Fluids*, page 290, in the Appendices for more about dehydration.

## Complications

In babies under three months of age, however, who have very immature immune systems, salmonellosis can sometimes be more severe. Salmonella infections can also be severe in children (and adults) who have sickle cell disease, who have no spleens, or whose immune systems are not normal and in elderly people who have other underlying chronic diseases.

In these children, the bacteria can spread out of the intestinal tract and multiply in the bloodstream. A baby with salmonella in his blood will have a fever over 101° or 102°F and become lethargic, cranky, and irritable. He may or may not have any diarrhea.

From the blood, salmonella bacteria can then invade other parts of the body. They can infect and grow in a baby's bones, causing osteomyelitis (inflammation of bone), or in a joint, causing septic arthritis. The area over the affected bone or joint becomes inflamed and swollen, warm to the touch, and painful to the baby. Salmonella bacteria can also infect the membranes (meninges) that cover a baby's brain and spinal cord, causing a life-threatening meningitis. For more about this serious disease, see *Meningitis*, page 183.

Such severe salmonella infections are very uncommon. At Children's Hospital we see about two or three babies a year with these complications of salmonellosis.

## CALL YOUR DOCTOR

- If your child has diarrhea and is under twelve months old.

- If your child of any age has any blood or mucus in his stools.

- If your child has diarrhea with abdominal pain for more than an hour or if your child has watery bowel movements more than ten times a day.

- If your child has any signs of dehydration: if he is not urinating as much as usual, if his mouth is dry, or if he is less active than usual.

NOTE: You do not need to call your pediatrician if your child just has a few loose bowel movements.

## Diagnosis

Whenever a child with diarrhea has any blood or mucus in her stools, we routinely have our laboratory test a sample of her stool for salmonella bacteria, as well as for the three other bacteria (campylobacter, shigella, and *Yersinia enterocolitica*) that most commonly cause diarrhea in children. Our lab cultures (grows) the bacteria in order to identify them. It may take up to five days to get the results.

If we suspect a baby may have salmonella growing in her bloodstream, we have the lab try to culture the bacteria from a sample of her blood. If we suspect she has a salmonella infection in a

bone or joint, a procedure can be performed to obtain a sample of bone or joint fluid for culture. If we suspect a baby has salmonella meningitis, a doctor may perform a lumbar puncture (spinal tap) to get a sample of spinal fluid for culture. For more about lumbar puncture, see "Diagnosis," page 185, in *Meningitis*.

## Treatment

If a child just has gastrointestinal symptoms, diarrhea, and vomiting, physicians usually do not prescribe antibiotics for salmonellosis. Antibiotics do not shorten the time a child has diarrhea, and they may actually make a child worse because they lengthen the time he carries the bacteria in his intestinal tract.

Whenever your child has diarrhea, whatever the cause, the most important treatment is to make sure that he takes in enough extra liquids to replace the fluid he is losing through frequent stools and through any vomiting or fever. If your baby is under a year, pediatricians advise that you give him special fluids called oral rehydration solutions. See *Fluids*, page 290, in the Appendices for more about these fluids, how to give them and what fluids to offer, and not offer, older children. See also "Treatment," page 57, in *Diarrhea* for information about what else to do and not do when your child has diarrhea.

Pediatricians usually do not advise giving babies or young children nonspecific antidiarrheal drugs. Some over-the-counter drugs reduce diarrhea by slowing muscle movements in the intestines; this slows the passage of wastes through the intestines. With salmonella infections, this could hurt a child by prolonging the time the bacteria remain in his intestines.

Diarrhea due to salmonella usually disappears on its own in a few days to a week, although occasionally it lasts longer. Many children, however, particularly children under five years, shed the bacteria in their stools for several months afterward. And a few people continue to shed salmonella—and can spread it to others—for more than a year.

If a child does develop a severe salmonella infection in his blood or bone or elsewhere, physicians usually prescribe a course of antibiotics. There are a number of different antibiotics available for the child. Children who have an infected area in a bone or joint may need to have it drained surgically.

For babies less than three months old and others at risk of developing severe infections, physicians may also prescribe antibiotics to prevent these complications.

## Hospitalization

At Children's Hospital we sometimes admit a young baby to the hospital for a few days even if she is not that sick and even if we only suspect she has salmonellosis. We give her antibiotics and monitor her condition with repeated blood cultures. We do not need to do this very often, perhaps five to ten times a year.

Salmonella infections kill about 500 Americans a year, according to the U.S. Public Health Service. However, it is very rare that an otherwise healthy child dies from salmonellosis. A number of the deaths in recent years have occurred among elderly people in nursing homes.

## *Prevention*

Salmonellosis is largely preventable, says the U.S. Department of Agriculture (USDA).

Remember that almost any raw food of animal origin may be contaminated with salmonella. However, you can easily kill any salmonella that may be present in a food by cooking it thoroughly. Salmonella bacteria do not survive, points out the USDA, when you cook meat to an internal temperature of 160°F or poultry to a temperature of 185°F.

Eggs should be refrigerated at a temperature of 40°F at all times to keep any salmonella bacteria from multiplying. Eggs also should be cooked thoroughly, the USDA advises. Cook scrambled eggs until they are firm throughout and not runny. Fry eggs for two to three minutes on each side, until the yolk begins to thicken, and cook soft-boiled eggs in boiling water for seven minutes. Children and adults at risk for severe salmonellosis, says the USDA, should eat only hard-cooked or firm eggs.

Pasteurization kills any salmonella, as well as other disease-causing organisms, that may be present in raw milk. Do not let your children drink raw, unpasteurized milk.

To keep from spreading salmonella and other germs in your kitchen, always wash your hands—and teach your children to wash their hands—before preparing or eating food. Wash your hands after you work with raw meat or poultry before you touch any other foods, objects, or surfaces.

Promptly wipe up any meat or poultry juices that spill on your counter. Thoroughly wash everything that raw meat, poultry, or eggs have touched—carving board, platter, knife, whisk, bowl—with soap and hot water before you use them for anything else. Do not use the same knife or cutting board to cut up vegetables for a salad without washing them first. Do not put cooked meat or poultry back on the same platter or board that held the raw meat; either scrub the platter first or use a different, clean platter for serving.

It is prudent to wash fruits and vegetables just before you serve them, particularly those you are going to eat raw.

For more tips about how to handle and cook various foods safely, see "Prevention," page 125, in *Food Poisoning*.

Remember, too, that bird and reptile feces may contain salmonella. Because young children are at increased risk for severe complications from salmonellosis, says the U.S. Public Health Service, children less than five years old should avoid contact with reptiles. Nor should ducklings and chicks be kept as household pets for infants and young children.

Reptiles should not be kept in day-care centers advises the Health Service, and people who have reptiles should always wash their hands after handling them or their cages. To prevent possible contamination of food, keep reptiles out of your kitchen, and do not use the kitchen sink for bathing them or washing their dishes, cages, or aquariums.

## Resources

For more information about preparing meat, poultry, and eggs, you can call the USDA's Meat and Poultry Hotline at 1-800-535-4555 or connect on the Internet to http://www.usda.gov.

# SCABIES

*Scabies must be treated by a doctor.*

## SYMPTOMS

- Very itchy, persistent rash
- Sometimes blisters, crusty sores

Scabies is a disease caused by tiny parasites called mites, which burrow into the skin. It is not a serious condition, but it is a very annoying one, for two reasons: the rash of scabies is intensely itchy, and the disease is contagious, so if your child gets it, other family members may also.

Scabies affects people of all ages, classes, income levels, and nationalities. Getting scabies has nothing to do with how clean your child is or with the cleanliness of your home or of your child's day-care center or school. You do not feel guilty when your child develops a viral upper respiratory infection, and you should not feel guilty if your child gets scabies.

Around the world scabies epidemics tend to occur in thirty-year cycles—fifteen-year-long outbreaks, then a fifteen-year-long gap. There can also be epidemics among people living in close quarters, as in hospitals or the military. However, scabies is common enough to be a problem at any time and in any season.

If you adopt a child from another country, especially Korea or Vietnam, you and your doctor need to be alert to any sign of scabies as part of your child's overall medical evaluation.

## Cause

Scabies is caused by the microscopic human itch mite, whose scientific name is *Sarcoptes scabiei.*

Mites are not insects but eight-legged relatives of ticks and spiders. The adult female mite has a rounded body and is about the size of a grain of sugar (see below). The mite burrows under your child's skin and deposits its eggs there—two or three a day. In ten days these eggs hatch to become adult mites. Someone who has scabies has, on average, eleven adult female mites on his body.

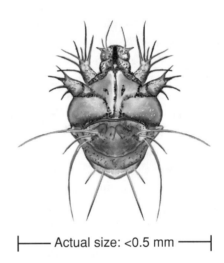

|— Actual size: <0.5 mm —|

*Scabies mite.*

## How It Spreads

In most cases your child gets infected with scabies mites by being in direct physical contact with someone who is himself infected. That contact might be holding hands in line at day-care with a child who has scabies; it might be playing with an adult neighbor or relative who is infected.

Your child can get scabies from someone who does not even know he has it himself because the infection usually does not cause any symptoms at first. In fact, by the time a person with scabies starts to itch, he probably has been infected for several weeks, giving him lots of opportunity to unknowingly transmit the mites.

Person-to-person contact is by far the most common way of getting scabies. However, although mites prefer skin contact, they can survive for three or four days on other surfaces. Therefore it is possible, though much less likely, to get scabies by being in contact with the clothing or bedding of an infected person. Your child could get scabies by wearing a hat or sweater that belongs to an infected playmate or by sleeping in that child's bed.

Scabies can also be transmitted sexually. However, a sexually active young person is more likely to get scabies from spending the night with a scabies-infected partner—that is, sleeping in the same bed—than he is from a brief sexual encounter with that person.

You cannot get *human* itch mites from your pets. However, a slightly different mite that also causes scabies can spread from animals to people. Dogs, especially puppies, are the major source of this type of scabies. Animal-transmitted scabies, unlike the more usual kind, clears up on its own in a few weeks, and there is very little risk of spreading it to other people. Even so, you should take your pet to a veterinarian for treatment.

## Incubation Period

Once mites are in your child's skin, it takes several weeks for a rash to appear—perhaps two weeks, more commonly four, and sometimes six or even more. However, from the time your child becomes infected, she is contagious, even when she has no symptoms.

If your child has had scabies before—and unfortunately, it is possible to get it more than once—symptoms will appear sooner, within a few days. On the positive side, the rash probably will not be as severe.

## Symptoms

The itchy rash of scabies is an allergic reaction to the mites, their excretions, and their eggs. Scabies causes very strong itching, especially at night because the warmth of lying in bed intensifies the feeling. As a result, a child with scabies may have a hard time falling asleep or may be awakened by itching in the middle of the night.

The type and location of the rash differ in younger children and older ones. Older children get many small, itchy, red, fluid-filled bumps or nodules (sometimes blisters, hives, and crusty sores as well). The rash typically occurs between the child's fingers and on the insides of her wrists, behind her elbows, in her armpits, around her breasts and genitals, along her waist at the belt line, and in her groin.

In infants and toddlers under two years of age, the bumps may be more scattered and isolated, and the rash often shows up in places where older children do not get it, such as on the palms of the hands, the soles of the feet, the scalp, face, neck, and lower back.

In all age groups the rash favors covered body parts, such as the genitals, groin, and armpits. Body folds—places where skin is in contact with skin—are especially likely places for the rash, but scabies can appear just about anywhere on your child's body.

## Complications

Children whose immune systems are not normal, such as those infected with human immunodeficiency virus (HIV), sometimes get an exaggerated kind of scabies called Norwegian or crusted scabies. Enormous numbers of mites are involved, increasing the risk of spreading the disease.

Scabies itself does not cause a fever. If your child does develop a fever while she has scabies, she probably has a secondary bacterial infection. This is uncommon, but it may happen if your child scratches so hard that she breaks her skin, allowing bacteria that normally live on the skin's surface, such as *Streptococcus pyogenes* (group A streptococcus) and *Staphylococcus aureus,* to enter her body. Other symptoms of a secondary infection are redness, warmth, pus, or tenderness out of proportion to the itch.

## CALL YOUR DOCTOR

- If your child has a persistant, itchy rash that you cannot identify.

- If your child has a rash and also has a fever (a temperature of 101°F or more) or other sign of bacterial infection.

- If other children or adults in your household show these signs of scabies.

## Diagnosis

If your child has scabies and you examine his skin with a magnifying glass, you may be able to see little black specks—the mites—but you cannot really be certain what they are until your doctor confirms it. You may also see thin gray or white wavy lines as fine as pencil marks where mites have burrowed into your child's skin. These burrows are most common between your child's fingers, inside his wrists and elbows, and on his penis. But once your child begins scratching, the lines are hard to see.

Many conditions that are common in children also cause itchy rashes, so to determine whether your child has scabies, your pediatrician must rule out such diseases as impetigo, eczema, dermatitis, psoriasis, and chickenpox.

Your physician may put a little oil or water on a place where your child has the rash and then gently scrape off a bit of skin. When she looks at that small sample of skin under a microscope, she should be able to see a mite, the mite's eggs, or its feces. There are other tests for scabies too, but usually looking under the microscope confirms the diagnosis. Many times scabies is suspected based solely on the time course of the rash and the appearance.

## Treatment

Scabies does not go away on its own. If your child is not treated, her rash may continue indefinitely, becoming worse over time and turning up over more and more of her body.

Your physician will suggest a cream or lotion, of a type called a scabicide, to kill the mites. You massage the scabicide into your child's body, leave it on for eight to fourteen hours, and then wash it off in the shower or bath. If the scabicide is properly applied, one treatment is usually enough. The key is to be thorough.

Your doctor will tell you to cover every bit of skin—not just places that have a rash—from your child's chin down to the soles of her feet. If your infant or toddler has scabies on her head, scalp, or neck, you need to cover those areas. Do not forget to coat her body folds, between her fingers and toes, under her arms, and on her genitals.

Make sure you cover every inch of the body, even applying the medication under her fingernails. If your child sucks her thumb, you need to put gloves on her so she does not get the medication in her mouth.

The drug of choice for treating scabies, according to the American Academy of Pediatrics, is permethrin, the same medication used in shampoos to treat head lice. The form of permethrin used for scabies is stronger than that used for lice. Your doctor may prescribe lindane instead of permethrin; however, lindane is not recommended for use in infants, young children, or pregnant women because it is readily absorbed into the skin.

You will probably want to apply the medication to your child when she goes to bed and then wash it off in the morning. Within one more day she will no longer be contagious, and she can go back to school or day-care.

Although you need to apply the medication thoroughly, that does not mean you should apply more than your pediatrician says. Permethrin comes in 15-gram and 30-gram quantities; the smaller amount is usually enough for the average child, the larger for the average adult.

Your physician may also suggest an oral medication such as an antihistamine to help relieve your child's itching. Younger children are often so preoccupied during the day that they are not terribly bothered by the itching but at bedtime, with fewer distractions, they may be unable to sleep. So an antihistamine like diphenhydramine is excellent because it is also a sedative. Or your doctor may prescribe a topical preparation for the itching.

The best way to prevent a secondary infection is to treat your child's scabies as soon as possible and to try to minimize your child's scratching—which is not easy. Cutting her fingernails and toenails and keeping them as clean as possible may help.

If your child does develop a secondary bacterial infection and the infection is not a major one, your doctor may not treat it because it will clear up during the treatment for the scabies. For a more serious infection, your doctor may prescribe an oral antibiotic.

## Treating Others

One of the nuisances of scabies is that you cannot get rid of it by treating only one person. It is so contagious that if someone in your home has it, most likely others do too. So you have to treat your immediate family and do it simultaneously. You must make sure that everyone who lives in your home—whether or not they have symptoms of scabies—is treated. Your doctor will prescribe medication for them as well as for the child with symptoms.

You should also advise anyone who has had frequent physical contact with members of your household that he needs to be treated. This includes any live-in help and regular babysitters; it may also include children or adults who sleep over, frequent visitors, and sexual partners. In deciding who should be treated, keep in mind that frequent and regular contact is the key element of risk. There is no need to treat someone, who saw your child for a day and picked her up once.

## Other Precautions

Because it is possible for mites to survive for several days off the human body, there is another annoying step in scabies treatment. You need to change your sheets and towels and wash the ones you are currently using, along with the underwear and clothing that people in your house have worn in the last few days.

Roll up these items—do not shake them because you may get the mites on you—and wash and dry them using the hot cycles of your washing machine and your dryer. If there is something you cannot machine-wash, either send it to the dry cleaner or store it in a plastic bag for four days; any mites on it will be dead by then. The plastic bag may be the best place for your child's favorite stuffed animal, for example.

Your child's rash and itching may start to improve as soon as he is treated, but often they do not go away completely at first. Your child may still itch several weeks after the treatment—not because the treatment did not kill the mites but because it can take that long for the allergic reaction to calm down.

Do not be tempted to give your child a second treatment of medication if your doctor has not told you to. This is a case where more does not equal better. Scabicides can hurt your child if they are not used properly. In fact, too much scabicide can itself cause a rash, which you might then mistake for a lingering bout of scabies.

Once in a while a second round of scabicide is needed, but this does not happen often. Let your doctor make that judgment if your child's itching has not stopped after a month.

## Prevention

Because scabies is so contagious, there is no way to prevent it completely. But you can minimize its effects by getting prompt treatment for your child and by making sure that everyone who is at risk gets immediate treatment too.

# SINUSITIS

The word *sinus* means "cavity," and *-itis* means "inflammation."

## SYMPTOMS

- Pain or pressure in the sinuses

- Headache

- Runny or congested nose

- Fever

- Mild sore throat and cough

We probably all have some degree of sinusitis—inflammation of the sinuses—every time we have a virus infection in the upper respiratory tract (a cold). A true bacterial infection in the sinuses, however, is much less common. If your child has bacterial sinusitis, he usually needs to take an antibiotic.

The sinuses are, literally, holes in the head. The sinuses are hollow spaces in the skull. Teenagers and adults usually have eight sinuses: four pairs arranged symmetrically on opposite sides of the nose (see figures page 243). Each pair of sinuses is named for the bone that encloses them. The frontal sinuses are just above the eyebrows, behind the forehead. The ethmoid sinuses are behind the bridge of the nose, between the eyes. The sphenoid sinuses flank the middle of the nose, back toward the ears. And the maxillary sinuses—the largest sinuses—are behind the cheeks, on both sides of the lower part of the nose.

Your infant has only two pairs of sinuses, the ethmoid and maxillary, which are extremely small at birth. The sphenoid sinuses do not start developing until your child is two or three years old, and the frontal sinuses are usually insignificant until he is six or eight. Your child is thus unlikely to develop sinusitis before he reaches the age of about two years, for the simple reason that children that young do not yet have much in the way of sinuses.

The sinuses do not become fully developed until your child becomes a young adult. In terms of developing sinusitis, however, your twelve-year-old or teenager's sinuses are probably not that much different from those of an adult.

Your child is most likely to develop a bacterial infection in his sinuses following a virus infection in his upper respiratory tract. The sinuses, like the nasal passages, are lined with membranes that constantly secrete mucus. This mucus normally drains out of the sinuses into the nasal passages via many tiny drainage channels, some no bigger than a millimeter across. To move the mucus along, the membranes are outfitted with microscopic brushes called cilia, which constantly sweep the mucus toward the throat, where it is eventually swallowed.

Virus infections in the upper respiratory tract—colds—actually damage these membranes and destroy these little brushes. The sinuses are normally sterile, without any germs in them, but with the little brushes off the job, bacteria can move along the drainage channels and invade the sinus cavities. The combination of the virus infection and this bacterial invasion cause the membranes to swell and become inflamed, clogging these drainage channels and trapping the bacteria inside. There they grow and multiply, and the sinuses—which are normally filled with air—start filling up instead with pus and mucus.

Children who have nasal allergies tend to develop bacterial infections in their sinuses more frequently than other people. This is because the allergic reaction also causes swelling and

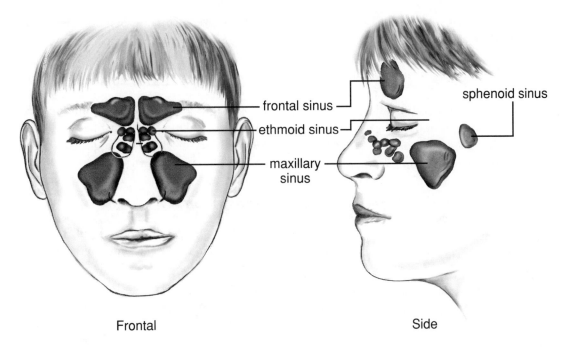

*Front and side view of sinuses.*

inflammation in their noses and sinuses, damaging the membranes and destroying the little brushes—and making it easier for bacteria to invade their sinus spaces.

And some children get sinusitis more often than others because of their anatomy. The sinuses vary considerably from person to person, both in size and in shape. If the anatomy of your child's sinuses is such that his drainage channels are smaller than usual or in some way kinked so that they do not drain as easily, they will be more easily blocked and he will be more susceptible to bacterial sinus infections.

## Causes

Three common organisms are responsible for most cases of bacterial sinusitis in both children and adults.

The number-one cause is a bacterium called *Streptococcus pneumoniae*, also known as the pneumococcus and sometimes strep pneumo for short. *Streptococcus pneumoniae* is also the most common cause of bacterial pneumonia in both children and adults, and it also causes meningitis and middle-ear infections in children. This is *not* the common strep bacterium that causes strep throats; that one is *Streptococcus pyogenes* (also called group A streptococcus).

A bacterium called *Haemophilus influenzae* is also a common cause of sinusitis. This name may sound familiar to you because your baby should have been immunized against hemophilus with a series of shots starting when she was about two months old; this is a vaccine that both the U.S. Public Health Service and the American Academy of Pediatrics recommend that all infants receive. However, this vaccine does not protect your child against sinusitis due to this type of hemophilus because the vaccine targets a different, more dangerous type of hemophilus (called type b) than the ones that cause sinusitis. The types causing sinusitis are also common causes of middle-ear infections in children. For more about this germ and information about the vaccine, see *Hemophilus Infections*, page 130.

In recent years physicians have more and more come to realize that a third bacterium, called *Branhamella catarrhalis*, is also a significant cause of sinusitis in children. It, too, also causes middle-ear infections.

Among the many other germs that also, less commonly, produce sinusitis are *Streptococcus pyogenes* (group A strep, the strep-throat strep), the bacterium *Staphylococcus aureus* (which also causes skin infections, food poisoning, and many other diseases), and rarely some fungi and certain bacteria, called anaerobes, that thrive in enclosed places (like blocked sinuses) where there is little or no oxygen.

## How It Spreads

Your child can catch any of the three bacteria that most commonly cause sinusitis from other people who are not sick at all.

These three bacteria are all ones that often live in our nasal passages and throats without causing us any infection or symptoms. About 25 to 50 percent of normal, healthy children thus carry *S. pneumoniae* without having any symptoms, and even among adults who have no contact with children, about 5 percent carry the bacteria. Even more children—some 60 to 90 percent—carry hemophilus bacteria in their noses.

People who are carriers shed these bacteria in the secretions that come from their noses and throats. If an infected person sneezes or coughs without covering his nose or mouth, he can spray bacteria directly on another person.

## Incubation Period

Because the bacteria that most commonly cause sinusitis are ones that often live harmlessly in the nose, their incubation periods are highly variable and not well known.

## Symptoms

Once bacteria spread from your child's nasal passages into her sinuses, they may settle down and grow in just one sinus or in all eight or in any number in between. And as pus and mucus accumulate in her sinus or sinuses, she develops some symptoms similar to those of an ordinary cold.

She has a runny nose. The secretions that drain out of her nose may be watery and clear, or they may be whitish or yellow with pus, or they may even turn green. Parents sometimes think the color of the drainage is the distinction between sinusitis and just a runny nose, but yellow or green drainage does not necessarily mean that your child has bacterial sinusitis. Most viral colds have at some point greenish or yellowish drainage from the nose.

Your child's nose may become congested and stuffed up, so much so that she may have trouble breathing through her nose. She may or may not have a fever; if she does, it is usually not high and usually does not last long. As the pus and mucus drip down the back of her throat—this is called a postnasal drip—it may irritate her throat and cause her to develop a mild sore throat and also cause her to have a daytime cough. When she lies down to sleep at night, pus and mucus may pool in her throat, and she may thus cough more at night. If she swallows much of the mucus, it may irritate her stomach and cause her to vomit. Her breath may smell bad.

Colds, however, go away by themselves, usually in ten to fourteen days or less. With bacterial sinusitis, however, your child's symptoms drag on longer. Traditionally, doctors use ten to fourteen days as the cut-off point. If a child has had a "cold" and daytime cough for that long, they start to suspect that he may have bacterial sinusitis. Also, sinusitis is suspected with fever, facial pain, and swollen face or eyes.

The hallmark of sinusitis—what really distinguishes it from a cold—is pain or pressure in the sinuses as pus and mucus accumulate in these usually empty spaces. Your child feels the pain or pressure in whichever sinuses are affected. If bacteria are growing in her maxillary sinuses, she may feel pain or pressure behind her cheeks. If bacteria are growing in her frontal sinuses, she may have a headache above her eyes. How sick your child feels and how much her energy level is down probably depends on how much pain or headache she feels.

Younger children do not often have a headache with sinusitis. That is the main difference between sinusitis in children and in adults. Younger children do not have headaches simply because they do not yet have sinuses up there behind their forehead. As you get older, you are more likely to have a sinus headache.

On the other hand, our sinuses vary so much from person to person, in both size and shape, that some 5 percent of adults do not have any frontal sinuses at all behind their forehead. These people thus can never have sinus headaches.

## Complications

Rarely, a bacterial infection can spread out of a child's sinuses and into other parts of his head, causing serious, even life-threatening complications.

The bacteria can invade the bones surrounding the sinuses and produce an infection called osteomyelitis (inflammation of bone). The child will have increased swelling and tenderness or pain around his sinuses.

Or a sinus infection can spread toward the eyes. In children the cavities containing the eyes (called the orbits) are separated from some of the sinuses by bones no thicker than a piece of paper. The bacteria can produce an abscess, a pocket of pus, in or near an eye, or they can cause orbital cellulitis, which is an inflammation of the soft tissues around the eye. The tissues, usually around just one eye, will become very red and swollen. The child's eye may bulge out, and he may have trouble seeing. He probably will have a fever and also pain around his eye.

Even more rarely, bacteria from the sinuses can spread to the brain and produce an abscess on or near the brain or an inflammation of the membranes surrounding the brain (meningitis). The child will have a severe headache and stiff neck and will become increasingly irritable. For more information about the symptoms of meningitis, see *Meningitis*, page 183.

Such complications of bacterial sinusitis used to be much more common before the introduction of antibiotics in the mid-twentieth century. Today these complications are so rare that at Children's Hospital we see only about five to ten children or teenagers a year who have them.

## Diagnosis

In deciding whether or not a child has true bacterial sinusitis and therefore needs an antibiotic, the first thing doctors look at is how long the child has had symptoms. As mentioned, ten to fourteen days is the traditional dividing line when doctors start to suspect bacterial sinusitis.

## CALL YOUR DOCTOR

• If your child—older than two years—
has a very runny nose and a daytime
cough for more than ten to fourteen
days, particularly if the drainage from
his nose is greenish and he also complains about a headache or a sense of
pressure or pain behind his cheeks or
forehead, or has facial swelling.

If your child has had symptoms for only a few
days, it is much more likely that he has a virus
infection or a combination of a virus and allergies. If your child has had a runny nose for two
weeks but is otherwise okay, however, he probably does not have bacterial sinusitis. If it was truly
bacterial sinusitis, he would be bothered by it more
than just having to blow his nose a lot.

If your child has had a runny nose and a fever
for two weeks, and the only symptom he has other
than the fever is a runny nose, maybe it is sinusitis, but maybe that fever has another cause.

Again, the color of drainage from your child's
nose is not a reliable sign. If the drainage is clear or
white, an infection is more likely to be due to a
virus, and if the drainage is yellow or green, an
infection is more likely to be bacterial sinusitis. But
there is considerable crossover between the two.

A major clue is the location of any pain or
pressure, whether it corresponds to the location
of any of the sinuses. Pain behind a child's cheeks,
for instance, suggests that he has an infection in
his maxillary sinuses. Pain behind his forehead
suggests an infection in his frontal sinuses. Your
pediatrician may tap or press gently on your
child's face, over his sinuses, to find out whether
he has any tenderness there.

Another possible cause of a persistent runny
nose is allergy. While true bacterial infections in

the sinuses are not all that common, nasal allergies are very common, affecting some 10 to 15
percent of all Americans. Nasal allergies are what
most people call hay fever and your doctor is
likely to call allergic rhinitis. (*Rhino-* means
"nose," and *-itis* means "inflammation," so *rhinitis* just means "inflammation of the nose," that
is, a runny nose.) Allergic rhinitis is not an
infectious disease but is caused by a person's sensitivity to some airborne substance or substances.

With allergic rhinitis, your child's runny nose
goes on and on, sometimes for weeks, much
longer than with a cold. His nasal secretions
remain clear and watery, and his nose or eyes are
often itchy. A big tip-off is if he tends to get
sinus problems at the same time every year. If
so, he may be allergic to certain pollens. The
peak seasons for pollen allergies are spring, summer, and fall—but not winter. Your child, however, could be allergic to other substances, such
as cat dander or dust mites, which could cause
him to have nasal and sinus symptoms the year
around. Allergic rhinitis is not common in children under about five years of age.

If your child's sinus symptoms do not
respond to antibiotic treatment or if he develops some complication, your physician may
suggest that he undergo testing.

The physician may have your child's sinuses
studied by CAT (computerized axial tomogra-
phy) scan. If he does have bacterial sinusitis,
his sinuses may appear totally white on the films
because they are completely filled with fluid. If
they are only partially filled, the bottom portions of his sinuses may appear white while the
upper portions, filled with air, remain dark. Or
the CAT scan may show some other problem,
such as a tumor or a congenital abnormality.

If the CAT scan does suggest that your child
has sinusitis, your physician may need to find

out whether there are indeed any bacteria or other organisms growing in his sinuses and, if so, what they are. To do this, she must obtain a sample of the pus from the child's sinuses and have the laboratory try to culture (grow) any organisms in the sample. It is rarely necessary to do this. A referral to an otolaryngologist (an ear, nose, and throat specialist) is necessary.

## Treatment

If your child has inflammation in his sinuses due to a virus infection or allergies, she does not need to take an antibiotic. Antibiotics do not help allergies or work against—that is, kill—any viruses.

If your child does have true bacterial sinusitis, she does need an antibiotic to kill the bacteria. There are many possible antibiotics that your pediatrician may choose for her. Physicians often prescribe amoxicillin (which is one of the penicillins) by mouth, usually for ten to fourteen days initially. If your child is allergic to penicillin, your pediatrician may instead prescribe trimethoprim-sulfamethoxazole.

While your child is taking the antibiotic, if she is still bothered by sinus pain or headache or has any fever, you can also give her acetaminophen. Acetaminophen can both relieve a child's pain and reduce her fever.

With bacterial sinusitis, your child probably will not feel sick enough to stay home from school. At most, she might want to stay home and rest for a day or two. You can be guided by how she feels and her general energy level.

If your child is coughing, a cough suppressant may help. The one that pediatricians most often suggest for children is dextromethorphan, which is also available over the counter. However, you do not necessarily want to suppress your child's cough completely. She is coughing

because excess mucus and pus are irritating and clogging her airways. Coughing is her body's way of getting rid of these excess secretions.

Give her a cough suppressant only if her cough is keeping her from sleeping. If your child's cough lasts more than three to five days or if it is getting progressively worse, you should call your doctor.

If your child does have nasal allergies that are contributing to her sinus problems, your pediatrician can advise you about how to avoid the substances causing her symptoms and also about allergy treatments. There are several different types of medications available that can prevent allergic rhinitis. Among the most commonly used are antihistamines. The antihistamines block a substance in the body called histamine, which is a main cause of allergic reactions. If your child has very severe allergies, your pediatrician may suggest allergy shots.

The sinus medicines that you can buy in your drugstore without a prescription generally contain various combinations of a pain and fever reliever (such as acetaminophen), a nasal decongestant, and sometimes an antihistamine. None of these ingredients can actually kill any of organisms that cause bacterial sinusitis.

Another consideration is that your child may not have all the symptoms that a given combination medicine targets, and it is never a good idea to take a medicine you do not need. It is an unnecessary expense, and all drugs can sometimes produce adverse effects.

Once your child starts taking an antibiotic for bacterial sinusitis, her symptoms should start to improve within the first few days. But sinusitis can go on for quite some time, even once you are on the antibiotics. Two weeks is probably an average length of time that it takes for a child to get better. Whenever your child's symptoms do disappear, your pediatrician will probably want her to take the antibiotic for five additional days to make sure the infection is completely cleared.

If your child's sinusitis does not respond to the antibiotic, your pediatrician may need to change the antibiotic. If your child has been taking penicillin, she may not respond because she is infected with a penicillin-resistant strain of bacteria; if so, she needs a different antibiotic that can kill these strains.

## Hospitalization

Occasionally a child needs to be hospitalized for bacterial sinusitis. At Children's Hospital, we need to admit about five to ten children a year for the treatment of sinusitis and its complications.

A child may need to receive antibiotics intravenously. In this case, his physicians probably would first have him undergo a CAT scan of his sinuses and would also obtain—via a needle inserted surgically into his sinuses—a sample of the pus in his sinuses in order to identify the responsible organism.

Sometimes a child may need to have pus drained surgically from one or more of his sinuses or from an abscess. Or an older child or teenager whose sinus drainage channels are not open enough may need surgery to create new, permanent drainage channels.

## Prevention

Since so many people carry the bacteria that most commonly cause sinusitis in their noses and throats without having any symptoms, you never know when your children might be infected with these germs and be shedding them in their nose and throat secretions.

Therefore, to reduce the chances of spreading these germs to others, teach your children to cover their noses and mouths whenever they need to sneeze or cough. And encourage your children not to share drinking glasses or soda cans with other children or adults or to eat from the same fork or spoon.

# SORE THROATS

Also called pharyngitis. *Pharynx* is the medical word for throat, and *-itis* means "inflammation."

## SYMPTOMS

- Pain in throat, ranging from mild to severe

- Fever

- Runny nose

- Cough

- Swollen glands

Most sore throats are caused by viruses and go away on their own. Whenever your child has a sore throat, however, the big question is whether or not she has a strep throat—that is, whether her sore throat is caused by *Streptococcus pyogenes* (group A Streptococcus; see page 254). If she does have a strep throat, she needs to take an antibiotic to prevent more serious disease. See *Strep Throat*, page 262.

In this section we will discuss the many sore throats your child will have that are *not* caused by streptococcus bacteria but by other germs.

## Causes

Apart from strep, the most common causes of children's sore throats are common respiratory viruses such as the ones that cause colds and flu.

Whatever your child's age, the most common culprits are the adenoviruses, so called because they were first found in adenoid tissue. There are dozens of different adenoviruses. Sore throats are the illnesses they most commonly produce, but they can also cause—in addition to colds—bronchiolitis, bronchitis, croup, and pneumonia.

Among the many other viruses that can cause sore throats are other common respiratory viruses: the parainfluenza viruses, the influenza viruses, and the enteroviruses.

Your child can develop a sore throat at any time of the year, but which of these viruses is the most likely cause depends upon the season.

In the winter the influenza viruses play more of a role, as do the parainfluenza viruses. Parainfluenza also plays a role in the fall. In the summer the enteroviruses are more common. And with the adenoviruses, there are so many different types, it is hard to generalize about their season.

In children over age ten and in teenagers, the Epstein-Barr virus can produce a bad sore throat that is one of the symptoms of infectious mononucleosis, commonly called mono. See *Mononucleosis*, page 188, for information about this disease.

Among bacteria, streptococci are the most common cause of sore throats. Your child is most likely to get a strep sore throat between the ages of five and ten years and during late fall, winter, or early spring.

Among the many other germs that sometimes produce sore throats are the herpes simplex virus (but this infection is more likely to be felt in the mouth than in the throat), and the measles and rubella viruses (which have more obvious, other symptoms). Diphtheria often starts with a severe sore throat, but these days this disease has virtually disappeared from the United States.

## How They Spread

When your child has a sore throat caused by one of the adenoviruses, the most common culprits among viruses, he sheds virus particles in the secretions that come from his nose and throat.

He can spray virus particles whenever he coughs or sneezes or blows his nose. These virus particles can get onto his hands, onto the tissue he uses to blow his nose, and onto any nearby surfaces: a dining room table, a kitchen countertop. If he sets the used tissue down on a bedside table, virus particles can get onto the table. From his fingers the virus can get onto anything else he touches.

When another child comes along and touches the table or countertop, she can get virus particles on her own hands. If she picks up his discarded tissue, she can also get virus on her hands. Then when she touches her nose—and we all touch our face more than we realize—she can infect herself.

An infected person can also deposit adenovirus on a drinking glass or a fork. If another person drinks from the same glass, he, too, can become infected.

Adenovirus particles can enter the body not only via the nose and mouth but also via the eyes. It may sound strange, but if you have adenovirus on your fingers, you can get a sore throat by rubbing your eyes.

Adenoviruses can also spread from person to person in poorly chlorinated swimming pools. Virus particles get into the water from an infected swimmer and presumably infect other swimmers through their eyes.

## Incubation Period

If your child is infected with adenovirus, it usually takes somewhere between two days and two weeks for her to develop symptoms.

## Symptoms

As virus particles multiply in your child's throat, they cause the tissues there to become swollen and inflamed. The soreness of his throat, as most of us know well, can range from a mere tickle or scratchy sensation to what feels like a lump so large he can hardly swallow. Your child can have a sore throat so painful that it is difficult for him to eat, particularly solid foods, or even to drink much liquid.

Children who are too young to say, "My throat hurts," may give you a clue by not eating as well as usual, by drooling a little more, or by acting a little more irritable when you try to feed them.

Along with his sore throat, your child may also have a fever ranging from fairly low to as high as 104° or 105° F. He may also have a runny nose and be coughing. If his sore throat is due to an adenovirus, he will often also have conjunctivitis (pinkeye), that is, reddened eyes. He may have a headache, he may be vomiting, he may have bad breath, and he may have pain in his abdomen. You may be able to feel or even see that the lymph glands (lymph nodes) in his neck are enlarged. He may be so sick that his energy level is way down, or the sore throat may be so mild that it barely slows him.

With an adenovirus, your child can have only a sore throat and no other symptoms. With the parainfluenza and influenza viruses, however, he probably will also have a fever and a runny nose. With these viruses it would be very unusual for him to have just a sore throat. He usually would also have other symptoms.

You can get a good view of a cooperative older child's throat by having him open his mouth wide and using a flashlight for better light, ask your child to say, "Ahhh," which will cause his throat to open up so that you get a better view. If you become familiar with how your child's throat looks when he is well, you will be better able to spot any changes that take place when he is sick.

When your child has a sore throat, you may be able to see that it looks red and inflamed. You

## CALL YOUR DOCTOR

- If your child has a very severe and very painful sore throat, particularly if it is so sore that it is affecting her appetite and she is reluctant to drink much or to eat solid foods.

- If your child has a fever (a temperature of 101°F or more) along with her sore throat.

- If you see pus (a white discharge) on your child's throat or tonsils.

- If your child has a rash along with her sore throat.

- If your child has a sore throat that has lasted for three days or longer without getting any better.

- If your child is sick enough with her sore throat that she must stay home from school and is not able to carry out her usual activities.

**CALL 911 or take your child to your hospital emergency room:**
- If your child has a very severe sore throat, is drooling, is having trouble breathing, and insists on sitting up with her head thrust forward. These are possible signs of epiglottitis, which is a medical emergency. See "Symptoms," page 106, in *Epiglottitis*.

may also see pus—a white discharge—on his throat and tonsils. Streptococcus infections may produce this pus. The adenoviruses and the Epstein-Barr virus can also cause it.

However, do not try looking in a very young child's throat or in the throat of a child who is uncooperative. It is not necessary for you to look because your doctor will do so.

Your child can also have a sore throat that is secondary to a virus infection of the nose, that is, a cold. At some time you have probably felt nasal secretions dripping down in back from your nose and irritating your throat. Physicians call this postnasal drip. Younger children cannot tell the difference, but an older child may be able to differentiate between this and an infection centered in his throat. Your child can also have infections in his nose and throat at the same time.

By contrast, if your child's sore throat is caused by a streptococcus infection, he is *not* likely to have a runny nose or much of a cough or reddened eyes. However, he may have a rash. For more information, see "Symptoms," page 262, in *Strep Throat*.

You do not always need to have your child see a physician when he has a mild sore throat. If your child says, "Oh, I have a sore throat," as an aside but has no fever and is doing his homework and eating and drinking fine, then it is very unlikely he has a strep throat. Or if his sore throat passes within twelve hours, if he is not complaining about it the next morning, then it was very unlikely that it was a strep.

Even if your child's sore throat is caused by a streptococcus infection, he does not necessarily have to start antibiotics the very first day. You have time to wait and see.

# *Diagnosis*

When the pediatricians at Children's Hospital suspect a child's sore throat is caused by streptococcus bacteria, they use a swab to get a sample of his throat secretions and send it off to the lab for testing. See "Diagnosis," page 264, in *Strep Throat.*

Otherwise the pediatricians usually do not attempt to find out what virus might be responsible because it makes no difference in the child's treatment. The actual identity of the virus is not important.

# *Treatment*

If tests on your child's throat secretions show that her sore throat is indeed caused by the group A streptococcus bacteria, your pediatrician will prescribe penicillin or another antibiotic. See "Treatment," page 265, in *Strep Throat.*

Otherwise, if your child has a garden-variety sore throat caused by a virus, she does not need antibiotics. Antibiotics do not work against viruses; they do not kill viruses.

Your pediatrician is likely to suggest that you give your child the following treatments at home:

## Gargling

Older children may be able to gargle with a solution of one teaspoon of table salt dissolved in one cup of warm water. Gargling with salt water is harmless for people who do not mind it. Some people find it helps relieve the soreness in their throat, but others do not think it helps much.

## Fluids

Be sure to encourage your child to drink extra fluids to keep her from becoming dehydrated. Whenever your child has a fever, she loses more

fluid than usual, and with a sore throat, she probably is not drinking as much liquid as usual. Cool, bland liquids are best; avoid citrus juices (such as orange juice) because they could irritate the inflamed tissues of her throat. See *Fluids*, page 290, in the Appendices for more information about what fluids to offer and not offer your child.

## Feeding

Your child may not want to eat much because her throat is painful. However, you do not need to worry about urging her to eat. If she loses a little weight, she will gain it right back when she is well again. Soft, bland foods usually meet with success, and ice cream is usually welcome. Avoid giving her very spicy foods because they could aggravate her throat pain. For an older child, hard candies may also relieve her throat pain.

## Humidity

Use a humidifier in your child's room to provide more moisture in the air she is breathing. The extra humidity helps soothe the inflamed tissues in her throat and keeps them from drying out. See *Humidity*, page 293, in the Appendices for more information about humidity and humidifiers.

## Warm Compresses

Your child's sore throat may feel better if you wrap a warm compress around the outside of her neck.

## Medications

For aches, pains, or fevers associated with a child's sore throat, you can give her acetaminophen.

The various over-the-counter sore throat lozenges do not contain any ingredients that can kill any of the viruses or bacteria that cause sore throats. If giving one makes your child's throat feel better and takes her mind off the sore throat, that is fine, but if you are giving it instead of seeing the doctor and finding out whether she has a strep throat, then it is not fine.

\* \* \*

Sore throats due to viruses are usually what physicians call self-limited. The soreness in your child's throat will disappear on its own, usually after two or three days. It will peak and tail off. It will usually take two or three days from the time it is at its worst until it is just lingering but not really slowing your child down much. If a sore throat lasts longer than this, it is a sign that something else is going on.

Your child may have some other disease. One possibility is that she is allergic to pollens or other airborne substances and a persistent postnasal drip is irritating her throat. In an older child another possibility is that she has mononucleosis. In that case she will probably also have a fever, swollen glands, and long-lasting fatigue. See "Symptoms," page 188, in *Mononucleosis*.

## Prevention

To help keep your child from spreading his sore throat to others, teach him to cover his nose and mouth when he sneezes or coughs. After he blows his nose, have him dispose of the used tissue in a place where the virus particles on it will not contaminate anyone else.

Since adenovirus and other viruses so often spread from person to person by hitching a ride on hands, encourage your children to wash their hands frequently, particularly after coughing into them or blowing their noses. Do not let a child with a sore throat share a spoon or fork, a can of soda, or a drinking glass with anyone else. Make sure he uses his own bathroom glass.

To prevent adenovirus particles from spreading from person to person in swimming pools, the American Academy of Pediatrics recommends "adequate chlorination of swimming pools." If your local swimming pool is having this problem, you might talk with the management about whether they are indeed chlorinating the pool sufficiently.

# STREPTOCOCCUS INFECTIONS

## SYMPTOMS

- Red, sore throat

- Fever

- Nausea

- Headache, malaise

- Abdominal pain

Streptococcus infections occur as a result of the presence of streptococci bacteria, of which there are many different kinds. One common strep is *Streptococcus pneumoniae* (also called pneumococcus), which is a major cause of conjunctivitis, meningitis, middle-ear infections, pneumonia and sinusitis. See the chapters about each of these diseases. Group B streptococci infections frequently cause blood infections in newborns and Group D streptococci are normally found in the stomach.

This chapter is about infections caused by another very common streptococcus called Group A Streptococcus (GAS), also known as *Streptococcus pyogenes*. The letter "A" refers to a classification of bacteria within the genus Streptococcus. The most common disease caused by GAS is a sore throat or "strep throat." Group A streptococci can be present in the throat or on the skin without causing any symptoms or they may cause infections that range from mild to life threatening. Certain strains of group A streptococci are more likely to cause severe disease than others are. Many other infections with which you are probably familiar are caused by

GAS: cellulitis (see page 256), scarlet fever (see page 260), and rheumatic fever (see page 258). These diseases (like scarlet fever) are not as serious or as common because treatment with antibiotics now prevents the strep infection from progressing or causing epidemics.

While most GAS infections are mild, sometimes the bacteria reach parts of body where bacteria are not usually found—in the blood, deep muscle, fat tissue, or lungs—and cause invasive infections. Invasive infections are more likely to happen when a person has sores, wounds, chickenpox, or other breaks in the skin that enable bacteria to enter tissue, while a healthy person can get invasive GAS disease but someone with a chronic illness or a compromised immune system is at higher risk. Not many people who come in contact with a virulent strain of Group A strep will develop invasive GAS disease. Many will simply develop a routine throat or skin infection. Most people, in fact, will be entirely asymptomatic (without symptoms).

In the United States, there are about 10 to 15,000 cases of invasive GAS disease each year, resulting in more than 2,000 deaths. The Centers for Disease Control and Prevention estimates between 500 to 1,500 cases of what has become known as "flesh-eating bacteria" and some 2 to 3,000 cases of toxic shock syndrome (TSS) annually. In contrast, several millions get strep throat and impetigo each year.

We have witnessed many epidemics of Group A streptococcal infections in our history. During the seventeenth century, scarlet fever raged throughout Europe. In a single year in the early eighteenth century, a scarlet fever epidemic killed 4,000 American colonists. Rheumatic fever was also epidemic, and during World War II, the United States military encountered repeated outbreaks of that disease.

## How It Spreads

GAS infections are spread when an infected person coughs or sneezes, sending contaminated droplets into the air. Another person inhales these secretions and gets the infection. Children are particularly susceptible because they may touch these secretions and as they frequently do, put their hands in their mouth or nose. You can also get a strep infection by contact with infected wounds or sores on the skin. The risk for spreading the infection is highest when your child is ill with active symptoms. Those who carry the bacteria but are asymptomatic are much less contagious. Once your infected child is treated with the appropriate antibiotic for twenty-four hours or longer, he is generally not contagious anymore.

## Incubation Period

The incubation period will depend upon the type of streptococci bacteria present.

## Symptoms

Most sore throats (approximately 85 percent) are caused by viruses. Approximately 20 percent of patients with a Group A strep infection will have a very red, sore throat, fever, and some drainage from the tonsils. Others are asymptomatic or have fever or a mild sore throat, or nonspecific symptoms like a headache, malaise, or nausea or tachycardia (rapid heart beat). Some children may have convulsions. Note that a cough, laryngitis, and stuffy nose are not characteristic of a strep infection. If your child is suffering from these symptoms, it is likely that another bacteria or virus is present or that there are complications. See *Sore Throats*, page 249.

---

### CALL YOUR DOCTOR

- If your child has a fever and very sore throat which persists for more than a day.
- If your child has fever and a skin wound.

---

## Diagnosis

If your child has a sore throat and fever, the doctor will take a throat culture with a swab to test for the presence of the strep bacteria. See "Diagnosis," page 264, in *Strep Throat*.

## Treatment

There are many different antibiotics used to treat a strep infection, but penicillin is often the preferred drug. While it is all right to wait for a positive culture proving GAS sore throats, it is important that your child complete the entire course of antibiotics as prescribed. See "Treatment," page 265, in *Strep Throat*.

It is particularly crucial to get early treatment in the case of an invasive disease. Early treatment may reduce the risk of death although it cannot, unfortunately, always prevent death.

## Prevention

While you may not be able to prevent a strep infection, you can reduce the chances of one occurring. Encourage your child to wash his hands frequently and thoroughly, especially after sneezing or coughing, before handling food, and before eating. If your child has a sore throat and fever, see your doctor, who will take a throat culture to test for strep throat. If strep throat is diagnosed, keep your child home until he has been on medication for at least twenty-four hours, during which time there has been no fever.

Any wounds should be kept clean and observed for signs of infection: increasing redness, swelling, drainage, and any pain at the wound site. See your child's doctor if a wound seems infected, especially if a fever develops.

# Cellulitis

**Cellulitis must be treated by a doctor.**

## SYMPTOMS

- Red, swollen, tender skin
- Chills
- Fever
- Sweats
- Swollen glands

Cellulitis is an infection of the skin that spreads on the body. It can affect any area of the body but most commonly appears on the face or lower legs. You will see cellulitis begin as an area of tenderness, swelling, and redness on your child's skin. The redness will start to spread, and your child may feel sick with fever, chills and sweats, and swollen glands near the infected skin. Cellulitis involves areas of tissue just below the skin surface and often begins in areas of broken skin, like a cut or scratch. It can also start in areas of intact skin, especially in children with diabetes or those who take medications that affect the immune system.

## Causes

Different types of bacteria can cause cellulitis, but the most common causes are Group A strep (*Streptococcus pyogenes*) and *Staphylococcus aureus*.

## How It Spreads

Cellulitis is not contagious.

## Incubation Period

Depending upon the type of bacteria present, cellulitis symptoms may take from an hour to several days to appear.

## Symptoms

Cellulitis generally starts with an area of the skin that is swollen, red, and tender to the touch. Your child may run a fever and have chills, sweats, and swollen glands near the infected skin area.

## CALL YOUR DOCTOR

- If your child's skin becomes red, warm, and painful, with or without fever and chills.

## Diagnosis

Your doctor can diagnose cellulitis by examining the area of skin that is affected. He may order blood cultures, particularly with a younger child, to check for blood poisoning (septicemia), which happens when bacteria from a skin infection spread into the bloodstream.

## Treatment

With antibiotic treatment, your child's cellulitis will clear up in seven to ten days. In addition to antibiotics, you can treat a mild case at home by applying heat or warm soaks to the affected parts of the body. Most likely, your doctor will want to examine your child after two to three days of antibiotics to make sure there is improvement.

A very severe case of cellulitis may require hospitalization so that antibiotics may be administered intravenously.

## Prevention

You can prevent cellulitis by protecting your child's skin from cuts, bruises, and scrapes—no easy task! Be sure that your child wears protective gear while biking, rollerblading, and playing soccer.

Be certain to wash any injuries well with soap and water. Cover the wound with an adhesive bandage. Always check with your doctor if your child gets any large wound, puncture, or bite (animal or human) because cellulitis can occur very quickly.

## Necrotizing Fasciitis and Toxic Shock Syndrome

*Necrotizing fasciitis or toxic shock syndrome is an emergency and must be treated immediately by doctors in a hospital.*

Necrotizing fasciitis is also known as the flesh-eating bacteria.

### SYMPTOMS

- High fever
- Rash
- Sore throat
- Dizziness
- Abdominal pain
- Severe pain and/or swelling at wound site
- Diarrhea or vomiting

Two of the most severe but least common of group A streptococcal (GAS) infections are necrotizing fasciitis ("flesh-eating bacteria") and streptococcal toxic shock syndrome (TSS). Keep in mind that when the tabloids coined the term flesh-eating bacteria, the public reacted because of the dramatic nature of the disease, not because of its widespread presence. While this is a serious, infectious disease that invades muscle and fat tissue, it occurs rarely.

Toxic shock syndrome is a rapidly progressing infection that causes shock and injury to internal organs such as the kidneys, liver, and lungs. TSS affects people of all ages, most of whom have no underlying disease that makes them susceptible to TSS. Complications can be serious. Infection in the soft tissue (the nonbony and noncartilaginous tissues of the body), shock, adult respiratory distress syndrome, and kidney failure are common.

These acute streptococcal infections can be primary, which means they invade normal tissue, or secondary, which means they invade tissue that has been compromised by trauma or some other disease. Primary invasions usually occur in the pharynx (throat). Secondary invasions can occur in previously normal skin or on skin or the tissue under it that has been traumatized by a wound or some other infection.

### Causes

These diseases may be caused by toxin-producing or invasive group A streptococcal infections that are particularly virulent. Other bacteria may also be involved.

### How They Spread

The organisms that cause these diseases are contagious. Toxic shock syndrome is actually caused by a toxin that is produced by the group A strep bacteria, which explains why two people could get the germ but only one might get TSS. It depends upon whether the toxin has been released. Caution is recommended because drainage and secretions may be infectious.

## Symptoms

Early signs of "flesh-eating bacteria" are fever, severe pain and swelling, and redness at the wound site. TSS symptoms may include fever, dizziness, confusion, a red rash, abdominal pain, and diarrhea. Unfortunately, there is no sign or symptom unique to TSS, and so it is sometimes difficult to differentiate from other illnesses.

## Treatment

Treatment of these infections requires hospitalization.

Despite modern treatments, approximately 30 to 70 percent of those with TSS die because the toxin is not inactivated by antibiotics and causes low blood pressure, shock, and vital organ failure. For necrotizing faciitis, intaveneous antibiotics are used in combination with surgery, which is required to open and drain infected areas and remove dead tissue.

## Prevention

There is no way to prevent these diseases, however, immediate attention to symptoms of strep infection is critical.

## *Rheumatic Fever*

***Rheumatic fever must be treated by a doctor.***

Rheumatic fever is so named because its symptoms—fever and pain in the joints—are similar to those of rheumatism. Rheumatic fever occurs particularly among children between five and

### SYMPTOMS

- Fatigue, fever
- Joint pain and swelling
- Nosebleeds
- Rash
- Heart murmur
- Twitching or abnormal movements of the hands, arms, or mouth

fifteen years old, although young adults in their early twenties are susceptible but less so.

If not treated properly, rheumatic fever can permanently damage the heart. The disease tends to recur and each subsequent attack may further weaken the heart. Rheumatic fever tends to run in families, perhaps because economic and environmental conditions (damp, cold climate) and poor hygiene habits may be contributing factors.

## Cause

Rheumatic fever is a complication of a group A streptococcal infection.

## How It Spreads

Rheumatic fever is not contagious, but the factors that contribute to it may cause outbreaks.

## Incubation Period

Typically, rheumatic fever occurs anywhere from one day to six weeks after an initial group A streptococcal infection occurred. The course of the disease generally runs from one to three months.

## Symptoms

The first symptoms of rheumatic fever appear one to four weeks after a group A strep infection (a "strep throat"). See *Strep Throat,* page 262. Its onset may be gradual or sudden, and symptoms may vary. Usually your child will first complain about fatigue and pain in his joints. He will have nosebleeds and a slight fever. In a more serious case, his fever will be high by the second day and continue for several weeks, generally subsiding in about two weeks.

Joint pain may develop at any stage and lasts from a few hours to several weeks. Your child's joints will swell and be tender to the touch. The swelling may simply stop in one area and then occur in another. As the pain subsides, the joints return to normal. There may be some twitching or rash. One of the most serious signs of this disease is the development of a heart murmur.

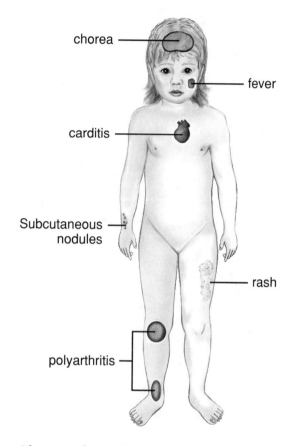

*Rheumatic fever may cause symptoms in various parts of the body.*

> ## CALL YOUR DOCTOR
>
> - If your child develops persistent joint pain and swelling.
> - If your child has a fever and swollen joints.

## Diagnosis

There is no single test to diagnose rheumatic fever. Instead, your doctor makes the diagnosis by looking at the group of symptoms manifested and the lab tests. Your doctor will take a detailed history and will examine your child to look for classic symptoms. He will do a throat culture to determine whether or not there is a group A streptococcal infection. Blood tests reveal information that helps to raise the suspicion of rheumatic fever.

## Treatment

Your child will need analgesic drugs to relieve the pain if it is severe. Good nutrition and bed rest are important parts of treatment. The doctor may prescribe steroids or other anti-inflammatory drugs to reduce the joint inflammation and penicillin if your child has been exposed to strep infection. Antibiotics are given to prevent recurrent attacks.

## Prevention

It is extremely important to treat any strep infection so that it does not develop into rheumatic fever. If rheumatic fever is diagnosed, antibiotics will be given to prevent damage to the heart.

# Scarlet Fever

***Scarlet fever must be treated by a doctor.***

Also called scarlatina.

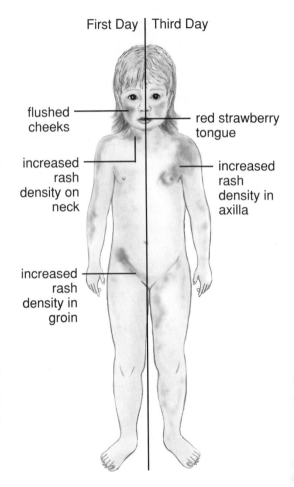

First Day | Third Day

flushed cheeks

red strawberry tongue

increased rash density on neck

increased rash density in axilla

increased rash density in groin

*Rash from scarlet fever: first and third days.*

## SYMPTOMS

- Fever
- Sore throat
- Swollen glands
- White coating on tongue turns to "strawberry tongue"
- Chills
- Nausea, abdominal pain
- Achy feeling
- Loss of appetite
- Rash (fine bumps; "sandpaper")
- Red streaks in skin creases

Scarlet fever, once a common, serious childhood disease, is easily treated now with penicillin. The disease gets its name from its characteristic scarlet red rash. Initially, the scarlet fever rash resembles severe sunburn. The rash (tiny red bumps that may be itchy) first appears on the neck and face, then spreads to the chest and back, and then to the rest of the body. You may see bright red streaks, called Pastia's lines, in the creases and folds of the skin—the underarms, elbows, and groin area. When you press on an area of the rash, it will turn white.

By the sixth day the rash usually has faded, but it leaves a rough, grainy feel to the skin, which may peel. For the first two days, the tongue has a heavy white coating (referred to as "white strawberry tongue"), and the papillae,

which are red and swollen, protrude. By the fourth or fifth day, the white coat sloughs off, leaving a characteristic red "strawberry tongue."

Generally, we see more scarlet fever during the winter and early spring. The children most frequently affected are between the ages of two and ten years.

## Causes

Scarlet fever is caused by an infection of group A streptococci bacteria (*Streptococcus pyogenes*), which produce a toxin that causes a rash in sensitive persons. We see this reaction in a small percentage of children with strep throat, but it is not typical. Therefore, scarlet feature is nothing more than a strep throat with a rash. See *Strep Throat,* page 262.

## How It Spreads

The group A streptococcal infections that cause scarlet fever are contagious. Strep bacteria can be passed through contact with the nasal or throat fluids of someone who has a strep throat infection or by touching infected skin.

Among school-age children, 15 to 20 percent may be asymptomatic carriers of strep bacteria, which means that they carry the bacteria but do not have any symptoms. If someone in the family has a strep throat infection, there's a 25 percent chance that someone else in the family will get it.

## Incubation Period

The incubation period for scarlet fever is usually two to four days after exposure. Generally the rash appears on the second day.

## Symptoms

Scarlet fever usually begins with a fever above 101°F, a reddened sore throat, and swollen glands. The tonsils and back of the throat may be covered with a whitish coating or appear red, swollen, and dotted with whitish or yellowish specks of pus. The tongue may have a whitish or yellowish coating. Later its surface sloughs off and it turns deep red, leaving the characteristic "strawberry tongue."

You child may also have chills and nausea. Some children complain of feeling achy all over. You will notice that your child will lose interest in eating—and no wonder, his throat is too sore.

While complications are rare, they can include otitis media (middle-ear infection), sinusitis, or an abscess on the tonsils.

### CALL YOUR DOCTOR

- If your child has a deep red rash that spreads down the body and is accompanied by fever.
- If scarlet fever symptoms do not subside twenty-four hours after treatment begins.

## Diagnosis

If your doctor suspects scarlet fever, he should always do a throat culture—a painless throat swab—to determine if group A strep is present. Some doctors use a "rapid" test that can confirm a strep infection within ten to thirty minutes during your office visit. The doctor will usually make a diagnosis from a physical exam, with a positive throat culture providing definitive information. The pattern of the rash's spread and the strawberry tongue are telltale signs of scarlet fever.

## Treatment

Your doctor will treat the infection with antibiotics (usually penicillin or, for penicillin-sensitive children, erythromycin) only if the throat culture is positive. Use nonaspirin pain reliever at the recommended dosage to treat your child's fever.

See that your child gets plenty of rest and lots of fluids. His throat will be very sore, so keep foods bland and soothing (soup, applesauce, mashed bananas, sherbet, fruit juices, ice pops or smoothies). Avoid foods that are rough or irritating, like citrus juices or spicy foods. A cool-mist humidifier to add moisture to the air will help soothe the throat passages. You can put a moist, warm towel around the neck—it can make swollen glands feel better. If your child is old enough, he may appreciate sucking on throat lozenges.

If the rash is itchy, trim your child's fingernails to prevent him from scratching and infecting his skin. Moisturizing cream will soothe the skin.

## Prevention

There is no way to avoid the strep infections that cause this disease. If your child is infected, keep her drinking glasses and eating utensils separate from those of the rest of the family. Wash them thoroughly in very hot soapy water. Be sure you wash your own hands frequently.

Keep your child home from child care or school at least until twenty-four hours after she begins antibiotic treatment and there has been no fever for twenty-four hours.

## *Strep Throat*

### *Strep throat must be treated by a doctor.*

Also called streptococcal pharyngitis. *Pharynx* is the medical word for throat, and *-itis* means "inflammation."

A strep throat is potentially one of the most serious kinds of sore throat your child can have. When he has a strep throat—that is, a sore throat caused by streptococcus bacteria—it is very important that he take antibiotics in order to keep him from getting rheumatic fever, a disease that can cause lifelong trouble.

When your child has a sore throat, however, streptococcus bacteria are only one of many possible microorganisms that may be responsible. Streps cause only about 15 percent of sore

---

## SYMPTOMS

- Severe sore throat
- Fever
- Headache
- Vomiting
- Swollen glands
- Abdominal pain

---

throats. See *Sore Throats*, page 249, for information about the many other throat infections he may have that are caused by other organisms.

Strep throat is primarily a disease of grade-school children. Your child is most likely to get a strep throat when he is between the ages of five and ten years. However, outbreaks sometimes occur among younger children who are attending day-care centers.

Like so many respiratory tract infections, strep throats are seasonal. Your child is most likely to get one in the late fall, winter, or early spring. During this time at The Children's Hospital of Philadelphia, we usually see about ten children a week who have strep throats.

## Cause

Strep throats are caused by a species of streptococcus bacteria called *Streptococcus pyogenes.* (A pyogen is a microorganism that produces pus.) This species of bacteria is commonly referred to as the group A streptococci.

There are more than eighty different strains of group A streptococci. Sore throats are the illnesses that they most frequently produce, but they also cause impetigo and other skin infections. The group A streps include the bacteria responsible for the so-called flesh-eating episodes that have received so much publicity recently, but these, fortunately, are extremely rare. See *Necrotizing Fasciitis*, page 257.

## How It Spreads

Your child gets a strep throat from another person who has a strep throat. People with strep throats shed streptococcus bacteria in the secretions that come out of their noses and throats.

When your child is infected, she can deposit the bacteria on anything she touches with her mouth: a drinking glass, a can of soda, a spoon, a fork, or the mouth of someone she kisses goodnight. She can spray the bacteria on anyone—a classmate sitting next to her at school—whenever she coughs or sneezes without covering her mouth or nose. If she does cover her mouth with her hand, she gets the bacteria on her fingers and can leave them on anyone she touches. She can also spray bacteria when she speaks; we all sometimes spit a little as we talk.

When a school friend or a sibling drinks out of the same soda can or uses the same spoon, he can get the streptococcus bacteria into his own mouth. Or if he gets the bacteria on his hands and then touches his face—and we all touch our faces more than we realize—he can get the bacteria into his nose or mouth. Once the bacteria get into his mouth, they settle down and start growing in the tissues lining his throat.

The reason strep throats are more common in the fall, winter, and spring is probably because that is when children that age are cooped up together in school. Just being all in the same place, they spread it among themselves more easily.

## Incubation Period

Your child usually will develop symptoms of a strep throat—if he is going to have any symptoms—some time between twelve hours and five days after he is infected with the bacteria.

## Symptoms

As the streptococcus bacteria multiply in your child's throat, they cause the tissues there to swell and become inflamed. A strep throat usually starts suddenly and is also usually more severe than sore throats due to other germs. A strep throat is typically very painful. You usually know it when you have it. Your child's throat may hurt so much when she swallows that she is reluctant to eat solid foods or drink much liquid.

Along with her sore throat, your child may also have a fever, which can range from 101° up to 104° or 105°F. She is likely to have a headache, may be vomiting, have abdominal pain, and may have bad breath. You may be able to feel or actually see that the lymph glands (lymph nodes) in her neck are enlarged. She may complain of pain in her abdomen. She can just feel lousy and be so sick that she has no choice but to stay in bed and home from school.

You can inspect an older child's throat by having her open her mouth wide and then gently depressing the back of her tongue slightly with the handle of a spoon. You can use a flashlight or a lamp to get more light into her throat.

When your child has a strep throat, you may be able to see on his throat and tonsils the pus that gives this streptococcus the *pyogenes* part of its name. Pus looks like a white discharge on the throat. A strep infection, however, is not the only possible cause of pus on your child's throat; a number of other germs can also cause this.

However, do not try looking in a very young child's throat or in the throat of a child who is uncooperative. It is not necessary for you to look because your doctor will do so.

There is a lot of variability in strep throats. Your child can have a strep throat that is very mild and causes few or no other symptoms. Many children have group A streptococcus infections in their throats and no symptoms at all.

With a strep throat, your child is not likely to have a runny nose or be coughing much or have reddened eyes. These symptoms are more typical of sore throats caused by viruses. In children under age five, however, strep throats can resemble viral sore throats.

## Complications

Occasionally a child with a strep throat also develops, within the first day or two, a fine red rash all over his body that feels like sandpaper. See the figure on page 260. This is the syndrome called scarlet fever. The rash just changes the name of the disease. In the early part of the twentieth century, before antibiotics, scarlet fever used to be a feared disease. Today its diagnosis and treatment are generally identical to those of strep throat. See *Scarlet Fever*, page 260.

If your child's strep throat or scarlet fever is not fully treated with antibiotics, however, she could suffer serious consequences. She could develop abscesses on or around her tonsils or in her nearby lymph glands. The bacteria could spread and also cause infections in her ears or in her sinuses.

The biggest danger of not treating a strep throat, however, is that your child could develop rheumatic fever. This infection can cause inflammation of the joints (arthritis) and can also permanently damage the valves inside the heart. For more about the symptoms, diagnosis, and treatment of rheumatic fever, see *Rheumatic Fever* page 258.

The main reason for treating your child with antibiotics when she has a strep throat, is to prevent her from developing rheumatic fever. The strep throat itself will most likely go away on its own within a few days.

An untreated strep infection could also attack your child's kidneys and produce a rare but serious condition called glomerulonephritis.

### CALL YOUR DOCTOR

- If your child has a very severe, very painful sore throat, particularly if it is so sore that he is reluctant to drink fluids or to eat solid foods.

- If you see pus—a white discharge—on your child's tonsils or the back of his throat.

- If your child has a fever of 101°F or more along with his sore throat.

- If your child has a rash along with his sore throat.

- If your child's sore throat has lasted for three days or more without getting any better.

- If your child's sore throat is cutting into his energy level so much that he must stay home from school and cannot go about his usual activities.

## Diagnosis

When your doctor examines your child's throat, he may be able to spot another classic but subtle sign of a strep throat: tiny purple dots on her palate. Doctors call these dots petechiae.

A physician cannot tell for sure, however, just by looking in your child's throat, whether her sore throat is caused by a streptococcus infection or by a virus, even if there is pus on the tonsils. A doctor can make an educated guess, but that is all. The infections can truly be indistinguishable.

At Children's Hospital, when we suspect a child may have a strep throat, we use a swab to obtain a sample of her throat secretions and then ask the hospital laboratory to test it for the presence of group A streptococci. The lab first does a rapid test, which takes only a few minutes, and we get the answer while the child is still in the office or the emergency department. If a rapid test is positive for group A strep, we prescribe an antibiotic for the child.

If the rapid test is negative, however, we need a second test. The rapid test can give a "false negative" answer, that is, fail to detect the presence of strep. So the lab then tries to culture (grow) the bacteria in order to identify them. A throat culture is a more sensitive, more reliable test, but it takes twenty-four hours, sometimes forty-eight hours, to get the answer. We will wait for a confirmed positive culture before starting drug treatment.

## Treatment

The standard treatment for a streptococcal infection of your child's throat is penicillin, either as a single shot or in the form of pills that your child must take by mouth two or three times a day (depending on the preparation) over the course of the next ten days. For children who are allergic to penicillin, physicians may give erythromycin or cephalosporin.

The advantage of a single shot is that you can be sure that your child got his full dose of the antibiotic, but the injection, of course, does hurt some. The advantage of the pills is that they do not hurt, but it is sometimes difficult to get some children to take so many pills. After a few days on the pills, your child's throat will feel better and it is easy to forget to finish the ten days of treatment. However, failure to complete the full treatment may result in the return of the strep throat.

And to prevent rheumatic fever, it is very, very important that your child take all the pills, for the full ten days, even after he feels better, to make sure the antibiotic kills all the group A strep in his body.

It is less important that your child start the antibiotic immediately. Studies show that antibiotics are effective at preventing rheumatic fever if you start them within the first nine days of a strep infection. So there is no tremendous rush. You are not putting your child at higher risk by waiting a day or so.

You should not let your child take antibiotics for a suspected strep throat without having him tested to make sure he does indeed have a strep infection. One reason for not taking an antibiotic if he does not truly need it is that the more penicillin he takes, the more likely he is to become allergic to it and therefore not able to take it when he does need it. A second reason is that the antibiotic may induce bacteria in his body to develop resistance to the drug.

In addition to an antibiotic, your pediatrician will probably suggest the following treatments.

### Fluids

Make sure your child drinks enough extra fluids to keep him from becoming dehydrated. He is losing more fluid than usual if he has a fever, and the soreness of his throat probably is also keeping him from drinking as much as usual. See *Fluids*, page 290, in the Appendices for more about dehydration and for information about what fluids to offer your child.

### Other Medications

If your child has a fever and is uncomfortable, you can give him acetaminophen. See also "Treatment," page 252, in *Sore Throats*.

To keep your child from giving his strep throat to anyone else, you should keep him home from school or from his day-care center for at least twenty-four hours after he starts taking his antibiotic—according to the recommendations of both the American Academy of Pediatrics and the U.S. Public Health Service—and also until he has no fever for twenty-four hours. During this time you should also keep him, if possible, away from having close contact with other children.

Strep throat is a disease that a person can get again and again throughout his lifetime, and children occasionally get repeated strep throats within a short period of time. There is no need for you to become alarmed about this. However, if your child has many strep throats over the course of a single year, he may need to have his tonsils removed surgically in the procedure called a tonsillectomy.

## Prevention

When your child has a strep throat, to help keep her from spreading the infection within your family, encourage her to cover her mouth and nose when she coughs or sneezes. When she blows her nose, have her dispose of the used tissue in a way that the bacteria on it will not spread to anyone else. Teach her to wash her hands frequently, particularly after coughing or sneezing into them or blowing her nose.

Do not let her share utensils, a can of soda, or drinking glass, not even the bathroom glass, with any of her brothers or sisters. And try to hold off kissing her on the mouth until she is well again.

And that spoon handle you used to look in her throat, make sure that you thoroughly wash it—as well as any other utensils, dishes, or glasses she has used—with hot water and soap before letting anyone else in your family use them.

# TETANUS

*A vaccine is available to protect your child against tetanus. See* **Vaccines,** *page 301, in the Appendices.*

*Tetanus must be treated by a doctor.*

## SYMPTOMS

- Stiff jaw
- Difficulty in swallowing
- Restlessness
- Irritability
- Severe muscle spasms
- Stiff neck, arms, or legs
- Headache
- Fever
- Sore throat
- Chills

Tetanus used to be a dreaded disease. Children were cautioned about the danger of rusty nails or rosebush thorns. Wounds from these might cause tetanus, or "lockjaw," another name for the disease. Today we do not worry about tetanus very much because it can be totally prevented through vaccination. Your child receives tetanus vaccine in combination with the diphtheria and pertussis (DTP) vaccine series given in infancy.

## Cause

When tetanus does strike, it is a very serious and frightening illness. In the United States most cases of tetanus develop from a cut or puncture injury.

Tetanus is caused by a type of soil bacterium called *Clostridium tetani.* The bacterium grows in a contaminated wound and produces a poison that affects the muscles and nerves. Sometimes the wound goes unnoticed or is so insignificant that the injured person does not even go to the doctor and the tetanus bacteria grows unobserved.

Tetanus begins gradually. Symptoms occur over a period of anywhere from one day to a week. Tetanus typically starts with muscle spasms that create a stiffness in the jaw (which explains the name *lockjaw*) and difficulty in swallowing and progresses to severe generalized muscle spasms. A person experiences stiffness or pain in the muscles of the neck, shoulder, or back, which soon spreads to the abdomen, upper arms, and thighs. These spasms may last for one week or more.

Tetanus is difficult to treat, but when the disease is diagnosed and treated very early, full recovery is possible. Recovery is slow, taking at least four to six weeks. Some of the types of wounds that lead to tetanus include burns, frostbite, ear infection, or surgical wounds.

Many developing countries have no effective prevention and immunization program, so the disease is much more prevalent in those locales than in the United States. Neonatal tetanus, another form of the disease that strikes newborns, is found mostly in developing countries and is caused primarily by birth under unsanitary conditions.

In the United States, tetanus may rarely occur in older patients or in those with unsuspected or undiagnosed immune dysfunction.

## How It Spreads

Tetanus does not spread from person to person.

## Incubation Period

It takes from three days to three weeks from the time of the injury until tetanus symptoms appear. On the average, however, symptoms appear on the seventh or eighth day. In neonatal tetanus, symptoms start within the first two weeks of life.

## Symptoms

The most frequent symptom is the characteristic stiff jaw. Other symptoms include difficulty in swallowing; restlessness and irritability; stiff neck, arms, or legs; headache; fever; sore throat; chills; and muscle spasms. As the infection progresses, the patient has trouble opening his jaws. One peculiarity of tetanus is that facial muscle spasms produce a characteristic expression with a fixed smile and elevated eyebrows.

A localized tetanus can occur with spasms of a group of muscles near the wound but without the characteristic lockjaw.

### CALL YOUR DOCTOR

- If your child gets a puncture wound and has not been immunized.
- If your child gets a puncture wound and exhibits any kind of muscle spasms or stiff neck or fever.

## Diagnosis

The wound should be cultured, but your physician can make a diagnosis from examining the wound and taking a history of how it occurred.

## Treatment

If your child gets a puncture or open-wound injury, call your doctor to determine the date of her last tetanus booster. For some wounds, your child may need a booster if more than five years have elapsed since the last dose. If she has not had a booster within the past ten years, she should receive a booster dose of vaccine or other medications to prevent tetanus disease.

If your child gets tetanus, she will be treated in the hospital. Her treatment will include antibiotics (penicillin G or tetracycline) to kill the bacteria and an antitoxin to neutralize the poison. She will take medicine to control muscle spasms and to stop the abnormal nerve activity that might otherwise cause disturbances in her heartbeat, blood pressure, and body temperature. Recovery usually takes at least four to six weeks.

Having tetanus disease does not make your child immune to the disease, so she will still need a full immunizing course of vaccine after recovery.

## Prevention

Your child should receive tetanus immunization as part of the DTP (diphtheria, tetanus, and pertussis) series, which is given in five doses beginning when your baby is two months old. See *Vaccines,* page 301, in the Appendices for a recommended schedule. Once the initial immunization series is completed, your child should continue to get a booster dose of tetanus vaccine every ten years for the rest of his life.

If more than five years have elapsed since your child's last dose of vaccine, a booster of Td (adult-type tetanus and diphtheria toxoids) should be considered if he is going to a summer camp or on a wilderness expedition where tetanus boosters may not be available.

Neonatal tetanus, caused by unsanitary conditions, can be prevented by making certain that all pregnant women have been immunized and that newborns are delivered in sanitary conditions.

# THRUSH

Also known as candidiasis.

## SYMPTOMS

- White cheeselike discharge in mouth
- Sore bleeding gums
- Persistent diaper rash

Candidiasis is an infection caused by candida, a yeastlike fungus. Candidiasis appears as oral "thrush" in 5 percent of newborns or more commonly as a diaper rash. We do not see thrush in older children and adolescents unless the immune system is compromised or there is a reaction to antibiotics or steroids.

Candida attacks parts of the mouth and throat, forming creamy white, cottage-cheeselike patches on the tongue and inside of the mouth. If you try to wipe off the patches, you will see that the area underneath looks raw and may bleed.

Thrush is relatively harmless and easy to treat. Usually there are no complications. In most people, a candidiasis infection flares up and then heals. But in newborns or persons with weak immune systems, this yeast can cause more serious or chronic infections. Infection usually begins on the tongue and cheek linings and may spread to the palate, gums, tonsils, pharynx, larynx, GI tract, respiratory system, and skin.

Many infants get thrush from their mothers during the birth process. In fact, some 5 percent of healthy newborns may suffer from thrush after being infected from a mother's vaginal yeast infection during delivery. After birth, babies get thrush from close contacts with family members who carry the infection on their hands. In older persons, antibiotics or inhaled steroids for asthma may upset the balance of microbes in the mouth, also resulting in thrush.

In healthy newborns, the most common form of candidiasis is a diaper rash. Thrush can make an existing diaper rash worse because this yeast thrives on damaged skin. Thrush makes the skin turn very red with sores that have a raised red border. Children who suck their thumbs or fingers may sometimes develop candida around their fingernails.

Although your child will outgrow thrush, she will not become immune to it. Adolescents and adults who experience an imbalance of candida may develop either vaginitis or lesions on the penis.

## *Causes*

Many candida species cause yeast infections; however, *Candida albicans* causes 90 percent of human yeast infections and is almost always the cause of thrush. These organisms are normally found in various parts of the body in healthy individuals and typically do not cause any symptoms. But certain conditions may upset the balance of microbes and allow an overgrowth of candida, which then causes the infection. An infant is probably predisposed to thrush because he gets the fungus early in life, before the normal bacteria that counterbalance it get established.

## *How It Spreads*

Thrush is spread from person to person. Newborns can acquire the organism in utero, during passage through the vagina, or after birth. A mild thrush infection is common in healthy infants.

If your child has persistent infections, your physician will request an evaluation to make sure there is no serious disease, since thrush can be a sign of abnormalities in the body's immune system.

## Incubation Period

It is difficult to pinpoint an incubation period because thrush is generally caused by a fungus that is already present. For newborns infected at birth, the infection usually appears within seven to ten days after delivery. Thrush is infectious as long as there are lesions present.

## Symptoms

Oral thrush appears as white cheeselike areas in the mouth that may bleed if you try to wipe them off. Your baby may have a sore mouth, which will become evident when he is fussy or cries when you try to feed him. A diaper rash that lasts three days or longer may be candidiasis.

### CALL YOUR DOCTOR

• If your baby fusses while feeding and has patches of white cheesy material on the inner cheeks and tongue.

## Diagnosis

Your doctor will probably diagnose thrush by examining your baby's mouth. Unless your child is sick or has an immune disorder, there is no need for any kind of test. If there is any question, your doctor may want to take a culture to look for yeast cells. She will scrape tiny patches of the yeast infection with a sterile swab. This may be a bit uncomfortable, particularly in a severe case, but your baby will fuss mostly because babies do not like to be "held down" during such a procedure.

## Treatment

Your doctor will commonly suggest a topical fungicide. Generally it takes about seven to fourteen days for most types of candidiasis to be cleared up in an otherwise healthy child.

You do not need to keep your baby home from the child-care center unless she is noticeably uncomfortable. However, parents and child-care providers should be meticulous about hand washing and disposal of tissues from children with thrush so they do not transmit it to other children.

If your child has diaper rash, change wet or soiled diapers often. Apply a topical nonprescription ointment such as zinc oxide. Your doctor may prescribe an antifungal cream or ointment.

## Prevention

Do not permit people to put their fingers in or near your newborn's mouth. Watch out for those doting aunts and uncles who think it is cute to let the baby suck on their fingers, which may carry a fungus. If you are bottle-feeding, be sure the nipples are sterile. Wash your hands before feeding your infant.

# TRICHINOSIS

*Trichinosis must be treated by a doctor.*

## SYMPTOMS

- Nausea
- Vomiting
- Abdominal pain
- Diarrhea
- Fever
- Muscle pain
- Swollen eyelids and face
- Poor vision
- Severe headache

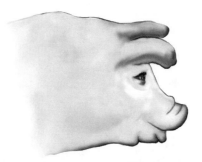

*One reason for the decline in trichinosis is that the worms are much less prevalent in pork than they used to be.*

Trichinosis is an uncommon but potentially serious form of food poisoning that can damage a person's muscles. It is one of the reasons you should always cook pork thoroughly before you serve it to your children and other family members.

During the late 1940s and early 1950s, about 400 people a year in the United States developed trichinosis, according to the U.S. Public Health Service's Centers for Disease Control and Prevention (CDC), and about ten people a year died from it.

Today trichinosis is much less common. Only a few dozen people in this country get it most years, and deaths are exceedingly rare. One reason for the decline in trichinosis is that the germs are much less prevalent in pork than they used to be.

However, occasional outbreaks do continue to occur. In a single year recently, fifteen people in Virginia got trichinosis from eating contaminated pork sold by one supplier, and in Des Moines ninety more people developed it from tainted pork served at a wedding reception.

## Cause

Trichinosis is caused by a worm named *Trichinella spiralis.* Trichinae, as these worms are also called, are no relation to earthworms but are a simpler—and much smaller—type of worm known as roundworms, nematodes, or sometimes helminths (from the Greek word for "worm"). Adult trichinae are only a few millimeters long.

Trichinella worms can infect virtually any warm-blooded animal, both farm animals and wild ones, particularly those that are carnivorous, that is, those that eat the meat of other animals. Infected animals have trichinella larvae embedded in their muscles, coiled inside calcified cysts (see page 272).

## How It Spreads

A person can become infected with trichinae and develop trichinosis if she eats raw or undercooked meat containing the larvae.

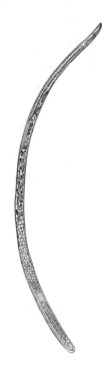

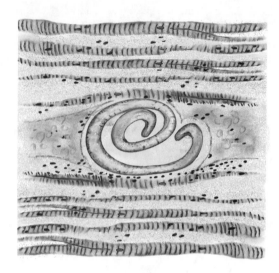

Trichinella spiralis *coiled in muscle.*

Trichinella spiralis.

People have contracted trichinosis from pork chops and roast pork, but the most common source is raw or undercooked pork sausage. The fifteen people in Virginia got it from pork sausage they ate raw, and the ninety people in Des Moines got it from a Southeast Asian dish called *som moo*, a type of pork sausage that is not cooked. Cooks making homemade sausage have contracted trichinosis by tasting the raw sausage to check its seasoning. People have also caught trichinosis by eating undercooked ground beef adulterated with pork or contaminated when it was cut by or ground in the same equipment used for pork.

Trichina worms are now much less prevalent in pork because since 1980 it has been illegal in the United States to feed raw garbage to pigs. Pigs used to become infected when they ate garbage containing scraps of raw pork and other meats. Today less

than 1 percent of the pork you buy contains trichinella cysts; surveys at slaughterhouses show that the proportion of pork containing the larvae ranges from 0 to 0.7 percent. Nevertheless, as the Virginia and Des Moines outbreaks show, some pork still does contain the larvae.

Although trichinae in pork have decreased, the larvae still infect many kinds of wild animals. People have also caught trichinosis from eating raw or undercooked bear, wild boar, cougar, and walrus.

## *Incubation Period*

It can take twenty-four hours to seven days from the time a person eats contaminated meat until he develops the first symptoms of trichinosis.

## *Symptoms*

How ill a person becomes varies depending on how many larvae he has ingested. A person may have no or very mild symptoms, or he may become severely sick.

The larvae burrow into the membranes lining the intestines and cause them to become inflamed. The person may have symptoms similar to those of many other gastrointestinal infections: nausea, vomiting, abdominal pain, diarrhea, and fever. This first, intestinal stage of trichinosis usually lasts a week or ten days.

In the intestines the larvae rapidly mature into adult worms, mate, and each female starts giving birth to hundreds or thousands of new larvae. These new larvae, in a second stage of the disease, migrate out of the person's intestines and into his bloodstream. From there they travel throughout his body, where—over a period of many weeks, as the females continue to produce new larvae—they embed themselves inside his muscles, coiling into cysts that eventually become calcified. The affected muscles become swollen, inflamed, and extremely painful.

The larvae first invade the muscles of a person's head and neck. His face becomes swollen and puffy, particularly around the eyes and eyelids. The person may develop blurred or double vision and become sensitive to light. His eyeballs may hurt whenever he moves his eyes. He may have difficulty chewing and speaking.

As larvae spread to other muscles, the person feels generally weak and tired. His muscles hurt and are tender to the touch. He may have a severe headache, and his fever may spike to 104° or 105°F. In severe cases the larvae can damage almost any organ, including the heart or brain. If they invade a person's respiratory muscles, he may have trouble breathing.

## Diagnosis

If physicians suspect a person has trichinosis, they have a laboratory test her blood for antibodies

### CALL YOUR DOCTOR

• If your child or anyone in your family has swelling in his eyelids and face, pains in his muscles, and a fever of 101°F or more, particularly if he has recently eaten raw or undercooked pork, wild game, or other meat.

to trichina worms. They may also perform a muscle biopsy, taking a small slice of muscle tissue, and have a lab study it under a microscope, looking for encysted larvae.

They have someone inspect the suspect meat itself, if it is still available, for trichinella larvae. They also attempt to track down anyone else who has eaten the meat and find out if they, too, are developing any symptoms of trichinosis.

## Treatment

If a person has severe trichinosis, she may need to be hospitalized. In the Virginia outbreak, nine of the fifteen people were sick enough they required hospitalization.

Physicians prescribe a type of medication called an anthelmintic for people who have trichinosis. (*Helminth,* you recall, means "worm.") One anthelmintic commonly used is mebendazole; people take it by mouth for ten to fourteen days. Another anthelmintic is thiabendazole, also taken by mouth for several days. To reduce the inflammation in a person's muscles, doctors sometimes also prescribe corticosteroids.

A person may continue to have swollen, painful, and stiff muscles and feel tired and weak for many weeks. In rare, severe infections, trichinosis can kill a person if the larvae damage the heart muscle and cause the heart to fail.

## Prevention

Remember that while there are fewer trichinae worms in pork sold in this country than there used to be, some pork does still contain the larvae. The U.S. Public Health Service warns that people should be aware of "the continued presence of Trichinella species in commercial pork and wild game in the United States."

However, you can readily kill any trichinella larvae—and any other germs—that may be present in pork or other meat by cooking it thoroughly before you serve it to your family. The U.S. Department of Agriculture recommends that you cook pork to an internal temperature of at least 160°F for medium or 170°F for well-done. The U.S. Public Health Service, on the other hand, simply recommends that you cook it to a temperature of 170°F.

Another reason trichinosis has become uncommon in this country, the U.S. Public Health Service points out, is that so many people have gotten and heeded this message about the need to cook pork thoroughly.

The widespread use of home freezers has also contributed to the decline of trichinosis. Freezing pork at a temperature of 5°F for twenty-one days (longer if the meat is more than six inches thick) also kills any trichinella larvae, says the U.S. Public Health Service.

Hunters, however, should know that freezing does not always kill trichinella larvae in wild game. The U.S. Public Health Service warns:

> All wild animal meat must be assumed to be infected with trichinae. . . Persons who consume meat from wild animals should be aware that freezing the meat may not eliminate the potential of trichinosis transmission. All wild animal meat must be cooked to 170 °F to safeguard against this disease.

## Resources

For more information about pork and other meats, how to store them, and how to cook them, you can call the Department of Agriculture's Meat and Poultry Hotline at 1-800-535-4555 or connect on the Internet at http://www.usda.gov.

# TUBERCULOSIS

***Tuberculosis must be treated by a doctor.***

Also known as TB.

## SYMPTOMS

- Cough

- Night sweats

- Weight loss

- Mild pneumonia symptoms (see *Pneumonia*, page 200)

- Persistant fevers

Tuberculosis is a progressive bacterial infection that can attack any part of the body but usually affects the lungs. If left untreated, TB can result in serious lung damage and even death. Fortunately, TB can be treated with antibiotics.

While TB was once very common (you have probably read descriptions of the sanatoriums where TB patients used to be sent), the disease is now quite rare, although there have been outbreaks. In the United States, TB is more common in populations that are medically underserved. Overall, TB in children younger than five years of age is rare. Many states require children to have a TB skin test before they can attend school.

## Causes

In order to understand TB in children, it is necessary to understand TB in adults. TB is primarily caused by the organism *Mycobacterium tuberculosis,* which is spread through the air when

an infected person coughs, sneezes, yells, or even sings. Another type of organism that causes TB in humans is *Mycobacterium bovis*. In parts of the world where milk is not pasteurized, the latter, bovine type is a common source of infection in children.

Although children may be infected, they do not transmit TB to others as easily as adults do. That is why children generally catch the disease from an infected adult. Fortunately, most kids can fight the bacteria. TB is especially dangerous for children younger than five and for children with weakened immune systems, such as those with AIDS.

There are two stages of a tuberculosis infection. If your child has a TB infection, she may have the germ in her without actually being sick. If she has active TB or TB disease, on the other hand, she is sick and has definite symptoms. If TB is left untreated, it can lie dormant for many years, surfacing during adolescence, pregnancy, or later. Certain infectious diseases (especially measles and pertussis) may activate tuberculosis that has been inactive. But active TB is preventable and curable.

Usually there are few complications with TB. The greatest risk is that the infection will spread into other organ systems, such as the kidney, liver, spleen, and brain. When this happens, your child will require hospitalization and drug therapy.

## *How It Spreads*

TB is usually spread when an infected adult coughs into the air and the germs are inhaled by a child who becomes infected. Children with TB of the lungs rarely infect other people because their cough is pretty ineffective and they tend to have few bacteria in their mucus secretions. Most children who are exposed to TB do not become ill because their immune system attacks the bacteria and prevents the disease from spreading. When a positive skin test indicates that there is a TB infection, that does not mean that the child has active TB. However, the infection must be treated to prevent a reactivation of the disease.

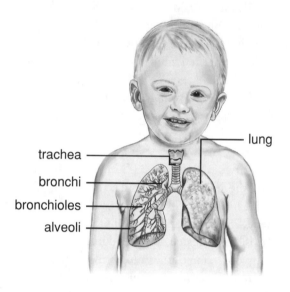

*Tuberculosis is a progressive bacterial infection that can attack any part of the body but usually affects the lungs.*

## Symptoms

TB can be asymptomatic or produce a variety of symptoms in children, including a cough that will not go away, night sweats, and weight loss. In general, only adults have the symptoms of coughing up blood, chest pain, and lingering fever. Most children will have mild pneumonia symptoms. Symptoms in children are so mild that parents usually do not seek health care until they see that their child is not gaining weight or is simply failing to thrive. Many times TB

infection is discovered on routine screening with a skin test or a routine check-up.

## Incubation Period

Tuberculosis can take anywhere from two to ten weeks from the time of infection to the onset of symptoms.

### CALL YOUR DOCTOR

- If your child has a lingering cough and fever.

- If your child has been exposed to an adult with known active TB.

## Diagnosis

TB is difficult to detect in young children. Often the only way to diagnose TB is through a positive skin test. Where you live, among other factors, determines how frequently the test will be done. The test is done with a small injection under the skin, usually on the forearm. If your child is infected, you will see a firm swelling in the area where the test was given. The test is read by your doctor two to three days later.

If your child's skin test is positive, your doctor will order chest X-rays. She may also order cultures of the secretions to determine whether there is active TB or simply exposure.

## Treatment

Treatment for TB usually lasts for months. To make a good recovery, your child will need plenty of rest so that his body's defenses do not become further compromised. You will have to pay attention to your child's diet to be sure that meals are nutritious. Your doctor will prescribe antituberculous drugs. Be sure to continue to use the drugs as directed. Your doctor will regularly see a patient to make sure all is going well.

One of the questions that parents commonly ask is "When can children with TB return to school?" Generally your child will be able to return to school or day-care soon after treatment begins. In general, children tolerate the treatment well.

## Prevention

The law requires physicians to report active TB to the local health department so that someone from there will contact the family for additional information. Health officials will try to determine the person who was the source of the disease. Preschoolers who have been exposed to adults with known active TB should receive preventive drug therapy while they wait to get a definitive skin test and chest X-ray results. When there is a case of TB in a school or day-care center, all family members and contacts should get skin tests.

It is critical to identify the source of a TB infection. Usually local health officials seek out everyone the child has had contact with—babysitters, housekeepers, school aides—and do a TB skin test on them. It is important to isolate the infected adult as much as possible, especially from young children who are susceptible, until treatment starts. All family members who have had contact with the infected adult are also treated, regardless of the results of their skin tests.

Keep your child's resistance high through good health habits, proper nutrition, and regular medical care. Never use unpasteurized milk, which can contain bacteria that cause tuberculosis.

# URINARY TRACT INFECTIONS

***Urinary tract infection must be treated by a doctor.***

Also known as UTIs.

## SYMPTOMS

- Fever

- Chills

- Burning sensation when urinating

- Sensation of always needing to urinate

- Strong odor in urine

- Blood in urine

- Wetting pants

- Low back pain

- In infants, fever, feeding problems, vomiting, diarrhea, abdominal distention

- In newborns, frequent or infrequent urination, strong odor in urine, irritability, diaper rash

Urinary tract infection is a common problem of childhood that is seen on a regular basis by pediatricians. Urinary tract infections comprise a group of illnesses that continue to confound parents and medical experts because in young children they often occur with few symptoms other than fever. The term *urinary tract infection* (UTI) encompasses a broad range of bacterial infections of the urinary tract. The urinary tract is comprised of the upper tract (kidneys and ureter) and the lower tract (bladder and urethra). When urine is produced in the kidneys, it passes into the urethra, a tube that contracts rhythmically to pass the urine to the bladder. From the bladder, the urine passes of the body through the urethra. The infection may be limited to the urethra (urethritis), the bladder (cystitis), or it may involve the kidney (pyelonephritis). With young children, it is often difficult to determine whether the infection is present only in the lower urinary tract or has spread to the upper tract.

The frequency of UTI varies by age and sex. In the newborn period, 1 to 2 percent of both girls and boys have UTIs. In infancy and child-

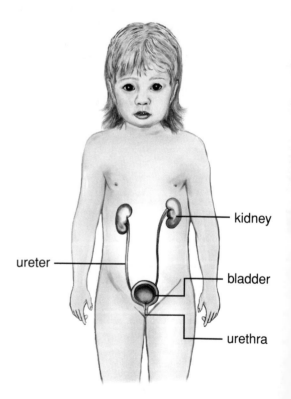

*Urinary tract.*

hood, UTIs are more common in girls than in boys, with approximately 1 percent of school-aged girls developing an infection yearly. Most infections of UTI are caused when bacteria from the bowel cross and travel up the urethra and grow in the bladder.

UTIs continue to occur more in girls than in boys throughout childhood and into adulthood. In fact, it is estimated that 5 percent of girls have had a UTI by the time they graduate high school and nearly 30 percent of females have at least one UTI in their lifetime. In contrast, the lifetime incidence of UTIs is approximately 1 percent in boys.

Several factors contribute to the development of UTIs. First, the short urethra in girls provides an easy pathway for bacteria. The longer urethra in boys prevents the entry of bacteria. Second, urine is sterile but if it sits in the bladder for extended periods of time, it encourages the growth of bacteria. Emptying the bladder completely and repeatedly flushes away bacteria before it can cause a problem. And third, use of antibiotics can change the "normal" bacteria allowing other bacteria to establish a foothold.

## Causes

One of the bacterial species commonly isolated from patients with UTIs is *Escherichia coli*, or *E. coli*, an intestinal bacterium. See *E. coli Disease*, page 97. Other intestinal bacteria can cause UTIs as well.

## How They Spread

UTIs are not contagious. Most infections are cured within one week with antibiotics. Recurrences are common.

## Incubation Period

The incubation period for a UTI depends upon the organism that is the culprit.

## Symptoms

The symptoms for a UTI depend upon the child's age and which part of the urinary tract is infected. Persistent bedwetting is not a symptom of an acute or chronic UTI unless there is a change from previous nighttime habits.

With a lower tract infection (also called bladder infection or cystitis), your child may have a fever and a burning or stinging sensation when she urinates. There is a sensation of increased urgency—she feels like she has to urinate frequently—and she may even lose control and wet her pants. Sometimes your child may produce only a small amount of urine and have low back pain or abdominal pain in the bladder area (below the navel and above the crotch). The urine may smell strong or be tinged slightly with blood.

An infection in the upper tract is called a kidney infection (pyelonephritis). With this kind of infection, the symptoms will be similar to those of a lower tract infection but may be accompanied by fever with chills, pain or ache in the side, or severe fatigue. This kind of infection is less common than cystitis. It frequently results from a lower urinary tract infection that travels up through the urinary tract.

In newborns and children under age two, symptoms are generally nonspecific and may be similar to those of a gastrointestinal infection: feeding problems, vomiting, diarrhea, abdominal distention, and jaundice. Newborns may have fever or sepsis (toxins in the blood). Your child may be voiding frequently or infrequently and may be constantly squirming and irritable.

Her urine may have a strong odor. A persistent diaper rash can be a sign of a UTI.

## CALL YOUR DOCTOR

- If your child was toilet trained and starts wetting the bed or having "accidents" during the day.

- If your child has a fever with chills, accompanied by back pain or discomfort with urination.

- If your child begins to urinate frequently either during the day or at night.

- If your child's urine smells strong or foul and is bloody or discolored (pink or tea-colored).

## *Diagnosis*

Your doctor will request a urine specimen to diagnose a UTI and to identify the bacterium causing the infection. For this simple procedure, your child urinates into a sterile container. It is important that the genital area be thoroughly cleansed before she voids into the container. Be sure to get specific instructions from your doctor. Samples obtained first thing in the morning are usually the most reliable. A urine specimen is relatively easy to obtain from a child who is toilet trained but much more difficult from a child who is not, in which case another method may be necessary. Your doctor may want to repeat this test after several days of antibiotic treatment to confirm that the bacteria is gone.

If your child is young and in diapers, your doctor may request that he be allowed to obtain a specimen of urine by inserting a tiny catheter up the urethra to the bladder. This is necessary to obtain an accurate urine culture, one not contaminated on the skin around the urethra.

## *Treatment*

Your doctor will want to treat a UTI by identifying the cause and eliminating or minimizing the potential for kidney damage. He will prescribe an oral antibiotic that should have your child feeling better within twenty-four to forty-eight hours. The kind of antibiotic prescribed and the length of treatment will depend on the type of bacterium causing the infection and the severity of infection.

If your child is less than six months old, she may be hospitalized, especially if she is vomiting. In that case she will need to be given fluids and antibiotics intravenously. Urine cultures may be repeated at certain intervals in the following months.

After the completion of antibiotics and the resolution of symptoms, further tests will be performed to determine if there is any abnormality in urine flow or genital-urinary anatomy. If there are certain anatomic defects or abnormalities, your child may need to be seen by a pediatric urologist (a doctor who specializes in urology; the genital-urinary system) who will help your doctor decide the best course of treatment. You may want to give her warm sitz baths for twenty to thirty minutes, three to four times a day, to relieve the symptoms of urgency, frequency, and mild urinary retention.

## *Prevention*

Encourage your child to drink lots of extra fluids. Discourage carbonated and caffeinated drinks; both have a tendency to irritate the bladder.

When you toilet train your daughter, teach her to wipe herself well after a bowel movement, wiping from the front toward the back to prevent intestinal bacteria from spreading to the urethra and the vagina. Buy your child loose-fitting cotton underwear rather than tight nylon panties. Change your infant's diaper immediately when there is a stool in it. Watch that your child does not become constipated because constipation may cause urethritis or poor bladder emptying and lead to a UTI.

# WARTS

Warts are one of the most common skin conditions that physicians see in their offices. Warts
were known long ago to the ancient Romans,
and they continue to interest researchers today.
This is largely because some scientists suspect
that a better understanding of the common wart
may clarify the relationship between viruses and
cancer, which remains unclear. Researchers also
continue to study warts because they are a frequent nuisance to physicians and their patients.
Nearly 50 percent of school-age children have
warts at some time or another.

Most parents recognize a wart when they see
one because they have probably had a wart themselves. Some children get a lot of warts, while
others get none or very few.

## Causes

While not serious, warts are infectious skin
tumors caused by a virus called human
papillomavirus (HPV). HPV produces an
increase in a skin protein called keratin. The rapidly produced skin cells form harmless tumors
or warts, easily recognizable hard bumps that
form on the skin's surface.

More than fifty different types of HPV have
been identified, but only a few of these (HPV
types 1, 2, 3, and 4) cause the three kinds of warts
that affect children most frequently—common,
plane (or flat), and plantar warts. Younger school-
age children often get common and plane warts,
while children twelve to sixteen years old are the
most likely age group to get plantar warts.

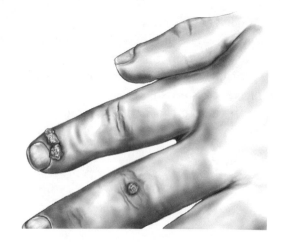

*Warts are a common skin condition.*

Warts can occur on any part of the skin but
most often appear on hands, fingers, and the soles
of the feet, apparently because these areas most
frequently come in contact with the virus. Warts
may collect stubbornly around the nails. They
can appear to be yellow, tan, grayish, black, or
brown. In some instances your pediatrician may
refer your child to a dermatologist (a doctor who
specializes in skin disorders) to have a wart
removed.

There is no known way to prevent warts.
There are three factors involved in infection:
exposure to the virus, an opening in the skin,
and individual susceptibility, which is probably
the most important and least understood. In
other words, your child's immune system determines whether or not he will get warts.

The typical wart, *Verruca vulgaris,* is the common wart. It is easily recognized by its rough,
cauliflowerlike appearance. Common warts
appear on the backs of the hands and fingers,
wrists, and around the knees. They are small,
hard, round, raised bumps with a rough surface approximately 1/8 inch in diameter. Sometimes these warts will appear in clusters, but

usually they are separate. The black specks sometimes present in the wart are caused by a tiny clot of blood in surface blood vessels. One variation of the common wart is the filiform wart, an elongated projection typically appearing on the face, eyelids, and nostrils. Occasionally common warts occur on the lips and in the mouth, probably as a result of the child biting on a wart.

Plane warts, *Verruca plantaris*, are small, smooth bumps around $1/16$ inch in diameter. Plane warts are less prominently raised than other warts and occur primarily on the face, hands, and shins. These warts are tan colored, flat, round, and grouped together.

Plantar warts appear on the plantar surfaces, commonly known as the soles of the feet. These are flat, rough warts that interrupt the natural skin lines. Unlike warts on other parts of the body, plantar warts cannot bulge outward and instead are pushed inward with every step a person takes. When plantar warts occur on pressure points, they can be quite painful. There may be a single wart or many.

Plantar warts are most common in people whose feet are moist. While there is no definitive proof, evidence suggests that plantar warts are spread by walking barefoot in showers, locker rooms, and around swimming pools. Plantar warts are difficult to eliminate.

## Diagnosis

Typically, your doctor will diagnose warts by looking at them. Plantar warts resemble plantar corns or calluses. Complications from warts are uncommon, but when one does occur, it is generally a consequence of treatment. For instance, some treatments produce scarring, which may be painful.

## How They Spread

Warts are spread by contact, either by touching someone else's wart, by touching something that a person with warts has just touched, or by touching your own wart and then touching yourself somewhere else. Generally breaks in the skin and moisture facilitate the transmission of warts.

Some children bite or chew on their warts, spreading them to other areas on their hands or to their face. Parents should discourage this behavior as well as scratching because it contributes to spreading the virus. You may want to cover a wart if it is in an area that is constantly being irritated. If that is the case, take your child to a dermatologist.

## Incubation Period

The average incubation period for warts is two to three months but can range to as long as eighteen to twenty months. Your child will be infectious as long as the wart is present.

## Symptoms

There are usually no symptoms associated with common or plane warts other than the unsightly bumps that distinguish them. Occasionally, a wart will produce a mechanical obstruction in the nostril or ear canal. Warts do not cause any illness, although plantar warts may be painful. Picking at warts may cause a secondary infection.

### CALL YOUR DOCTOR

- If you notice pus around your child's wart or if it constantly bleeds or is very painful.

# Treatment

Warts are essentially harmless. In children most warts on the hands, feet, arms, or legs, if left untreated, will generally disappear in a couple of years. In fact, 65 percent of warts will disappear within two years. It is not clear why warts disappear spontaneously, but it has been suggested that their disappearance can be linked to an acquired immunity caused by a buildup of antibodies.

Warts are best treated with benign neglect because, unfortunately, treatment sometimes spreads the warts. Most warts are removed simply because a child becomes upset about the cosmetic implications.

There is no specific medicine to kill the virus that causes warts; however, there are medicines and techniques to get rid of warts. But no treatment can guarantee remission or prevent recurrence. Instead, the aim of treatment is to destroy the warts with minimal discomfort or scarring.

With any method that your doctor tries, several treatments may be required, especially if your child has many warts. The small flat warts that children commonly develop are difficult to manage. Since they disappear spontaneously, your physician may choose not to treat them. If you want to treat your child's flat warts, it is best to treat them with daily use of topical acne agents, including vitamin A to promote healing.

Plantar warts are generally treated by paring down the wart (some physicians use formaldehyde to facilitate this step), followed by the application of strong acids, coupled with daily home use of 40 percent salicylic acid plasters. Sometimes pads or special shoes are recommended to ease pressure on the various pressure points. Aggressive therapy should be performed carefully because scarring on the bottom of the foot is extremely painful.

Many over-the-counter medications exist—try these first. Some of the medicines that you can use against common or plantar warts include Occlusal, Occlusal-HP, Trans-Ver-Sal, Duofilm, Duoplant, and Viranol. These medicines contain salicylic acid, which loosens and destroys hard tissue so that it can be scraped away. Most of these medicines instruct you to soften the wart with warm water and then apply according to directions. A couple of times a week, remove the dead parts of the warts with an emery board. Some physicians suggest using ordinary corn plasters that contain salicylic acid.

A more aggressive method of removing warts involves freezing the warts either with dry ice (solid carbon dioxide) or liquid nitrogen and then lifting out the wart and a bit of surrounding skin. This method is moderately painful and sometimes must be repeated several times because the warts often recur. Parents concur that most young children are not likely to sit still for this treatment.

Some doctors use electrosurgery—destruction with an electric current—to eradicate warts. This treatment may cause scarring, so you may want to wait and see if the warts go away by themselves.

People have always searched for charms or cures to deal with warts. The success of folk "cures," such as rubbing the warts with earwax, rely largely on the power of suggestion. Mark Twain wrote of several methods of curing warts in *Tom Sawyer,* including one that requires putting some blood from the wart on half a bean and then burying the bean at the crossroads on a moonless night at midnight.

If you wish to have your child's warts removed and are not successful with over-the-counter medications, consult your physician. Keep in mind that if there is a single lesion in an accessible location where a small scar will not matter, then removal may be worth the effort. It is probably better to leave clusters of warts alone. As a parent, you will have to weigh the different factors—your child's embarrassment versus the pain, cost, and likely outcome—before deciding to treat warts.

## Prevention

You can teach your child to prevent warts by avoiding contact with someone else's warts or by avoiding touching his own so the virus does not spread. He should keep his skin dry to prevent the transmission of warts.

# WHOOPING COUGH

*There is a vaccine to protect your child against whooping cough. See* Vaccines, *page 301, in the Appendices.*

***Whooping cough must be treated by a doctor.***

Also known as pertussis.

## SYMPTOMS

- Runny nose
- Fever
- Loss of appetite
- General malaise
- Spells or fits of coughing that are prolonged, sometimes ending with a whooping sound
- Vomiting after a coughing spell
- Lethargy

Pertussis, or whooping cough as it is more commonly called, is a serious, highly infectious disease that affects the lungs and airways.

Whooping cough gets its name from the characteristic crowing, or "whoop," sound as air is drawn back into the lungs after coughing. Infants may not whoop as loudly as older children. It can be frightening to see your baby's lips turn blue as she struggles to get her breath back. The coughing spells are so severe and last so long (often more than a minute) that your child may vomit afterward. However, between spells your child will seem fine and most likely will resume normal activities.

Whooping cough strikes children under the age of one hardest. Half of the whooping cough cases

in the United States occur in that age group, and more than half of these infants must be hospitalized. Only 15 percent of whooping cough cases occur in children older than fifteen. Because adolescents and adults tend to have milder symptoms, diagnosis is more difficult because whooping cough looks like other upper respiratory infections.

A child with whooping cough can be sick for some time. The disease generally begins with one to two weeks of common cold symptoms, including a mild cough. For the next two to six weeks, your child will experience increasing bouts of severe coughing, as many as fifteen attacks in a twenty-four-hour period, more frequently at night. After that, there is a convalescence of three to four weeks, during which the coughing occurs less often. In some children this final stage lasts for months.

Complications may include an earache or viral infections, but pneumonia (see *Pneumonia,* page 200) is the greatest risk of whooping cough.

## Causes

*Bordetella pertussis,* the bacterium that causes whooping cough, was first described by Jules Bordet, physician, bacteriologist, and immunologist, and Octave Gengou, a bacteriologist, in 1900. Six years later, these Belgian researchers were able to cultivate the bacterium and study the disease. Their work led to the development of a vaccine to immunize against whooping cough. The vaccine has reduced the annual number of deaths in the United States to fewer than twenty. That is remarkable when you consider that whooping cough killed five to ten thousand people in this country each year before the vaccine was available.

In the United States, the highest recorded number of pertussis cases occurred in 1934 when more than 260,000 cases were reported. With the introduction of the pertussis vaccine, the number of cases dropped to an all time low of 1,010 cases in 1976. However, since the 1980s, the reported cases have steadily increased to 6,586 cases in 1993.

## How It Spreads

Pertussis is very contagious and is spread most commonly by close contact with discharges from the nose and throat of an infected person. If someone in your household has whooping cough, there is a 90 percent probability that the family members who have not had the vaccine will get the disease. That is why your physician will prescribe a prophylactic (disease-preventing) antibiotic or booster doses of the vaccine for family members of the infected person, even if they have previously been inoculated.

## Incubation Period

The time between exposure to whooping cough and the first symptoms of the illness is usually seven to ten days, but it can be as long as twenty days.

## Symptoms

Pertussis has three stages. During the first two weeks your child will exhibit the symptoms of a common cold: runny nose, slight cough, low-grade fever, and perhaps some loss of appetite or general malaise. The next two to six weeks his coughing spells will become much more frequent and severe. It is during this time that your doctor first suspects a possibility of pertussis. You may see your child cough five to ten times, get red in the face and stop breathing for an instant, then hear the characteristic whooping sound as he draws air back into his lungs (in children less than six months, there may be no whoop). He may

vomit, turn blue, or be exhausted after a coughing spell. The coughing spells often exhaust the infant and results in a weight loss. The final stage of the disease can last six to eight weeks. During this time, the coughing and vomiting decrease.

### CALL YOUR DOCTOR

- Immediately if you think your child has whooping cough.
- If your child has prolonged coughing spells that make him turn red or blue; that are followed by vomiting; or that occur with a whooping sound when your child breathes in.
- If your child has been exposed to someone with whooping cough, even if he has had all of his scheduled DTP or DTaP shots. (For more about these vaccines, see "Prevention" below.)

## Diagnosis

Your physician will confirm a diagnosis of whooping cough by taking samples of your child's respiratory fluids—from the nose. Additional diagnostic tests may include blood tests and a chest X-ray to detect a pneumonia. There are some new tests that are promising because they are more rapid and more accurate, but they are available only in research labs at the present time.

## Treatment

The drug most often used to treat pertussis is the antibiotic erythromycin. When given early in the course of the disease, it will decrease the number and severity of coughing spells. Treatment is continued for fourteen days. If treatment is started one or two weeks into the course of the disease, it will not improve the symptoms but it will prevent the spread of the infection to others.

Coughing spells can leave a child exhausted so rest is essential. A calm, quiet environment is helpful. Additionally, keep the environment free of factors that promote coughing such as dust, smoke, or sudden changes in temperature.

Infants and children who are congested and exhausted may not be interested in drinking and eating. Making sure your child has adequate fluids will help clear thick mucous and prevent dehydration (see *Fluids*, page 290). Also, adequate nutrition is important to prevent weight loss. Small feedings given frequently are usually successful. If your child vomits after eating, wait a few minutes and try to offer additional food.

If your child feels better, he can return to school or the child-care center five days after starting antibiotic therapy. Pertussis is a reportable disease so someone from your local health department will probably contact you.

## Hospitalization

Infants with whooping cough often require hospital care. The hospital staff will monitor your child's breathing and heart rate, and occasionally oxygen may be needed. Your child will probably be isolated from other patients for five days after antibiotics are started, and staff and visitors may have to take special precautions, such as wearing masks, to prevent the spread of infection.

## *Prevention*

Fortunately, this disease can largely be prevented by the pertussis vaccine, which is part of the DTP (diphtheria-tetanus-pertussis) immunization routinely given in five doses before your child's sixth birthday. Usually your child will receive this shot at two, four, six, and eighteen months and five years of age. Most states have laws requiring schoolchildren to be immunized. The vaccine protects 70 to 90 percent of immunized children against pertussis and also makes the disease milder for those who do catch it. About half of the children who get the vaccine experience some mild side effects, including fever, irritability, and soreness at the injection site. DTaP is a type of pertussis vaccine that is different from that used in the standard DTP shot and results in milder or less local reactions. DTaP is now being used routinely in lieu of DTP for all doses.

# Appendices

# GENERAL TREATMENTS FOR CHILDREN

## *Fluids*

When your child is sick, it is very important—as we have emphasized throughout this book—that you make sure that she takes in plenty of extra fluids in order to prevent dehydration. Dehydration can be very dangerous, even life-threatening, for children—particularly for small babies.

If your child has a fever, she is losing more fluid from her body than usual by evaporation from her warmer skin and, because she is breathing faster, from the tissues lining her respiratory tract. She also needs more fluid when she has a fever because the fever causes her metabolic rate to rise. If she has a very runny nose, she is also losing extra fluid in the mucus and other secretions coming from her nose.

And anytime a child does not feel well, particularly if she has a fever, her appetite is likely to be down and she may also not be drinking as much liquid as usual. If she has a sore throat, especially, and it is painful for her to swallow, she is probably drinking less.

The greatest risk of dehydration, however, comes when a child has a gastrointestinal infection and is losing large amounts of fluid through diarrhea and may also be vomiting repeatedly.

The reason that dehydration is particularly dangerous for babies is because they are so small; they have a larger surface area of skin in relation to their body mass than older children do. And, of course, a baby cannot tell you when she is thirsty. This means that a baby can become dehydrated much more rapidly than an older child—and the smaller a baby, the more quickly it can happen.

When a child becomes dehydrated, water is pulled out of her body tissues. She tends to breathe faster; her heart beats more rapidly and may beat erratically. With severe dehydration, the volume of blood can drop to the point where it becomes unable to supply the needs of the vital organs.

Dehydration from diarrhea can kill a child in a short time. It kills 300 to 500 children in this country every year, according to the U.S. Public Health Service's Centers for Disease Control and Prevention in Atlanta. Eighty-five percent of these children are babies in their first year of life.

## Preventing Dehydration

If you have a baby under a year old, you should not give her plain water. In babies this young, the kidneys are still immature. This means that they not only are losing water but may also be losing essential salts (called electrolytes), including sodium, potassium, and chloride. You need to give your baby a liquid that replaces these essential salts.

Pediatricians therefore advise that you give babies special fluids called oral rehydration solutions. These special solutions generally contain glucose (sugar) for energy in addition to these essential salts. Some of the common brands of oral rehydration solutions are Pedialyte, Rehydralyte, and Ricelyte. These are available over the counter, without a prescription, in drugstores.

*The U.S. Public Health Service's Centers for Disease Control and Prevention recommend that all families with infants and small children keep a supply of oral rehydration solution at home at all times. Having oral rehydration solutions on hand could be life-saving.*

# HOW TO TELL IF YOUR CHILD IS DEHYDRATED

**The following are signs that your child may be becoming dehydrated:**

- He is not urinating as often or as much as usual or, if a baby, is not wetting as many diapers as usual.

- His mucous membranes, particularly the inside of his mouth, are becoming dry. The inside of his mouth may feel sticky or tacky rather than moist, and his lips may be a bit cracked.

- His eyes may look sunken in.

- The fontanels (soft spots) on a young baby's head may be sunken down.

- He is breathing faster, and his heart is racing.

- He does not shed any tears when he is crying.

- The most important sign is if your child is not behaving normally: if he is very irritable or less active than usual, is sleeping more, and is not playing as much.

**If your child develops any of the above signs of possible dehydration, call your pediatrician promptly.**

**Dehydration usually does not develop so fast that it requires a middle-of-the-night phone call to your pediatrician, but if your child is listless and lethargic, CALL YOUR DOCTOR IMMEDIATELY, whatever the time of day or night.**

**The younger your baby, the less able he is to tolerate dehydration, and the sooner you should call your pediatrician.**

When your baby has a gastrointestinal infection and has diarrhea and is vomiting, administering these special rehydration solutions is not easy. You need to give her very small amounts at a time. Otherwise she is likely to vomit the solution back up. You can use a medicine dropper, spoon, or bottle to give her just one or two ounces. Then wait for 20 minutes or so to allow the solution to pass through her stomach and into her intestines. Then give her another one or two ounces and wait another 20 minutes. Then another few ounces, and so forth.

At Children's Hospital, when we see an infant who is dehydrated, we evaluate the degree of his dehydration and calculate how much oral rehydration solution he needs, depending on his weight and state of dehydration. We then give his mother a specific goal: try to get him to drink a certain number of ounces of rehydration solution over the next so-many hours.

If a mother cannot accomplish this—and it can be difficult if her baby is having frequent watery bowel movements and is also vomiting—we can give the baby fluid intravenously in our emergency department. If a child is more severely dehydrated, we can admit him to the hospital for intravenous fluid. We then measure the actual amounts of the various essential salts he is losing and make up a rehydration solution specifically for him.

If you are breastfeeding your baby, you can continue to give her fluids by nursing her, even when she has a gastrointestinal infection. However, if you are feeding your baby a cow's milk infant formula and she has a gastrointestinal upset, your doctor may advise that you stop giving her the formula for a short time. See *Feeding*, below right.

\* \* \*

With older children, toddlers to teenagers, whose kidneys are mature, you can be more liberal with the fluids you offer. You can give an older child whatever liquids he likes and is used to drinking: fruit juices, punches, soft drinks, freezer pops, water ices, sherbets, sports drinks, broths, soups. Offer him a variety of liquids, and you can even include treats, such as flavored ice. Whatever you can get your child to drink is okay.

However, if an older child has a gastrointestinal problem, there are some liquids that you need to avoid. Doctors usually advise that a person with a stomach upset drink only clear fluids, and the main nonclear fluid to avoid—as with babies—is milk. Milk and milk products are harder to digest than clear liquids and can make diarrhea worse and cause more gas in the intestines. So hold off not only on milk but also on cream soups, ice cream, and other dairy products until your child is well again.

Also, when your older child has an upset stomach, the carbon dioxide bubbles in carbonated soft drinks can irritate his stomach and intestines. You can overcome this by first stirring out the bubbles to make the drinks flat. And too much of fluids with high sugar content—such as apple juice or some soft drinks—can make diarrhea worse. But if those are the only things your child wants to drink, let him. Any type of clear fluid is fine.

When your child has a sore throat, cool fluids such as flavored ice may soothe his throat a little bit, while citrus juices or other acidic beverages may irritate the inflamed membranes in the throat. Similarly, if he has mumps, citrus or acidic drinks may increase the pain in his swollen salivary glands.

## Are You Giving Your Child Enough Fluids?

You can get a good idea about whether your child is getting enough extra fluid by paying attention to her urination. If she is urinating as often and as much as usual—or if she is a baby, she is wetting her diaper as often—you are probably giving her enough.

## *Feeding*

When your child is sick, if he does not have a fever—and if he has a cold, he may well not have a fever—his appetite will usually remain good. However, if he *does* have a fever, he probably will lose his appetite some. This is because a fever causes the activity of the stomach to slow down and a person digests food more slowly.

Parents often become very concerned when their child loses his appetite, and they sometimes focus on the fact that he has lost half a pound or so. However, you really do not need to worry about this, neither about his loss of appetite nor his loss of weight.

Just continue to offer your child whatever foods he likes to eat and is used to eating. If he does eat them, fine, but if he refuses the food, you do not need to try to force him to eat it. When your child is sick, encouraging fluids is far more important than pushing food.

If your child has an upset stomach, however, and has diarrhea or is vomiting, there are certain types of foods that could make his symptoms worse and that you should avoid giving him. Milk and other dairy products may cause him to have more diarrhea, as may foods with a high sugar content. Foods that are high in fat (such as french fries) are harder for him to digest, and spicy foods (such as pizza) may irritate his stomach. Offer your child bland foods instead; they are easier for a queasy stomach to digest.

If you are breastfeeding a baby, you can continue to nurse her even when she has an upset stomach; breast milk is very easy for babies to digest. However, if she is on a cow's milk formula, pediatricians may advise that you stop giving her the formula for a short time while she is sick and while you are giving her the oral rehydration solutions, see "Fluids," page 290. Cow's milk is very different in composition from human breast milk, and it is more difficult for a baby's immature digestive system to digest. If she has diarrhea, cow's milk or other milk products are likely to make her diarrhea worse, and she may have even more trouble with gas in her intestines and be more uncomfortable. You should get her back on her regular diet, however, in twenty-four hours.

A baby who has started to eat some solid foods may, when she has a queasy stomach, begin refusing these foods. Again, you do not need to worry about this. As soon as you can, however, try to get her back on solid foods. Again, start with bland, easy-to-digest foods. A diet that pediatricians often recommend for very young children is bland and includes bananas, rice, applesauce, and toast. But then do try to get your child back on her regular diet, again, within twenty-four hours.

Any weight that your child may lose while she is sick is only a temporary loss. As soon as she feels well again and her appetite returns, she will gain the weight right back again.

# Humidity

Whenever your child has a respiratory infection, you can use a humidifier in his room to increase the moisture content of the air that he is breathing. During winter particularly—which is both the respiratory-virus season and the heating season—the air in our homes often becomes very dry.

When your child has an upper respiratory infection (a cold or the flu) with a very runny or congested nose, the mucous membranes lining his nasal passages and throat become swollen and inflamed. More moisture in the air that he breathes will help moisten and soothe these tissues, and it will also help liquefy and loosen the excess mucus and other secretions clogging his nose.

If your child has an infection in his lower respiratory tract (his lungs), such as bronchiolitis or pneumonia, more humidity may also be helpful. The extra moisture will not reach down as far as the inflamed tissue in his lungs, but it will help alleviate any upper respiratory symptoms he may also have.

If your baby or toddler develops croup (a barking cough caused by inflammation in the lower throat), mist therapy—that is, extra humidity—is the main treatment, both at home and in the hospital. See *Croup*, page 46.

Electric humidifiers are available in a wide range of prices and types. There are portable tabletop models that can humidify just one room and also larger models that can add moisture to the air throughout a whole house. Some humidifiers produce moisture by boiling water and thus emit warm mist or steam; other models produce moisture by evaporation and emit a cool mist. You can find information about models and prices of humidifiers in *Consumer Reports* magazine, which from time to time publishes evaluations of the various brands.

We suggest that you choose a cool-mist humidifier rather than one that emits a warm mist. This is so that there is no danger that your child will scald himself if he happens to tip the humidifier over.

Humidifiers do need regular care and attention. You need to refill the water tank periodically, and some humidifiers require distilled water. All humidifiers need to be cleaned and disinfected regularly because they can become a breeding ground for bacteria and particularly molds. Indeed, if a family member is allergic to molds, allergists advise that you not use a humidifier.

Extra humidity in a sick room is less important for older children, teenagers, and adults than it is for younger children. Because older children have larger air passages, they do not become congested as easily when they have a respiratory infection. However, a humidifier may provide some relief even for an older child.

# WHEN TO KEEP YOUR CHILD HOME

You do not need to keep your child home from day-care or school—nor does a child-care center need to exclude a child—every time she has a minor illness. "Most infections do not constitute a reason for excluding a child from child care," says the American Academy of Pediatrics.

Most children do not need to be excluded for mild respiratory illnesses, says the academy. Exclusion of "children with respiratory symptoms associated with the common cold, croup, bronchitis, pneumonia, sinusitis and/or [a middle-ear infection] probably will not decrease the spread of infection."

However, definitely do keep your child home from her child-care center, says the Academy of Pediatrics, in the following circumstances—both to help her get well and also to keep her from spreading a disease to others.

- Whenever your child has a fever—that is, a temperature of 101°F or above. Keep her home as long as she continues to have a fever. See *Fevers*, page 109.

- If your child is having any difficulty breathing. Breathing difficulties can be potentially life-threatening. She needs to be evaluated by a pediatrician.

- If your child has an illness that keeps her from participating comfortably in the activities of the day-care program.

- If your child is irritable, lethargic, or crying persistently. These could be signs of severe illness.

- If your child has diarrhea and her stools contain blood or mucus. She should stay home until she is over her diarrhea.

- If your child has vomited two or more times in the previous twenty-four hours, unless your pediatrician has determined she does not have a communicable disease and is not in danger of becoming dehydrated.

- If your child has a rash plus a fever or a change in her behavior, unless your pediatrician determines she does not have a communicable disease.

- If your child develops pink or red eyes accompanied by a white or yellow discharge, until her pediatrician approves her return with treatment. See *Conjunctivitis*, page 42.

- If your child has mouth sores and is also drooling, unless your physician determines she is noninfectious. She could be infected with herpes simplex type 1 or another virus, which she could spread to others via her saliva. See *Herpes Simplex Type 1*, page 144.

If your child has been diagnosed with and is being treated for any of the following infectious diseases, the Academy of Pediatrics recommends that you keep her home from day-care or school—again, to keep her from spreading the disease to others—for the specified period of time.

**Chickenpox (Varicella):** Until the sixth day after your child's rash first appeared. If she has a mild case, however, she can go back to school earlier if all her lesions have dried and are crusted over.

If your child has shingles (a reactivation of vari-cella virus infection, also called herpes zoster), she should stay home if her lesions cannot be covered by her clothing or with a dressing. For more informa-tion about chickenpox and shingles, see page 30.

***E. coli*** **0157:H7 Disease:** Until your child has re-covered from her diarrhea and also has had two nega-tive cultures from her stools. See page 97.

**Head Lice:** Until after you have given your child the first treatment with a lice-killing medication. See page 161.

**Hepatitis A:** Until at least one week after your child began developing jaundice or other symptoms. See page 136.

**Impetigo:** Until twenty-four hours after your child has started taking the oral or topical antibiotic that your pediatrician prescribed. See page 147.

**Measles:** Until six days after your child's rash first broke out. See page 179.

**Mumps:** Until nine days after the salivary glands in your child's cheeks began to swell. See page 191.

**Rubella (German Measles):** Until seven days after your child's rash first appeared. See page 225.

**Scabies:** Until after you have treated your child with the medication that your pediatrician suggested. See page 237.

**Shigella Diarrhea:** Until your child has recovered from the dysentery (bloody diarrhea) and has also had two negative stool cultures. See page 72.

**Strep Throat (Streptococcal Pharyngitis):** Until your child has been taking the oral antibiotic pre-scribed by her pediatrician for at least twenty-four hours and also until she has been without any fever for twenty-four hours. See page 262.

**Tuberculosis:** Until your pediatrician or local health department has determined that your child is no longer infectious. This will be soon after she has started taking the prescribed antituberculosis medi-cations. See page 275.

**Whooping Cough (Pertussis):** Until your child has been taking the erythromycin that her pediatrician prescribed for five days and also until she feels well enough to go back. See page 286.

# RECOMMENDATIONS FOR DAY-CARE PROVIDERS

Young children—particularly infants and toddlers who are not toilet trained—spread disease-causing microorganisms far more readily than do older children and adults. Babies and toddlers also get sick more often for reasons we discussed in the introduction to this book. They then shed the germs in the secretions from their nose, their saliva, and particularly in their stools, and they are not old enough to be careful about where they leave these secretions.

It should be no surprise, then, that young children who attend child-care programs—where they are in contact with many other young children—catch infectious diseases more often than do children who are cared for at home. Children who go to day-care get more colds, have more diarrhea, and develop more middle-ear infections, and they also frequently carry germs home and infect their families and neighbors.

People who provide day-care for young children must therefore take precautions to prevent the spread of disease-causing organisms in their facilities, both to protect the children and also to keep from becoming infected themselves. "Child care programs that provide infant and toddler care," emphasizes the American Academy of Pediatrics, "need to give special attention to infection control measures."

The U.S. Public Health Service's Centers for Disease Control and Prevention and the American Academy of Pediatrics have both set forth detailed recommendations for reducing the spread of infectious diseases in child-care centers.

The U.S. Public Health Service's recommendations are published in a 139-page spiral-bound handbook called *The ABC's of Safe and Healthy Child Care.* This book also discusses many other topics in addition to how to prevent infectious diseases, including safety, first aid, medications, and toilet training. If you provide child care for other people's children, you should be familiar with this book. You can order a copy for $19.00, plus shipping, from the National Technical Information Service, 5285 Port Royal Road, Springfield VA 22161. Or you can order the book by phone from National Tech at 1-800-CDC-1824. You can also download this book from the Internet at http://www.cdc.gov/ncidod/hip/abc/contents.htm.

The recommendations of the Academy of Pediatrics are published in a thick paperback titled *Red Book: Report of the Committee on Infectious Diseases,* commonly just called the *Red Book.* Written for physicians and other health professionals, this volume includes technical information about diagnosing and treating infectious diseases of children. The academy updates the *Red Book* periodically; the most recent version is 764 pages and costs about $80.00 at medical bookstores.

All fifty states license child-care centers that are over a certain size, and each state and some cities (including Philadelphia) have their own rules and regulations about health and safety. In Pennsylvania, for instance, the Department of Public Welfare is responsible for the licensing and registration of child-care facilities. If you are thinking about taking care of children in your home, you need to find out what the regulations are in your community. There may even be zoning issues involved.

The following discussion highlights some of the many specific recommendations from the

U.S. Public Health Service and the American Academy of Pediatrics.

Child-care providers, in addition to having parents' home and work addresses and telephone numbers, should also know the names, addresses, and phone numbers of each child's doctor and hospital. The Academy of Pediatrics advises that each child-care program also have its own health-care consultant.

## *Vaccinations*

All the children in a day-care program should be up-to-date on their vaccinations. Both the Academy of Pediatrics and the U.S. Public Health Service currently recommend that all children routinely be immunized against ten diseases: chickenpox, diphtheria, hemophilus infections, hepatitis B, measles, mumps, poliomyelitis, rubella (German measles), tetanus, and whooping cough (pertussis). See the *Vaccines* section, page 301, for the recommended schedule for these shots. Also see the chapters on each of these diseases.

In addition, many states have their own requirements for vaccinations for children in child-care programs. All fifty states, for instance, require that children attending day-care centers be immunized against diphtheria.

Adults who take care of children in day-care centers also need to be vaccinated against some diseases, both to protect themselves and to protect the children in their care. The U.S. Public Health Service recommends that all adults—whether they are taking care of children or not—be immune to measles, mumps, and rubella. All adults also need to be vaccinated against diphtheria and tetanus every ten years.

All child-care providers, says the Health Service, should also be vaccinated against influenza; this is a shot they need to get every year.

Day-care workers who have not had chickenpox should consider getting vaccinated against this disease. People working with children who are not toilet trained should be fully immunized, with four doses of vaccine, against poliomyelitis. This is because young children who have been vaccinated with oral polio vaccine shed live vaccine virus for several weeks. See "Prevention," page 211, in *Poliomyelitis.*

The U.S. Public Health Service does not routinely recommend hepatitis A and hepatitis B vaccines for all child-care workers. However, hepatitis A vaccine may be indicated if the risk of the disease in a community is high, says the service, and those who may have contact with blood or blood-contaminated body fluids should be immunized with three doses of hepatitis B vaccine. For more information, see *Vaccines,* page 301, and the chapters on each of these diseases.

People who are beginning work as child-care providers, the U.S. Public Health Service and Academy of Pediatrics further recommend, should also take a skin test for tuberculosis and repeat the test every two years. Anyone who turns out to have active tuberculosis should not be allowed to take care of children.

\* \* \*

When the children arrive at a day-care center each day, the staff should check the health of each child, advises the U.S. Public Health Service. And because young children can become sick very quickly, the staff should continue to monitor their health throughout the day. For information about when to send a sick child home—and when not to admit him to the center in the first place—see *When to Keep Your Child Home,* page 295.

# Hand Washing

The single most effective practice that a child-care center can implement to minimize the spread of disease-causing organisms, emphasize both the U.S. Public Health Service and the Academy of Pediatrics, is frequent hand washing. As we have discussed throughout this book, both adults and children can be carrying and shedding germs without showing any signs of illness themselves.

Day-care workers—and also the children, when they are old enough—should wash their hands when they arrive at the day-care center, before and after eating any food, after using the toilet, after handling pets, whenever their hands look dirty, and before they go home at the end of the session. Toddlers and older children should have access to sinks that are at their own height, with soap dispensers and paper towels. The staff should also wash their hands after changing a child's diapers and before handling, preparing, or serving food. "Caregivers who prepare food for infants," emphasizes the Academy of Pediatrics, "should be especially aware of the importance of careful handwashing."

\* \* \*

Many germs can stay alive on inanimate surfaces for long periods of time, some for weeks and some even for months. The staff of a child-care center should clean and disinfect tables and floors regularly. Spills of saliva, vomit, urine, feces, and other body fluids should be wiped up immediately with a freshly prepared solution of detergent or disinfectant.

Day-care providers need to be particularly careful about any spills of blood or body fluids containing blood. Some very serious diseases can spread in blood, particularly acquired immunodeficiency syndrome (AIDS) and hepatitis B. A child in a day-care program could be infected with either of these viruses, and the staff might not necessarily know about it. It is better to be safe and assume that all blood is infectious.

The person who cleans up the blood should wear disposable gloves and prepare a fresh solution of 1:64 household bleach (¼ cup of bleach diluted in 1 gallon of water). She needs to apply the solution to the bloody area for two minutes and then rinse it off and dry the area with disposable towels. Afterward, she needs to wash her hands thoroughly and place any blood-contaminated material in a plastic bag with a secure tie for disposal.

Children in a day-care program should not share bedding, warns the U.S. Public Health Service. Each child should have his own sleeping mat, crib, or cot and blankets labeled with his name. Infants' sheets, pillowcases, and blankets need to be cleaned and sanitized every day and their mattresses every week and whenever they become wet or soiled. All bedding—cribs, cots, mattresses, blankets, sheets—should be cleaned and sanitized before being reassigned to another child.

Nor should babies and toddlers share toys, says the Health Service. Children who are still in diapers should have only toys that can be washed. Any toy that one child puts in her mouth or otherwise contaminates should be washed and disinfected before another child touches it. The toys that infants and toddlers play with need to be cleaned and disinfected every day. Toys that older children play with should be cleaned weekly and whenever they become soiled.

# Food Preparation

Day-care centers should have separate areas for preparing food and for changing diapers.

Ideally, different people should prepare food and change diapers or help older children go to the bathroom, both U.S. Public Health Service and the Academy of Pediatrics advise. Tables and countertops used for preparing and serving food should be cleaned and sanitized between uses and before and after eating. For more recommendations about how to keep disease-causing organisms from spreading in food, see "Prevention," page 125, in *Food Poisoning*.

## Diapering

Diaper-changing areas should be used only for changing diapers. "Diaper changing areas should never be located in food preparation areas," the *Red Book* emphasizes in boldface type, "and should never be used for temporary placement of food." Diaper-changing surfaces should be smooth and nonporous (not wood) and cleaned and disinfected after each diaper change. It is best to use diapers with outer covers that are waterproof and can contain liquid stools or urine or use plastic pants, says the Health Service, and make sure that children always wear clothes over their diapers.

Diapers and clothing soiled with fecal material should not be washed or rinsed at the day-care center, says the U.S. Public Health Service. It is okay to dispose of stools in a toilet, but soiled diapers and clothing should be put in a plastic bag and sealed to await pickup by the child's parents or guardian at the end of the day.

For older children, the Academy advises using child-sized toilets or modified toilet seats rather than potty chairs. If potty chairs are used, "they should be emptied into a toilet, cleaned in a utility sink, and disinfected after each use."

Afterward, even more important than at home, staff members should wash their hands thoroughly. There should be handwashing sinks right next to each diapering and toileting area, and these sinks should never be used for food preparation.

# VACCINES

A vaccine consists of an inactivated or killed germ—a bacterium or virus—or a piece of one. When a vaccine is introduced into a child's body, usually as a shot, it stimulates the immune system to make antibodies that can overcome that germ and protect the child from catching that disease. There are currently ten vaccines that both the U.S. Public Health Service and the American Academy of Pediatrics recommend that *all* children routinely receive, to prevent them from catching the following diseases:

## Chickenpox

Until 1995, when the vaccine was introduced, nearly every child in this country caught chickenpox. Usually it means an itchy rash lasting a week or so, with some fever and malaise. However, complications of chickenpox put 9,300 people a year into the hospital and killed 50 to 100. For more information, see page 30.

## Diphtheria

Diphtheria is potentially a very severe disease. Up through the 1920s, it killed about 15,000 people a year in the United States, most of them children. Today diphtheria is rare in this country, thanks to vaccination, but it is still prevalent in developing countries and kills up to about 10 percent of the people who contract it. See page 80.

## Hemophilus Infections

Before hemophilus vaccine was introduced in 1985, infections with *Haemophilus influenzae* type b bacteria caused serious, life-threatening diseases, most commonly meningitis, particularly in babies and toddlers. These infections used to kill 600 to 900 children a year in the United States. See page 130.

## Hepatitis B

Hepatitis B virus multiplies in a person's liver and can produce chronic liver disease, including cirrhosis and liver cancer, conditions that kill 4,000 to 5,000 Americans a year. The risk of developing chronic liver disease is highest if a child under the age of five catches hepatitis B virus. Vaccination against hepatitis B has been recommended for all babies since 1991. See page 140.

## Measles

Measles also used to be so prevalent that nearly every child got it. Usually it means a fever, cough, red eyes, and a rash lasting a week or so. However, measles is a far more dangerous disease than many people realize; worldwide, it still kills about a million people a year, most of them children. See page 179.

## Mumps

Mumps also used to be so common that virtually every child caught it. A person's salivary glands and face become swollen, and she is sick for a week or two. However, in males past puberty—teenage boys and men—mumps can cause sterility, that is, make them unable to father children. See page 191.

## Poliomyelitis (Polio)

In the late 1940s and early 1950s, tens of thousands of people in this country caught polio every year, as people now in their fifties and older remember all too well. If a person survived the disease, it could leave him crippled or paralyzed for life. See page 211.

# Rubella (German Measles)

Rubella is generally a mild rash disease if a person catches it as a child, but if a woman becomes infected with rubella virus while she is pregnant, it can cause severe birth defects in her baby. A baby could be born deaf or blind or with a deformed heart or damaged brain. See page 225.

# Tetanus

Infection with tetanus bacteria causes severe muscle spasms, particularly of the jaw, and kills 45 to 55 percent of its victims. Thanks to vaccination, it is now rare in this country. The threat of tetanus, however, is virtually everywhere around us because the bacteria are widespread in soils. See page 267.

# Whooping Cough (Pertussis)

Whooping cough bacteria multiply in the respiratory tract, and a person typically has bouts of convulsive coughing that may persist on and off for months. Thousands of Americans, most of them children, still catch whooping cough every year, and the number has been increasing in recent years. See page 286.

* * *

Parents sometimes ask—since these diseases are now so rare in the United States—why we still need to have our children vaccinated. The answer is simple. The bacteria and viruses that cause these diseases are still around, and still cause outbreaks from time to time. If we do not vaccinate our children, these diseases could make a come back and wreak their havoc again. From 1989 through 1991, for instance, measles did come back in the United States; over 55,000 people, mostly preschool children, caught the disease. These diseases are prevalent in developing countries, and the germs could return to this country at any time on a plane coming from abroad.

Your baby needs to start receiving some of these vaccines shortly after birth. Some of these vaccines are usually combined into a single shot: children take a so-called MMR shot containing vaccines against measles, mumps, and rubella and a DTP shot with vaccines against diphtheria, tetanus, and pertussis (whooping cough). Some of the other vaccines are also sometimes combined.

The schedule for these shots as recommended by the U.S. Public Health Service and the American Academy of Pediatrics is shown on page 303.

The U.S. Public Health Service also recommends that adolescents who have neither had chickenpox nor been vaccinated against it receive chickenpox vaccine at age eleven to twelve. Since chickenpox vaccine has been available only since 1995, many adolescents are still susceptible to the disease.

Similarly, since the hepatitis B vaccine has been recommended for all babies only since 1991, many young people are still susceptible to this disease. The Public Health Service recommends that adolescents age eleven to twelve be vaccinated against hepatitis B virus.

The Health Service also recommends that adults who are not immune to measles, mumps, and rubella get vaccinated against these diseases.

Women in their child-bearing years should be immune to rubella before they become pregnant. About 10 percent of American women this age, according to the U.S. Public Health Service's Centers for Disease Control and Prevention, remain susceptible to rubella and thus at risk of having a baby with severe birth defects. See "Prevention," page 228, in *Rubella*.

The protection from diphtheria and tetanus vaccines wears off in time, and the U.S. Public Health Service recommends that all of us receive

| Vaccine | Age | | | | | | | | |
|---|---|---|---|---|---|---|---|---|---|
| | Birth | 1 Mo. | 2 Mos. | 4 Mos. | 6 Mos. | 12 Mos. | 15 Mos. | 18 Mos. | 4-6 Yrs. |
| Hepatitis B | Hep B-1 | | | | | | | | |
| | | Hep B-2 | | | Hep B-3 | | | | |
| Diphtheria tetanus pertussis | | | DTP | DTP | DTP | | DTP | | DTP |
| *Haemophilus influenzae* type b | | Hib | Hib | Hib | Hib | | | | |
| Polio | | | Polio | Polio | Polio | | | | Polio |
| Measles-mumps-rubella (MMR) | | | | | MMR | | | MMR | |
| Chickenpox virus | | | | | Chickenpox | | | | |

■ Range of Acceptable Ages for Vaccination

*Recommended vacine schedule.*

booster shots of these two vaccines every ten years for the rest of our lives. Physicians usually administer these two vaccines together in a single shot.

Children and adults who have asthma and certain other chronic diseases, as well as adults over the age of sixty-five, need to be vaccinated against influenza (flu) every year. See "Prevention," page 156, in *Influenza*. Similarly, children with sickle cell anemia and other chronic diseases and adults over age sixty-five need to be vaccinated against *Streptococcus pneumoniae* (pneumococcus) bacteria, which cause pneumonia, meningitis, and other diseases. See "Prevention," page 209, in *Pneumonia* and page 187 in *Meningitis*.

If you and your family are traveling abroad to developing countries, the U.S. Public Health Service recommends still other vaccines, depending on the countries you plan to visit. For many countries, including Mexico, the Health Service advises that you get a shot of vaccine or gammaglobulin to protect you against hepatitis A. See "Prevention," page 138, in *Hepatitis A*.

## Resources

You can find out which vaccines are currently recommended for the places you plan to visit by phoning the U.S. Public Health Service's Centers for Disease Control and Prevention (CDC). The CDC provides an automated Traveler's Hotline at 1-888-232-3228. You can either listen to the information or receive it by fax. You can also obtain it by connecting to the CDC on the Internet at http://www.cdc.gov.

Scientists are constantly improving vaccines and devising new ones, and the U.S. Public Health Service periodically modifies these recommendations. Your physician will know about any recent changes to the recommendations. You can also obtain up-to-date information about vaccines directly from CDC by phoning 1-800-CDC-SHOT. Again, you can either listen to the information, receive it by fax, or get it from the Internet at the above Web site.

All vaccines, like all medicines, may sometimes produce side effects, most of them minor, such as a passing fever or some soreness at the site of an injection. However, there is a National Vaccine Injury Compensation Program to help people who experience rare, serious, adverse reactions. If you think your child has been harmed by a vaccine, you can get information about this program by calling 1-800-338-2382.

Remember, however, that the risk of experiencing significant side effects from a vaccine is far less than the risk from catching the disease. "Vaccination is safer than accepting the risk for the diseases these diseases prevent," the U.S. Public Health Service emphasizes. "Failure to vaccinate increases the risk to both the individual and society."

# INDEX

## A

Abdominal pain or distension, diseases possibly causing, xvii

Acetaminophen, 3, 25, 28, 89, 145, 153, 181, 218, 224, 228, 247, 265

Acyclovir, 33

Adenoidectomy, 92–93

Adenoviruses, 35, 249–50

AIDS
    and pneumonia, 202
    and tuberculosis, 275

Air sacs (alveoli), diagram of, 21, 22, 200

Allergic rhinitis, 37–38, 246

Alveoli. *See* Air sacs

Amantadine, 156

American Academy of Pediatrics, 20, 39, 45, 60, 66, 76, 79, 86, 91, 93, 107, 108, 112, 128, 133, 153, 156, 163, 177, 194, 209, 240, 253, 266

Amoxicillin, 89, 247

Animal-borne diseases, 2–13
    Cat scratch disease, 2–3
    Psittacosis, 5–6
    Rabies, 6–9
    Toxocariasis, 9–11
    Toxoplasmosis, 11–13

Anthelmintic, 273

Antibiotics, as treatment, 3, 57, 76, 82, 89, 91, 100, 107, 108, 124–25, 148, 175, 186, 207, 235, 245, 259, 261, 268

Antihistamine, 33, 40, 155, 240, 247

Antimotility drugs, 57

Antitoxin, 82

Anus, diagram of, 55

Appendix, diagram of, 55

Arboviruses, 103

Armpit termperature, taking, 112

Arthritis. *See* Lyme disease

Aspirin, avoiding. *See* Reye's syndrome

Asthma, 37

Athlete's Foot, 14–15, 159
    causes of, 14
    diagnosis of, 15
    prevention of, 15
    symptoms of, 14–15
    treatment of, 15
    when to call doctor, 15

## B

B19 virus, 115

Baby measles. *See* Roseola

*Bacillus cereus*, 120, 121, 122

Back pain, low, diseases possibly causing, xvii

*Bartonella henselae* bacteria, 3

Bats, infection from. *See* Animal-borne diseases

Bell's palsy, 173

Benadryl, avoid combining with Caladryl, 33

Bites, from infected wild animals. *See* Rabies

Blisters
    mouth, diseases possibly causing, xviii. *See* Hand, foot, and mouth disease; Herpes Simplex Type I; Impetigo
    skin, diseases possibly causing, xix

Body temperature, normal, 109

Borrel, Amédée, 171

*Borrelia burgdorferi*, 171

Botulism, 16–20, 120. *See also* Food poisoning
    cause of, 16
    diagnosis of, 18
    incubation period of, 18
    prevention of, 19–20
    spreading of, 16–18
    symptoms of, 16, 18
    treatment of, 19
    when to call doctor, 18

Brain, diagram of, 183

*Branhamella catarrhalis*, 87

BRAT diet, 59

Breastfeeding, 58, 67, 93, 230

Breathing difficulty, diseases possibly causing, xvii

Breathing rapid, diseases possibly causing, xvii

Bronchial tube, 21, 22

Bronchioles, diagram of, 21, 22, 200

Bronchiolitis, 21–26, 36. *See also* Common colds; Respiratory syncytial virus (RSV)

305

Bronchiolitis, (*cond.*)
  causes of, 22
  diagnosis of, 23–24
  incubation period of, 23
  prevention of, 26
  spreading of, 22
  symptoms of, 21, 23
  treatment of, 24–25
  when to call doctor, 24
Bug-transmitted disease. *See* Arboviruses
Burgdorfer, Willy, 171
Burning sensation when urinating, diseases possibly causing, xvii

# C

Caladryl, avoid combining with Benadryl, 33
Calcification in the brain, 12
California encephalitis (CE), 103
Campylobacter diarrhea, 53, 60–63, 75, 119
  causes of, 60
  diagnosis of, 62
  incubation period for, 61
  prevention of, 62–63
  spreading of, 60–61
  symptoms of, 60, 61–62
  treatment of, 62
  when to call doctor, 62
Candidiasis. *See* Thrush
Canned foods, improperly processed. *See* Botulism, 16
Cat, infection from. *See* Animal-borne diseases
CAT scan, 89, 218, 246, 248
Cat scratch disease, 2–3
  causes of, 3
  diagnosis of, 3
  incubation period of, 3
  prevention of, 3

symptoms of, 2, 3
  when to call doctor, 3
Cellulitis, 256–57
  diagnosis of, 256
  prevention of, 257
  spreading of, 256
  symptoms of, 256
  treatment of, 256–57
Cerebrospinal fluid (CSF), 104
Cerumen. *See* Ear wax
Cheeks, swollen, diseases possibly causing, xvii
Chest pain, diseases possibly causing, xvii
Chewing trouble, diseases possibly causing, xvii
Chickenpox, 30–33, 202, 217, 295–96, 301
  causes of, 31
  diagnosis of, 32
  incubation period of, 32
  prevention of, 33
  spreading of, 31–32
  symptoms of, 30, 32
  treatment of, 32–33
  vaccine, 301
Chills, diseases possibly causing, xvii
*Chlamydia psittaci* bacteria, 5
*Chlamydia trachomatis*, 202
Chlorination, 63, 67, 138
Cholesteatoma, 93
Chorioretinitis, 12
Chronic, definition of, 142
Cirrhosis, 140, 142
Clark, Fred, 72
*Clostridium botulinum*, 16, 20, 121
*Clostridium perfringens*, 120, 121
*Chlostridium tetani*, 267
Clothing, for fever, 113
*Coccidioides immitis*, 202
Cochlea, diagram of, 84

Codeine, 89
Cold sores. *See* Herpes Simplex Type I
Colds. *See* Common colds
Colon, diagram of, 55
Coma, diseases possibly causing, xvii
Common colds, 34–41
  complications of, 36–37
  diagnosis of, 37–38
  incubation period of, 35
  prevention of, 41
  spreading of, 35
  symptoms of, 34, 35–36
  treatment for, 38
  when to call doctor, 37
Confusion, diseases possibly causing, xvii
Conjunctiva, diagram of, 42
Conjunctivitis, 42–45
  causes of, 42
  diagnosis of, 43
  incubation period of, 43
  prevention of, 45
  spreading of, 42
  symptoms, 42, 43
  treatment of, 44–45
  when to call doctor, 44
Constipation, 18
Convulsions, diseases possibly causing, xvii
Cooperative Extension Service, 20, 178
Cooties. *See* Lice
Coronoaviruses, 35
Corticosteroids, 50, 168, 215, 229
*Corynebacterium diphtheriae*, 80–81
Cough, about, 40
  diseases possibly causing, xvii
  suppressant, 40, 155, 247

# F